PREVENTING MEDICATION ERRORS and IMPROVING DRUG THERAPY OUTCOMES

A Management Systems Approach

PREVENTING MEDICATION ERRORS and IMPROVING DRUG THERAPY OUTCOMES

A Management Systems Approach

Charles D. Hepler
Richard Segal

CRC PRESS

Boca Raton London New York Washington, D.C.

Library of Congress Cataloging-in-Publication Data

Hepler, Charles D.
Preventing medication errors and improving drug therapy outcomes / Charles D. Hepler and Richard Segal.
p. cm.
Includes bibliographical references and index.
ISBN 0-8493-1576-X (alk. paper)
1. Medication errors. I. Segal, Richard. II. Title.

RM146.H47 2003
615.5'8--dc21 2002041401

Direct all inquiries to CRC Press LLC, 2000 N.W. Corporate Blvd., Boca Raton, Florida 33431.

Visit the CRC Press Web site at www.crcpress.com

International Standard Book Number 0-8493-1576-X
Library of Congress Card Number 2002041401
Printed in the United States of America 2 3 4 5 6 7 8 9 0
Printed on acid-free paper

Foreword

The quality of health care in America is much lower than it could be. Such a statement once would have shocked some people who thought (wishfully?) that American health care was the best it could be, that is, before the Institute of Medicine's Committee on the Quality of Health Care in America issued its two reports: *To Err Is Human* and *Crossing the Quality Chasm*. Now some of the evidence is out in the open. In its final report, the Committee wrote:

> The U.S. health care delivery system does not provide consistent, high-quality medical care to all people. Americans should be able to count on receiving care that meets their needs and is based on the best scientific knowledge — yet there is strong evidence that this frequently is not the case. Health care harms patients too frequently and routinely fails to deliver its potential benefits. Indeed, between the health care we now have and the health care we could have lies not just a gap, but a chasm.[1]

Drug therapy may be the most frequently used mode of therapy. For example, about two thirds of office visits to American physicians resulted in new or renewed prescriptions.[2] Drugs also may be the most studied therapeutic modality, perhaps because of drug marketing laws in developed nations. Consequently, drug therapy often can rest on a solid scientific basis.

The purpose of drug therapy should be to improve the length and quality of people's lives. Availability of safe and effective drug products has improved the management of both acute and chronic diseases. Reaching both clinical and quality-of-life objectives is often less expensive and less painful because drug therapy is available.

Toward this end, most nations have developed elaborate procedures for evaluating the safety and efficacy of drug products and for controlling their use, for example,

- New drug approval procedures based on proof that a drug is safe and effective
- Prescription-only and pharmacy-only distribution
- Product label restrictions
- Professional supervision

In addition, many health care finance programs may seek the safest and most efficient (cost-effective) drug products from among those deemed safe and effective by government. They may encourage prescribers to use them instead of less efficient or less safe alternatives.

However, it is well documented that drug products often fail to improve quality of life and may injure patients. Most importantly, in the judgment of some investigators, patient injury and death often could have been avoided. Mismanaged drug therapy may result in additional medical care, e.g., physician office visits, emergency room visits, hospital admissions, and increased length or complexity of hospitalization. Some people die from drug injury. These significantly reduce the overall effectiveness of drug therapy and increase total costs of care. Because drugs are the treatment of choice for many diseases, problems with drug therapy obviously can reduce the overall effectiveness of medical treatment.

This phenomenon, which we call preventable drug-related morbidity (PDRM), has provoked various explanations of how it occurs and how it could be prevented in the future. The commonly assumed causes of PDRM are inherently unsafe drugs, errors by a professional, errors by the patient or caregiver, or random accident. In simple language, the usual suspects in PDRM are the "four bads": bad drugs, bad prescribing, bad patients, or bad luck.

The majority of attempts to correct the problem have, logically, attempted to correct the four bads. This results in calls for stricter drug laws, more stringent drug testing, negligence lawsuits (including patients' contributory negligence), and professional sanctions. Sometimes the result is despair that bad things happen to good people. Such simple explanations may have succeeded up to a point, but little research exists to support their effectiveness for improving outcomes.

Simple explanations (and their corresponding correctives) are limited at best, and occasionally harmful. This has led some researchers and scholars from simple cause-and-effect models to a new perspective or paradigm of systems models, specifically comprehensive drug therapy management,[3] pharmaceutical care,[4] and medicines management.

This paradigm shift is consistent with broader changes that are going on in technology assessment. The framework of technology assessment is changing, in many fields, from a view of technology as part of a process to a view of technology as a means to an outcome. This always broadens the perspective of assessment, and usually pushes the perspective toward the systems paradigm.

A familiar example is the difference between assessing aircraft safety and air transportation safety. For a long time, the focus was on the safety of the product, i.e., the aircraft. Then, when most aircrafts were well designed and safe, emphasis shifted to pilot error. Then the emphasis shifted to the air traffic control system, including airport location and design. Most recently, emphasis is on the whole air transportation system including passenger behavior.

That's about where drug product technology is today. Most nations in the industrialized world now manage to keep ineffective and unsafe drugs off the market. In America, these changes have often followed public outrage. American drug safety requirements followed the marketing of sulfanilamide in a toxic vehicle. Efficacy requirements followed the thalidomide disaster. Medicines, however, still injure and kill their intended beneficiaries.

We are now moving through the "pilot error" phase, in which we* blame the doctor. When a drug injury occurs, we may also blame the patient, family members, and other professionals. It is time for us to move on to the "air travel system" level of understanding. It is, perhaps, time for the American people to become outraged again. This time, however, more stringent drug marketing laws will not solve the problem. Everyone involved in medications use should understand this complicated process. Beyond standards for the safety and effectiveness of drug products, we need new standards for how doctors, pharmacists, patients, and family members use medications.

Moving from a product perspective to a system perspective profoundly changed air travel. Likewise, moving from a drug product perspective to a medications use** perspective can profoundly influence how drug products are assessed and used. The outcomes of drug therapy depend not only on the basic technology, but also on the information processing system. Although this is becoming well recognized with air travel, many stakeholders tend to oversimplify and trivialize the system in which drug products are used.

This book will describe a systems perspective for medications use. After an introduction, it will loosely follow a problem-solving outline: present the data that suggest a problem (research findings about PDRM), analyze the causes, define the problem, identify and evaluate alternative solutions, and propose means for implementing solutions and following up. In the process, it will present medications use systems ideas, terminology, and applications.

A systems view may seem, at first, to mystify a simple subject or to make an already complex subject even more complex. The systems view is a holistic alternative interpretation of the facts. It requires different research methods and management tools. These may be unfamiliar at first. The systems view, however, does not complicate a simple reality — quite the opposite. It is the reality of medications use that is complex, and we cannot improve it with simplistic models. A systems view should provide a means of understanding medications use and then, perhaps, simplifying it. The systems view (eventually) provides insights that are well worth the initial inconvenience.

In the old story of the three blind men touching the elephant, one felt the leg and said that the elephant was like a tree, another felt the trunk and said that the elephant was like a huge snake, and the third felt its side and insisted that the elephant was like a wall. Each was correct, but none could place his observations into a holistic perspective. The real elephant was, in fact, a living, learning, changing organism, much more complicated than a tree, a snake, and a wall. So is medications use more than the sum of its parts.

---

* Essentially, "we" is everyone with an interest in medications use, especially the politicians, judges, consultants, researchers, program managers, and health policy makers who could promote needed change if they recognized the need and a way to do it.

** A preparation used to diagnose or treat diseases or symptoms. The terms *medication* and *medicine* are synonymous. *Medication use* is more common in the United States, while *medicines use* is more common in Canada, the U.K., and in international English usage.

Why Read This Book?

This book is for anyone with an interest in medications use: students preparing for health professions or careers in health service management; graduate students and researchers; practicing health care professionals; pharmacy managers; insurance program managers; health care purchasers. Patients or family members may read this book to gain a better understanding of how their insurance program, doctor, and pharmacist should cooperate so that medications already on the market can be used more safely and effectively. Although it is not about government policy or research methods, the systems perspective may interest policy makers, insurance executives, and health service researchers.

Read this book in order to learn:

- That the industrialized world has a "second drug problem": drugs approved as safe and effective frequently injure the patients they were intended to help.
- How large the problem is.
- Why medications often fail to produce the desired result and how to avoid such failures.
- New ways to think about drug product safety and effectiveness.
- How the main participants in a medications use system can improve outcomes.
- How professional and personal values, attitudes, and ethical reasoning fit into drug therapy.
- What a properly designed and managed drug therapy system would look like — specific components, how the components should fit together into a system, and how the system can be maintained and improved.
- Ways to evaluate medications use systems, how to recognize ineffective system operations, how to identify missing system components, and how to correct them.
- How the environment of medications use affects systems operations and patient outcomes, and why standards must change to improve drug safety and effectiveness.

A Reader's Guide

This book explores medications use from a social systems perspective. A systems perspective encompasses many participants on at least four levels:

patient, patient care, clinical management (governance), and whole societies. Its preoccupations are how these levels interact and how various participants' beliefs, decisions, communications, and actions combine to produce results.

This is not a book about drug uses and doses, i.e., clinical pharmacology. Understanding a clinical therapeutic system, however, is a necessary complement to understanding the clinical pharmacology of a prescription. To someone who is unwilling to settle for the common circumstance of "right" therapy and "wrong" result, understanding the use system is no less important than understanding pharmacology. A health professional who tried to treat a patient without understanding pathophysiology and pharmacology would be irresponsibly risking failure or even injury to the patient. A health professional who tries to treat a patient without understanding his *social* circumstances is taking a similar risk.

The Preface and Chapters 1 to 3 are the basis upon which the rest of the book is built. Please read them, even if you are an accomplished student of this topic. Some readers may want to move directly from Chapter 3 to Chapter 6, where the main argument of the book resumes, and then return to Chapters 4 and 5 later.

Chapters 4 and 5 have two purposes. First, they introduce some basic problems in medications use in familiar language (e.g., cost, access, and quality). For example, Chapter 5 explains the cost-effectiveness of drug products in detail. It describes federal drug regulation and shows why federal law is incapable of solving the problem by itself. Second, Chapters 4 and 5 provide clarity about terminology and subject matter that is made fuzzy by common usage. Quality of life is a good example. Chapter 4 describes it as a precise (and fundamentally important) aspect of health care outcomes. Readers who are familiar with the differences between medical and "folk" views of disease and illness, and who understand quality of life, may wish to skim over Chapter 4. Readers with a good background in cost, access, and quality of drug products may skim Chapter 5.

Most people first think of prescribing improvement when they decide to improve medications use. Most health care programs spend considerable time and effort to influence prescribing. Chapter 6 discusses this topic. It also reviews the literature on the unintended consequences of direct prescribing restriction programs and discusses them as an example of quick-fix approaches. The chapter concludes that much of the time and effort spent on prescribing restrictions may be unproductive or counterproductive, at least in the U.S. managed care system.

Chapter 7 continues the theme of continuous quality improvement, introduced in Chapter 4, and describes the information components needed for medications use systems. Chapter 8 outlines two basic systems and describes how they fit together in principle. Chapter 9 further develops a theory of medications use systems with evidence from both a simulation and published research.

Chapter 10 describes a pharmaceutical care system in detail. Readers who already understand pharmaceutical care or who are interested only in the big picture may be able to skim over Chapter 10 and come back to it later. Chapter 11 pulls most of the ideas of the book together to show what a medications management system would look like from the "top floor" of a managed care organization to a "corner pharmacy." Chapters 12 and 13 describe various managed care provisions that affect medications use. Readers who understand the details of managed care may be able to read these chapters quickly. Chapters 14 and 15 describe paths and barriers to creating medications use systems. Chapter 14 considers the problem from a marketing perspective, and Chapter 15 describes changes that need to occur at all levels of the health care enterprise.

Two Dilemmas

This book requires some knowledge from many subject areas. This creates some difficulties. On the one hand, I have used the book for 3 years with pharmacy students and entering graduate students. Many students — and I assume many other readers — need an introduction to the basics before they can understand the real significance of a systems approach. On the other hand, some specialists may feel that discussions of basic concepts, such as quality of life or cost-effectiveness, interfere with the "plot" and slow down progress toward describing medications use systems. Both readers are important; however, to make the book more accessible to nonspecialists, I chose to introduce the necessary basics and to beg the indulgence of more sophisticated readers.

A second dilemma is that if the book covers the respective subjects in depth, it may obscure the essential connections of the system's view. If the topics are only introduced, to keep the connections clear, then experts in the respective topics may feel that the coverage of their topic is superficial and that important detail has been omitted.

Again, I have chosen to risk the second way. This book is not intended to be a compendium on health care quality, pharmacoeconomics, quality of life, prescribing research, patient behavior, clinical practice, or even systems theory. It is intended to describe a personal synthesis of research, to provide an idea of what might comprise a safe and effective medications use system. References to more detailed works are liberally provided. The more one understands of these subjects, the more one may get out of this book.

References

1. Institute of Medicine, *Crossing the Quality Chasm: A New Health System for the 21st Century*, National Academy Press, Washington, D.C., 2001.
2. Cherry, D.K. and Woodwell, D.A., 2000 Summary Advance Data from Vital and Health Statistics, 328, 6-5-0002.

3. Williard, R.L., Tresolini, C.P., and O'Neill, E.H., Characteristics, importance, and implications of comprehensive drug therapy management, *Am. J. Health Syst. Pharm.*, 53, 623, 1996.
4. Hepler, C.D. and Strand, L.M., Opportunities and responsibilities in pharmaceutical care, *Am. J. Pharm. Educ.*, 53 (Suppl.), 7s, 1989.

Preface

> **LaStima, Katherine.** PITTSFIELD. Katherine, 13, died suddenly on Thursday, July 3, 1997, at Hale Memorial Hospital. Beloved daughter of Carl and Joanne LaStima and sister of Steven. Private funeral services will be Monday, July 7, at Sacred Heart Church.

Katherine LaStima* was a normal schoolgirl with normal physical, mental, and social development, healthy except for chronic bronchial asthma. According to her parents, Katherine had asthma since she was a baby. She was in the care of Dr. Michael, a Belchertown allergist who had been caring for her since 1986. He considered her asthma to be "moderate, with occasional severe exacerbations." She had been admitted to Hale Memorial Hospital on five occasions over the past 10 years with acute respiratory distress.

On July 2, 1997, Katherine went to the Pittsfield County Fair with some friends and Mary Reilly, an adult friend of the family. According to Ms. Reilly, while at the fair, Katherine began to have trouble breathing, but was able to get relief from her albuterol inhaler. Ms. Reilly recalled seeing her use the inhaler a few times but did not think anything of it, as it seemed to be helping and Mrs. LaStima had made certain that Katherine took it with her when she left home that morning. Toward the end of the afternoon, Katherine told Ms. Reilly that she was having a lot of trouble breathing and wanted to go home. However, she was not able to walk to the parking lot. Ms. Reilly phoned the city ambulance service, which transported Katherine to Hale Memorial and notified Mr. and Mrs. LaStima.

The duty physician at the Hale Memorial Emergency Room, Dr. J.S., diagnosed severe acute asthma based on Katherine's appearance and history. He began intranasal oxygen and emergency medications, ordered blood gas determinations, and admitted her. Dr. Michael arrived shortly thereafter and confirmed Dr. J.S.'s orders. Katherine appeared to respond initially but entered respiratory failure at 7 P.M. and died despite appropriate emergency measures. The cause of death was cerebral anoxia secondary to respiratory arrest from status asthmaticus.

---

* The story of Katherine LaStima is based on facts taken from *Penelope A. Cafarelle and Ralph M. Cafarelle, Jr. as mother and father of Jennifer Lynne Cafarelle, and as administrators of the Estate of Jennifer Lynne Cafarelle vs. Brockton Oaks CVS, Inc.* Memorandum of decision and order on defendant's motion for summary judgement. Commonwealth of Massachusetts Superior Civil Action No. 94-0414a.:1-20, 1997. We have changed the names of people involved and the locale, and updated some of the facts. The obituary notice is fictional, as we imagine it might have been. The story is accurate in its essentials.

Acknowledgments

Over the years that the ideas for this book have been fermenting, many events have taken place that influenced and — I hope — improved it. The Harvard Medical Practice Study was published. Prominent and not-prominent people died because of medications misuse. Newspaper reporters wrote hard-hitting stories of injury and death, from among whom I wish to single out Richard Knox of the *Boston Globe* and Steve Twedt of the *Pittsburgh Post-Gazette.* Lucian Leape, David Bates, and other members of what became known as the Adverse Drug Event Prevention Study began their enormously influential series of research reports on systems analysis of Adverse Drug Events in hospitals. The Institute of Medicine Committee on the Quality of Health Care in America issued its two reports, one on medical error and one on what America should do to improve the health care delivery system.

More than 10 years ago, pharmaceutical societies around the world had adopted a new vision of cooperative pharmaceutical practice called pharmaceutical care, which soon became a theory of how physicians, nurses, pharmacists, and patients could form cooperative microsystems that would make drug therapy safer and more effective. This vision completed (perhaps) the changes in pharmaceutical education that the clinical pharmacy movement had begun. John Gans, Henri Manasse, Mary Ann Koda-Kimble, and Dick Penna (among thousands of others) made that happen. Bob Cipolle, Linda Strand, Peter Morley, Cal Knowlton, and Dick Penna wrote books about how to practice it and how to teach it.

Something is missing, however. The basic drug therapy arrangements available to the vast majority of Americans remain the same, perhaps a bit worse because everybody is busier. The media are still preoccupied with good drugs and bad drugs and cheap drugs and expensive drugs, but not with a safe way to use them. We are managing costs instead of care, and it is not working. It is clear to me that a book about the medications use system might help.

About 400 second-year Pharm. D. students read early drafts of this book and showed me what they understood (or not) from earlier versions. About 10 graduate students and a few patient colleagues explained how I could improve the book. David Angaran (who kept asking good questions), David Brushwood, Judy Cantrill, Richard Faris, Tobias Gerhard, Neil MacKinnon, Brian Sauer, Richard Segal (who contributed Chapters 12 and 13), and Michael Taylor were particularly helpful. However, I am responsible for the ideas in my chapters and the way that I expressed them.

Charles D. Hepler
Gainesville, Florida

The Authors

Charles D. Hepler, Ph.D., is distinguished professor in the Department of Pharmacy Health Care Administration and director of the DuBow Family Center for Research in Pharmaceutical Care at the University of Florida. He is also visiting professor in the School of Pharmacy and Pharmaceutical Sciences, University of Manchester, England.

Professor Hepler received a B.S. in pharmacy from the University of Connecticut and M.S. and Ph.D. degrees from the University of Iowa. He completed a pharmacy residency at the University of Iowa Hospitals. He has been a faculty member of the University of Iowa College of Pharmacy and the Medical College of Virginia (VCU) School of Pharmacy.

Professor Hepler was principal investigator of the Therapeutic Outcomes Monitoring project, which developed a practical system for pharmaceutical care in community pharmacy. He has consulted on pharmaceutical care projects in Denmark, Spain, and British Columbia. He is currently studying the development and application of quality indicators for medications use and their application to continuous quality improvement in community pharmacies.

He has written more than 80 research, scholarly, and professional articles; 14 book chapters; and 3 books, and he has presented more than 60 professional papers at professional meetings in 15 nations, including strategic planning exercises for the Department of Health in the United Kingdom and the Council of Europe. He chaired programs on pharmaceutical care in community practice, offered by the International Pharmaceutical Federation (FIP) from 1993 to 1996 in Tokyo, Lisbon, Stockholm, and Jerusalem. In spring of 1997, he completed a six-city lecture tour of New Zealand, promoting discussion of drug therapy optimization among pharmacists and general practice physicians.

He was co-recipient (with Linda Strand) of the 1997 Remington Medal, awarded by the American Pharmaceutical Association (APhA). He has also received the 1997 FIP Pharmaceutical Practitioner of the Year; the 1997 American Society of Health-System Pharmacists (ASHP) Award for Sustained Contributions to the Literature of Pharmacy Practice in Health Systems; the 1992 Research Achievement Award in Economic, Marketing and Management Sciences from the American Association of Pharmaceutical Scientists; the 1991 and 1998 APhA Research Awards in Social, Economic and Administrative Sciences; the 1989 ASHP Research Award; and the 1986 ASHP Award for Achievement in the Professional Practice of Hospital Pharmacy. He has been designated a distinguished alumnus by the University of Connecticut College of Pharmacy (1998) and the University of Iowa College of

Pharmacy (1999). He is a corresponding (honorary) member of the Swiss Pharmaceutical Society and has received the Award of Distinction from the College of Pharmacy of Gipuzkoa (Spain).

Richard Segal, Ph.D., is research foundation professor and chair of Pharmacy Health Care Administration at the University of Florida College of Pharmacy.

Dr. Segal received his B.S. in pharmacy from the University of Connecticut in 1976, completed a residency at Saint Mary's Hospital/Mayo School of Health Sciences, received his M.S. in hospital and clinical pharmacy from the University of Iowa in 1981, and received his Ph.D. in pharmaceutical outcomes research from the Virginia Commonwealth University in 1983. Also in 1983, he joined the Ohio State University as an assistant professor and was promoted to associate professor in 1988. In 1988, he joined the faculty at the University of Florida and was promoted to professor in 1994.

Dr. Segal's research interests include disease management; outcomes research; pharmacoeconomics; quality improvement, particularly in the areas of drug prescribing; pharmaceutical care; drug use evaluation; and total quality management. In addition, he has authored a number of manuscripts in the areas of the sociobehavioral aspects of drug therapy and the psychology of the medications use process.

Dr. Segal is widely recognized for his work in explaining why clinical practice is so often inconsistent with evidence-based best practices. During the past 5 years, Segal has led a research team that has developed and tested evidence-based clinical practice guidelines for managed care organizations in the private and public sectors. These projects have resulted in one of the most successful research streams in disease management originating in academic pharmacy. An example of this work includes the development of innovative methods for implementing best-practice guidelines for dyspepsia to improve patient outcomes and to reduce overall health care costs.

Dr. Segal, along with other members of the DuBow Family Center for Research in Pharmaceutical Care, has also developed tools for implementing pharmaceutical care. The thrust of their research is aimed at detecting why preventable drug-related morbidity (PDRM) occurs and developing, implementing, and evaluating interventions intended to reduce PDRMs. Their internationally recognized program, called Therapeutics Outcomes Monitoring (TOM), provides pharmacists with a system for detecting problem patients and guidelines for resolving pharmaceutical problems experienced by patients. This program has been implemented in the United States and in other countries located in North America, Europe, and Africa.

Dr. Segal has been recognized for his contributions to the research literature, receiving best-paper awards from the two largest pharmaceutical associations in the United States. He is also the recipient of numerous regional and national awards recognizing his work in clinical research and the mentoring of students. He has authored or co-authored more than 90 published papers and has received awards for his research in the areas of clinical research, hospital practice research, and pharmacoeconomics.

Contents

1 **The Second Drug Problem** ... **1**
Why Do These Problems Persist? ... 4
Thesis — A Systems Approach ... 7
The Way Forward ... 8
References ... 10

2 **Morbidity and Mortality from Medication Use** ... **11**
Review of Research Data on Adverse Outcomes of Drug Therapy ... 12
Adverse Drug Reactions ... 13
Preventable Adverse Outcomes ... 13
Medical Record Review ... 13
Selected Examples ... 15
Hospitalization ... 15
Emergency Department Visits ... 18
Inpatient Studies ... 18
Drug-Related Deaths ... 19
Indicator (Large Sample) Studies ... 20
Possible Significance of PDRM ... 22
Cost of PDRM ... 22
Summary ... 24
References ... 25

3 **Understanding Adverse Drug Therapy Outcomes** ... **29**
Changing Attitudes toward Adverse Outcomes of Drug Therapy ... 29
Causal Attributions of DRM: From the Four Bads to System Failure ... 31
The Medicines Use Process Causes Adverse Outcomes ... 33
A Model of the Medications Use Process ... 35
The Adverse Outcome ... 39
Adverse Drug Reactions ... 39
Drug-Related Morbidity and Adverse Drug Event ... 40
Errors, Drug Therapy Problems, and System Failures ... 42
Errors ... 42
Drug Therapy Problems ... 47
System Failures ... 49
Preventability ... 53
Preventability in Medical Record Reviews ... 53
Proposed Definition of Preventability ... 54

PDRM Indicators......56
Summary (Preventability Definition)......57
Preventability Depends on Assumptions and Paradigm......58
Active Errors and Theoretically Perfect Systems......60
Summary of the Preventable DRM Model......61
Where Do Medications Use Systems Fail?......63
Hospital Admissions Studies......63
Inpatient Studies......66
Chapter Summary......67
Conclusion: Looking Forward to Systematic Medications Use Management......67
References......69

4 People and Purpose in Medication Use......73
Introduction......74
The People in Medication Use......75
Environment of Medication Use......76
Objectives of Medication Use......76
Professional Objectives......77
Personal Objectives......78
Medicines as Instruments......79
Quality of Life......79
Three Basic Relationships......83
Paternal Relationship......83
Consumer Relationship......84
Therapeutic Relationship......85
Authority......85
Caring......85
Competence......86
Example......86
Two Main Perspectives on Drug Therapy: Illness and Disease......88
Sickness and Legitimization......90
Models of Disease and Therapy......91
Clinical Negotiation......92
Summary......92
References......93
Appendix 1: How to Get the SF-36 and SF-12......95
Appendix 2: How to Get the Living with Asthma Questionnaire......96

5 Access, Cost, and Quality Issues in Medication Use......97
Introduction......97
Relationship of Access, Cost, and Quality......98
Accessibility of Care......99
Physical Access......99
Financial Access......100

Costs of Drug Therapy 103
Efficiency 107
Calculating Efficiency 109
Which Choice Is Optimal? 111
Sensitivity Analysis 113
Finding a Common Ground for Deciding 114
Balancing Values 114
Suboptimization and Values 114
Finding a Common Ground 115
Quality of Care 116
Quality Domains 117
Quality Components 117
Quality Standards 119
Joint Commission on Accreditation of Healthcare Organizations 119
Example of Quality Improvement 120
Coming Full Circle 121
Quality Assessment 121
Six Methods of Quality Assessment 122
Two Remaining Issues in Quality Assessment 125
Evidence vs. Professional Consensus 125
Market Forces 126
Summary on Quality 127
Patient Satisfaction with Care 128
Why the Interest in Satisfaction? 128
Satisfaction with Drug Therapy 129
Critique of Satisfaction Measures 129
Consumer Focus 129
Measurement Issues 130
Drug Law: Quality of Drug Products as Legal Requirements for Safety and Efficacy 131
Regulatory Perspective on Drug Product Quality 131
Major Provisions 133
Worthless Drugs 133
Unsafe Drugs 134
Unapproved and Off-Label Uses 135
Drug Enforcement Administration 136
Nonprescription Drugs and Nutritional Supplements 136
State Law 138
Drug Products vs. Drug Use 138
Effectiveness and Efficacy 139
Evaluating Effectiveness and Safety in Use 140
Drug Product Withdrawals 140
Chapter Summary 147
References 147
Appendix 1: Orphan Drug Law 150
Appendix 2: Steps in Cost-Effectiveness Analysis 152

6 **Prescribing and Prescribing Influence** 155
Prescribing in Medications Use 156
Criteria for Prescribing Appropriateness 158
Philosophical Basis of Prescribing Quality 158
Proposed Criteria for Appropriate Prescribing 159
Understanding the Prescribing Process 162
Characteristics of Inappropriate Prescribers 163
The Social Psychology of Prescribing 163
Active Problem Solving 165
Reasoned Policy and Rules 168
Unreasoned Rules and Habit 168
Psychological Models and Prescribing Improvement 169
Sociology of Prescribing 170
Networks and Relationships 171
Stages of Adoption 173
Issues Influencing Adoption 175
Willingness to Adopt 176
Sociological Models and Prescribing Improvement 177
Methods of Influencing Prescribing 178
Educational Approaches to Prescribing Influence 178
Mass Communications 178
Individual and Small Group Education 179
Prescribing Restrictions 180
Review of Literature on Prescribing Restrictions 180
Conclusion from Literature Review 184
Examining the Prescribing Influence Anomaly 184
Is the Research Flawed? 184
Formulary Terminology Is Vague 185
Effectiveness May Depend on Environment 185
Balance and Burden of Proof 186
Suboptimality by Design? 186
Promoting Products of a Favored Manufacturer 187
Cost Shifting to Consumers 188
Summary: Toward Systematic Improvement of Prescribing 188
Conclusion 190
References 191
Appendix: Examples of Prescribing Studies 194

7 **Medications Use System Performance Information** 197
Performance Database 198
Performance Guidelines 198
Performance Indicator 200
Standards 200
Types of Indicators 201
Process and Outcome 201
Sentinel vs. Rate Based 201

Minimum Information Needed for an Indicator 201
Examples of Medications Use Indicators 202
Criteria for Indicators 204
Reliability 205
Validity 206
Feasibility 208
Medications Use System Performance Indicators 209
Indicator Development Process 209
Examples of Indicators 210
Delphi Panel 210
Data Collection and Results 211
Further Validation 211
Application 212
Pharmaceutical Care and Medications Use Management 213
Summary and Conclusion 214
References 214

8 **Outline of a Medications Use System 217**
Pharmaceutical Care and Pharmaceutical Care System 218
Principles of Pharmaceutical Care 219
Relationships Diagram 223
Flow Diagrams: Pharmaceutical Care and Medications Management Systems 224
Drug Therapy Process 224
Pharmaceutical Care System 225
Medications Management System 226
Performance Indicators 227
Concepts in the Systems Paradigm 228
System Model of Error Prevention 229
Systems and Processes 232
System Components 232
Inputs and Outputs 233
Processes (Transformations) 233
Purpose 233
Control 234
Environment 235
Connective Summary 235
References 236
Appendix: Medications Use Paradigms: Product, Process, or System .. 238

9 **Effect of Pharmaceutical Care Systems on Outcomes and Costs 245**
Simulation Model of Medications Use 246
Simulation Results: Total Cost Function and Risk of DRM 249
Total Cost of Care 251

Summary ... 253
Review of Research Evidence ... 253
Connective Summary ... 260
References ... 261

10 A Pharmaceutical Care System ... 263
Need for a Consistent Process ... 264
Drug Therapy Problems ... 273
Classification of DTPs ... 273
Theoretical and Actual DTPs ... 274
Documentation: Problem-Oriented Medical Records and SOAP Notes ... 276
SOAP Notes ... 276
Documenting the Eight Steps ... 277
Professional Dialog ... 278
Example ... 279
Background ... 279
Commentary ... 281
Summary ... 281
References ... 284

11 Medications Management System ... 285
Pharmaceutical Care and Medications Management ... 287
Elements of Systematic Improvement in the Quality of Medications Use ... 287
Example of Medications Management on the Program and Practice Levels ... 288
Introductory Note ... 288
Acme Zenith Health Plan ... 289
Goals and Objectives of Medications Management ... 290
Process of QI: FOCUS ... 290
Find a Process to Improve ... 290
Organize a Team to Study the Problem ... 292
Clarify the Team's Understanding of the Process ... 293
Understand the Root Causes of Variation in the Output ... 293
Organization of Causes: Ishikawa (Affinity) Diagram ... 294
Select the Improvement ... 296
Plan, Do, Check, Act ... 297
Plan ... 297
Do: Implementation of Plan ... 298
Check ... 301
Act ... 304
Connective Summary ... 305
References ... 306

12 Managed Care **307**
Introduction: Scope of Managed Care 308
History of Managed Care 308
Types of Managed Care Organizations 309
Preferred Provider Organizations 310
Health Maintenance Organizations (HMOs) 310
Point-of-Service (POS) Plans 314
Recent Managed Care Trends 315
Shifting Enrollments 315
Medicare Managed Care 315
Medicaid Managed Care 316
Medical Groups 316
Costs 316
Performance Measurement in Managed Care 318
Conclusion 319
References 320

13 Managed Care Strategies to Influence the Cost, Access, and Quality of Medicines Use **323**
Medication Carve-Outs and Pharmacy Benefit Managers 323
Drug Formulary 325
Critique 327
Utilization Controls on Patient Behavior 327
Deductibles and Copayments 327
Tiered Copayments 328
Rx to OTC Switch 329
Drug Caps 329
Improving Prescription Information Exchange between Providers 330
Critique 330
Utilization Controls on Physicians 331
Promotion of Best Practices 332
Conclusion 335
References 336

14 A Market Perspective **339**
Professions as Marketing Mechanisms 340
Stakeholders in the Market for Medications Use Systems 342
Adoption of Medications Use Systems 343
Recognition of Unmet Need or Problem 344
Advantages of MUSs over the Status Quo 345
Perceived Risk of Change 347
Compatibility of the Innovation with Current Values, Norms, Beliefs, and Procedures 349
Competition on Quality 349

Emerging Concept of Value ... 350
New Accreditation Standards for Medications Use ... 350
Possibilities for the Future ... 351
Complexity: The Ease of Understanding and Using the Innovation ... 351
Divisibility: Required Degree of Commitment ... 352
Communicability of Results ... 353
Summary of the DoI Analysis ... 353
System Learning Disabilities: Psychological Barriers to System Improvement ... 354
Denial, Justification of Status Quo ... 354
"I Am My Job (Profession ...)" ... 355
The Root Cause Is "Out There" ... 355
Proactive Reaction ... 356
Acquiescence, Adjusting Expectations, Accepting the Unsatisfactory ... 356
Fixation on Events ... 357
Delusion of Self-Correcting Experience ... 357
Myth of the Management (Health Care) Team ... 358
Summary: Performance Indicators Are Crucial ... 358
References ... 358

15 Finding a Way Toward Medications Use Systems ... 361
Organizational and Environmental Context of PDRM ... 362
Lack of Response ... 362
Managed Care ... 366
ERISA: A Shield for Employers and Managed Care? ... 368
Getting the Problem and Solutions in the Open ... 369
Managed Care Is an Essential Part of the Solution ... 370
A Vision of Medication Use on the "High Plateau" ... 370
Rule 1: Care Is Based on Continuous Healing Relationships ... 371
Old ... 371
New ... 371
Rule 2: Care Is Customized according to Patients' Needs and Values ... 371
Old ... 371
New ... 372
Rule 3: The Patient Is the Source of Control ... 372
Old ... 372
New ... 372
Rule 4: Shared Knowledge and Free Flow of Information ... 372
Old ... 372
New ... 373
Rule 5: Decision Making Is Based on Evidence ... 373
Old ... 373

New 373
Rule 6: Safety Is a System Property 373
Old 373
New 374
Rule 7: Transparency Is Necessary 374
Old 374
New 374
Rule 8: Needs Are Anticipated 375
Old 375
New 375
Rule 9: Continuous Decrease in Waste 375
Old 375
New 375
Rule 10: Cooperation among Clinicians 376
Old 376
New 376
Moving Forward 377
Model-T Era 377
Change at Every Level 378
Patients 379
What Should Physicians and Pharmacists Do? 386
Pharmacists as Part of the Solution 387
Managed Care 389
Purchasers 391
Accreditors and Regulators: Quality Standards 392
An Incrementalist's Concerns 395
Safety and Quality Are Different 397
Conclusion 398
Recommendations 398
References 401

Glossary 403

Index 419

1

The Second Drug Problem

> How is it possible that modern medicine still does not provide care of known benefit sufficiently and correctly? Quite simply, deficiencies in medical quality are due to inadequacies of organization, delivery, and financing systems.
>
> **Bernard Bloom**

Drug therapy may be the most common modality of therapy in the industrialized world. In the United States, just under two thirds of all physician office visits include one or more prescriptions. The frequency of prescription use increases slightly with age (Figure 1.1).[1]

Doctors and patients intend drug therapy to improve the quality of peoples' lives, by curing or controlling disease. However, this is too often not the outcome of drug therapy. Research data show that preventable injury and death from drug therapy are major public health problems in most industrialized nations. Their costs, both human and financial, are major burdens on everyone. The billions of dollars that are spent to correct preventable drug-related morbidity (PDRM) could be used to prevent it, thereby gaining not only better quality of care but also reduced costs and improved access.

Adverse effects of drug therapy may be the fourth leading cause of death in the United States, according to a literature review in the *Journal of the American Medical Association*.[2] Lazarou et al. estimated that in 1994 there were from 76,000 to 137,000 deaths from adverse drug reactions (ADRs) in U.S. hospitals. Even with the lower estimate, ADRs would be the sixth leading cause of death. This ranks mortality rates from ADRs among those caused by heart disease, cancer, stroke, and accidents. A recent report of the Institute of Medicine (IOM) reviewed the prevalence and significance of human error in health care and its implication for patient safety. The report found that medication-related errors are "one of the most common types of errors ... substantial numbers of individuals are affected, and it accounts for a sizeable increase in health care costs."[3]

Chapter 2 will show that the prevalence of preventable hospital admissions caused by drug therapy rivals those from myocardial infarctions, cancer,

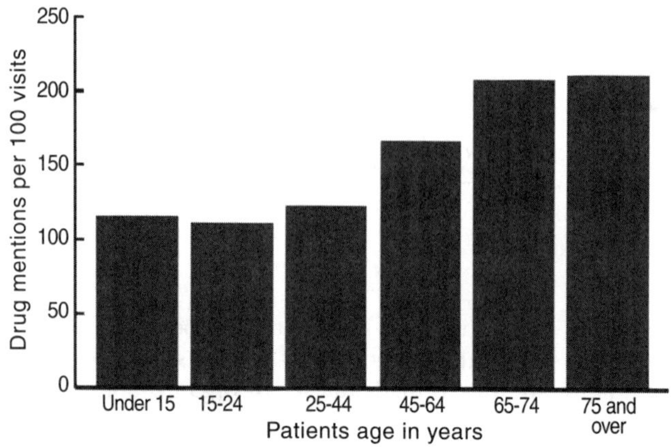

FIGURE 1.1
Number of prescriptions (mentions) per 100 physician office visits in the United States in the year 2000 (National Ambulatory Medical Care Survey).

diabetes mellitus, and asthma. Comparisons to diabetes and asthma are ironic, by the way, because drug therapy is such an important part of their management, and we know that mismanagement of drug therapy is a cause of hospital admission for patients with those diseases.

The money spent to correct preventable office visits, emergency department visits, hospital days, etc., may approximate $100 to $300 annually for each man, woman, and child in the United States. The news media now refers to the intentional abuse of drugs as "the drug problem." Preventable drug-related morbidity is then the industrialized world's "second drug problem." It lags drug abuse in popular coverage but may well cause more human misery and waste more money than drug abuse. Clearly, we should prevent adverse outcomes of drug therapy from a clinical and humanitarian viewpoint. Moreover, by preventing them, we may make health care much more efficient.

Stories about real people add human meaning to the statistics. When we consider the tragedy of Katherine's death (see Preface) in the context of research, we see that it is not a rare occurrence. There are many more stories of avoidable injury and death from mismanaged drug therapy. They shock and offend, and make many people seek simple explanations and quick solutions. Katherine LaStima's death is shocking and offensive, but is actually one of the less dramatic and more commonplace examples. Her story is rather a tragic symbol of how ordinary this problem really may be in community health care.

The death of Katherine is a symbol of a pervasive and major public health problem — adverse outcomes from the mismanagement of routine drug therapy. Although people die of asthma, nearly all asthma deaths are preventable.[4,5] If Katherine had been murdered or killed by a drunk driver, we would be outraged. We should be even more outraged by a death due to inadequate medical care. The mismanagement that killed Katherine LaStima exemplifies many important points found in research literature, but perhaps most of all, her death illustrates the banality of evil and the wisdom of Edmund Burke's admonition, "The only thing necessary for the triumph of evil is for good men to do nothing."

Two reports from the IOM on the quality of medical care in America produced a flurry of activity recently and some continuing effort to correct the problem.[3,6] But still, there is no consensus to improve the overall system of medication use.

Preventing PDRM should be directed at root causes. The sheer number of potentially significant root causes, however, suggests that preventing PDRM by separate, specific remedies might be impossibly complicated, especially considering the thousands of drug products available. Furthermore, few studies show that changing one element in medications use affects outcomes. Theoretically, reengineering the medications use system could address many root causes for many drugs, providers, and patients. This has in fact been confirmed by several studies that improved outcomes and reduced total costs, as described in Chapter 8.

Dramatic improvements in patient outcomes are possible when physicians, patients, and pharmacists cooperate in systematically managing outcomes. This promising research has been accumulating for nearly 20 years, yet somehow it has not yet been followed up by many health care professionals and researchers, and continues to be ignored by many new mandarins of managed care. Meanwhile, literally thousands of lives and millions of dollars are wasted by PDRM. So, there are two problems: the basic problem of PDRM, and the secondary problem that society has been so slow to respond to the primary problem.

This situation should provoke strong motives to do whatever is needed to make drug therapy safer and more effective. Health professionals and managers in North America and Europe are among the best educated in the world. Given the significance of the problem, their response has been absurdly inadequate. A preventable disease is endemic to most or all of the industrialized world. Its prevalence and cost rank with major diseases like diabetes and heart disease. We have some evidence about how to prevent or at least ameliorate this disease, but we do very little with it. This is surely not the way the world of health care is supposed to work.

Most citizens of the United States, Canada, U.K., and other countries known to have high prevalence of PDRM seem to take great pride in the quality of their medical care, but seem to accept such failure. Many are shocked by the facts. We could not have the PDRM problem some people say. It must be confined to subpopulations like the elderly, poor, or teaching hospital patients or rural backwaters. Furthermore, people have faith in their doctors and pharmacists. If we had the PDRM problem, would not the doctors, pharmacists, and hospitals know about it and fix it? The short answer is no.

Why Do These Problems Persist?

These problems exist, and persist, because the technology of drug therapy has far outstripped society's traditional ways of thinking about it and customary arrangements to control it. The United States and many other Western societies have demanded that marketed drug products be safe and effective. Then, in effect, they have sent those safe and effective drug products into an unsafe and ineffective system of use.

In the days of tinctures and fluid extracts (roughly until the 1940s), the list of effective drug products was shorter and, the rate of pharmaceutical innovation was slower than today. Professionals and patients had time to develop experience with drugs. Concerns involved drug purity, potency, and consistency. The pharmacist's job was to obtain high-quality crude drugs and to prepare them properly. A pharmacy smelled like, and in many ways was, an apothecary shop. One-way communications from physician to pharmacist through a prescription were sufficient.

Making drug products has now been taken over mainly by the pharmaceutical industry. This has led to many new drug products, safer and more effective. Drugs, dosage forms, and their potency are now standardized. Most nations closely regulate the pharmaceutical industry. Manufacturers have to prove the safety, effectiveness, purity, potency, and consistency of drug products.

Drug products make billions of dollars for their manufacturers. Consequently, they are articles of commerce as much as professional instruments of care. The industry has become a powerful force. It advertises directly to consumers. It contributes to political campaigns and funds research. Only the naive would believe that the industry does not influence the interpretation of research results.[7]

Consumers and purchasers, especially third-party payers like insurance companies, are keenly aware of drug products as expensive articles of commerce. Total expenditures for drugs are rising rapidly. Higher prices and higher total expenditures for drug products are a real worry, but they must not be allowed to draw attention away from how well those expensive medicines are used. The proper use of medications can lower total costs of care, and misuse can increase it by more than the cost of the drugs themselves.

The list of drug products numbers into the thousands, and innovation (real or apparent) is rapid. The complexities of dosages, drug interactions, and allergies are mind-boggling. Nonetheless, the family physician is expected to manage therapeutics single-handedly. Communication to the pharmacist is still mostly one-way, through a prescription, although the biggest questions now may concern the effect that the prescription is having on the patient. Community pharmacists, freed from drug preparation, have become part of a commercial distribution system.

In short, reality today is quite different from when drug controls were set up. Traditional thinking about drug therapy, however, has outlived the galenical era. The concepts and language that stakeholders* use to talk about drug therapy, adverse effects, and treatment failures may be the basic problems. How we think about medications use surely determines how speak about it and what we do about it.

The medications use system is poorly understood. The conventional wisdom about how to provide safe, effective, and efficient drug therapy sometimes lacks a basis in fact, and is therefore often wrong. For example, unsafe drug products and inappropriate prescribing are not the leading cause of patient injury in ambulatory care, and sometimes have nothing to do with causing injury. Yet managed care organizations spend more money to influence prescribing than on any other aspect of medications use.

Like many others, Katherine LaStima did not die of an adverse drug reaction, toxicity, or side effect. Despite being in the care of a specialist, she died of the natural course of her disease, asthma. She died in part from exposure to an overload of allergens at the county fair and in part because her doctor, pharmacist, parents, and even Katherine herself did not control her drug therapy, and therefore did not control her asthma.

Overuse of albuterol, an asthma "rescue" medicine, is rarely harmful and did not kill (or even directly harm) Katherine. Frequent inhaler use, however, is a useful marker to show that asthma is slipping out of control. The extra albuterol helped Katherine to breathe while her disease was getting worse. Also, she was using too little "preventer" medicine (a steroid-like cortisone) that fights the cause of asthma symptoms. In effect, Katherine was fighting her symptoms instead of her disease. When she went to the fair, she may have been extremely vulnerable to the allergens that she encountered there.

Many people seem to focus on the drug product instead of the manner of its use. Perhaps some patients and providers value convenience and reassurance more than competent care and a disciplined, full understanding of how to use medicines. The effects of the preventer medication would not have been apparent to them, so perhaps Katherine and her parents did not fully understand that it was essential.

We have to change the normal arrangements of community practice. These arrangements do not permit enough coordinated attention to drug therapy. In particular, interprofessional cooperation is usually inadequate. A patient, physician, or pharmacist cannot manage drug therapy alone. Katherine's pharmacist obviously emphasized his function as a dispenser of medicines rather than his potential role as a co-therapist in the management of Katherine's asthma.

When something goes wrong and a patient is injured, the tendency is to look for simple solutions: the drug product itself or the people involved. While professional errors cause some heart-wrenching injuries, very few patient

* Many kinds of people have an interest in how medications are used: regulators, purchasers, providers, professionals, patients, and family members.

injuries are caused by errors, at least as most people would understand the term. In this instance, the physician and pharmacist were sued.

People like Katherine are not supposed to die of asthma, so it would have seemed that somebody must have made a mistake, for example, the doctor or pharmacist who treated Katherine. She had been repeatedly hospitalized in the past, and her pattern of medication use just before she died showed that she probably was beginning another exacerbation. Court records show that Dr. Michael and the pharmacist, Mr. Merchant, knew the possible adverse consequences of her medication use pattern. They said that they had warned her mother, Joanne, more than once. Her death could have been prevented by any of the participants in her care, even by Katherine herself.

The point is not to exculpate the doctor or pharmacist. Of course people should be held accountable when they fail to meet their responsibilities. Accountability, with or without punishment, seems just and may provide some measure of meaning and closure to a tragic event. Nevertheless, there are two problems with the approach of blame and liability. The first is that apportioning blame among all the participants in drug therapy, given their rights to defend themselves, can be cumbersome and expensive at best. Since blame is retrospective, the second problem is that blame seldom leads to preventative measures. Risk management may emphasize money rather than causes.

Long court battles are likely, one case at a time. Some, perhaps most, will be settled with no finding of blame and with confidential agreements. Possibly, professionals can be sanctioned by their regulatory boards. Neither outcome is likely to reduce the risk of the next tragedy. No penalty that a court could have imposed on Dr. Michael, Mr. Merchant, or the LaStimas would have reduced the likelihood of *another* patient being injured by inadequate management. Such tragedies are repeated again and again by different people.

Perhaps more importantly, changing our view from blame toward prevention would allow us to think about this problem more productively. More sophisticated, professional practice standards in Massachusetts might have prevented her death. Hale Hospital should have known the significance of Katherine's prior admissions for asthma. A computer at the insurance company could have flagged her inappropriate prescription refill patterns. The mass media could have done a better job of informing the public about the dangers of medications use. None was to blame. Outside the structure of error and blame, however, each of them could have contributed to a safer system of medication use. (As it happened, the insurance company that paid for Katherine's albuterol might have objected to her overuse, had it known about it. Mr. Merchant concealed the timing of some refills so that the LaStimas would not have to pay for them out of pocket. But the insurance company did not object to Katherine's *underuse* of preventer medication, which probably contributed as much to her death as her overuse of albuterol.)

Instead of apportioning blame through litigation, our legal system could have interpreted Katherine's long-standing misuse of medications as demonstrating systems' failure. Perhaps failure of a single component or participant could have been detected and corrected before her final asthma attack.

We must question the basic arrangements for providing therapy.

Most Western medical systems tacitly hold that the doctor will be responsible for "everything," but PDRMs are invisible to many physicians. For example, a California study of drug-related hospital readmissions found that fewer than a fifth of the drug-related admissions identified by medical audit had been coded as drug related by the admitting physician. The magnitude of this problem is hidden from the very people who are expected to detect it.

Health care programs lack adequate mechanisms for assessing, directing, and controlling actual medications use (as contrasted to drug prescribing, which is often used as a surrogate measure). Without valid and reliable feedback on performance, consistent improvement is impossible.

Some health care policies may worsen the problem. For example, efforts to control expenditures include pressure on professional fees. To maintain their incomes, physicians and pharmacists may feel pressure to see more patients and fill more prescriptions. Pharmacists are not held to standards requiring them to participate in managing drug therapy outcomes. High prescription volumes and low professional service expectations may further degrade system performance.

Finally, many pharmaceutical and medical societies have addressed the problem, but no professional or consumer body has made this problem its major priority or taken the responsibility to solve it.

Thesis — A Systems Approach

A systematic response to the PDRM problem would recognize that most adverse outcomes are caused by system failures — for example, a combination of nonresponse to symptoms, inappropriate prescribing, basic pharmacology, insurance provisions, package labeling, dispensing errors, inadequate patient cooperation, and idiosyncrasy. Real improvement will not be possible by blaming parts of the system or by removing a few scapegoats. Real improvement will be possible only by changing how the delivery of drug therapy is organized, provided, regulated, and financed and how individuals behave in specific cases.

The professionals, academics, and consumers of the industrialized world need to evaluate the safety and effectiveness of medications use in their respective populations and to change their assumptions about drug therapy. They need to develop more systematic ways of providing drug therapy. Consistent with recommendations from the IOM, this will mean:

- Reengineered care processes: more information and faster flow among patients, physicians, and pharmacists
- Fuller use of information technology in planning care and in evaluating quality

- More focused and frequent attention to practice-wide and population-wide results
- Development of effective teams: more responsible cooperation among patients, physicians, and pharmacists
- Coordination of care across patient conditions, and type and location of service
- More management of outcomes

This would increase the efficiency of drug therapy and consequently of medical care itself. The problems that killed Katherine LaStima are endemic. We need a new way to understand the safe and effective *use* of safe and effective *medicines*. And then we need to construct new, cost-effective systems. But most of all, we need to act.

The primary care marketplace is evolving too slowly and painfully. Insurance companies and managed care organizations are preoccupied with minimizing the cost of specific services, e.g., physician visits and drug product costs. This must be replaced by a marketplace in which payment conditions require all providers to participate in delivering coordinated, cost-effective care.

At present, disease management is a familiar idea of how to coordinate care. Disease management is often an important and welcome step toward "vertically" integrating the steps in medication use. However, *disease* management appears incomplete from a medication systems perspective. Disease management should be seen as an intermediate stage on the path toward pharmaceutical care, that is, *patient*-centered medication use management. A patient may have more than one disease that affects his quality of life and his consumption of health care resources. If one imagines a disease management program for many diseases, one arrives at the idea of "horizontal" integration — coordinated care of multiple patient problems.

Further, disease management may emphasize objective aspects but minimize a patient's subjective "illness" experience. It might then fall short of improving a patient's overall health-related quality of life and may therefore not sufficiently influence demand for health care services or patient satisfaction.

The Way Forward

We can see the health care system in a four-level framework.[8] Improving the quality and increasing the overall cost-effectiveness of drug therapy requires change on all four levels:

1. *Patient-centered pharmaceutical care* by individual health professionals to individual patients.
2. *Pharmaceutical care in microsystems.* Drug therapy is often necessary, difficult, and dangerous. Therefore:
   a. Direct patient care microsystems should include pharmaceutical care subsystems. These are described in detail in Chapter 10 and elsewhere in this book.
   b. Pharmaceutical care systems require cooperation by a pharmacist and physician, as well as other caregivers and the patient. This cooperation can be left to chance. However, it also can be structured by developing collaborative practice agreements among pharmacists, physicians, and clinical nurses, and by explaining the collaborative practices to patients in a way they can understand. In short, health professionals can construct specific systems for their own practices and their patients.
3. *Organizational medications management systems.*
   a. Professional practices, hospitals, nursing homes, and other provider organizations should institute appropriate practice management systems, including a formative performance appraisal and quality improvement (QI) systems. These are described in Chapters 5, 7, and 11.
4. *Environment that supports medications use management.* To sustain safe and effective medications use, professionals should promote changes in professional standards and regulations. Professional organizations should promote quality standards for themselves and managed care organizations.
   a. Cost management (e.g., drug product cost control) should optimize the costs of outcomes. Minimizing payments for components like drugs, professional services, etc., may lead to higher total costs and poorer quality. Influential purchasers of health care services, e.g., employers and governmental agencies, have the sophistication to demand total value for cost. Often, quality of drug therapy is free.
   b. Managed care organization (broadly speaking, whether private or governmental) should routinely collect, organize, and interpret data on the safety and effectiveness of the medications use systems under their influence. They should encourage pharmaceutical care system development, e.g., through reimbursement policies.

The "sharp end" is level 1. Levels 2 to 4 have value — and deserve support — only to the extent that patients receive the best outcome possible. At the same time, the environmental realities (level 4) powerfully influence the behavior of institutions (level 3) and practice groups (level 2). The merits of laws, policies, and rules must be judged by their ability to encourage appropriate patient care and acceptable patient experience.

References

1. Cherry, D.K. and Woodwell, D.A., 2000 Summary Advance Data from Vital and Health Statistics, 328, 6-5-0002.
2. Lazarou, J., Pomeranz, B.H., and Corey, P.N., Incidence of adverse drug reactions in hospitalized patients, *JAMA*, 279, 1200, 1998.
3. Kohn, L.T., Corrigan, J.M., and Donaldson, M.S., *To Err Is Human: Building a Safer Health System,* National Academy Press, Washington, D.C., 2000.
4. Fletcher, H.J., Ibrahim, S.A., and Speight, N., Survey of asthma deaths in the Northern region, 1970–85, *Arch. Dis. Child*, 65, 163, 1990 [see comments].
5. Hindi Alexander, M.C. and Middleton, E., Jr., Asthma deaths: are they preventable? *N. Engl. Reg. Allergy Proc.*, 7, 462, 1986.
6. Institute of Medicine, *Crossing the Quality Chasm: A New Health System for the 21st Century,* National Academy Press, Washington, D.C., 2001.
7. Mundy, A., *Dispensing with the Truth: The Victims, the Drug Companies, and the Dramatic Story behind the Battle over Fen-Phen*, St. Martin's Press, New York, 2001.
8. Berwick, D.M., A user's manual for the IOM's Quality Chasm Report, *Health Aff.*, 21, 80, 2002.

2

Morbidity and Mortality from Medication Use

> I find the medicine worse than the malady.
>
> **Beaumont and Fletcher, 1647**

A fundamental objective of professional practice is to help individual patients or clients solve problems. Specifically, professionals apply *general* knowledge, e.g., scientific knowledge, to *specific* circumstances, governed by the principle of beneficence.[1] Further, the objectives of beneficent action are, in order of priority:

1. To do no harm
2. To prevent harm
3. To remove harm
4. To promote good

The first principle is to do no harm. However, this is seldom a satisfactory goal. A professional can avoid committing errors or doing harm by doing nothing. To be worth his fee, so to speak, the professional must act to prevent harm, to remove harm, or even to promote good. To promote good is both a professional aspiration and a motivation.

Drug therapy would appear near the top of most people's lists of how a health professional might remove the harm of disease or promote good. More than half of all physician office visits result in one or more prescriptions. The ideal objective of drug therapy is to improve the quality of a patient's life.[2] In part because of legal requirements for the licensing of new drugs, drug products have more rigorous scientific evidence regarding safety, basic efficacy, and often, physiological effects than any other mode of therapy. It seems that drug therapy would exemplify the idea of applying scientific knowledge to improve people's lives. This very often occurs. One need only cite antibiotics to establish this.

Furthermore, an elaborate procedure to regulate drug marketing has developed over the years in response to various disasters, such as the use of a toxic vehicle for sulfanilamide and the birth of thalidomide babies. Almost every nation requires rigorous clinical trials to establish safety and efficacy, and limits claims regarding safety and effectiveness. So, on the one hand, the dangers of drug products are widely recognized. On the other hand, effectiveness and safety exist in a balance. The drug products marketed in the United States and other developed nations are arguably as safe as they can be without sacrificing access to effective drugs.

Premarketing clinical trials are carried out according to strict procedures (research protocols) that were approved by the Food and Drug Administration (FDA). These protocols define the population, especially the diseases to be treated; comorbidities (concomitant diseases) to be excluded; the manner of drug use; and the required clinical testing and reporting. Some populations (e.g., elderly, children, pregnant women) tend to be excluded from drug trials unless it is absolutely necessary to include them. This is for their protection, but it means that scientific studies of drug use in those populations may be scant or slow to appear.

After marketing, drugs may be used for many more indications and for more types of people than those that were included in the clinical trials. This so-called "off-label" use is possible because the states control the practice of medicine. The FDA is specifically prohibited from interfering with the practice of medicine. Doctors often need the flexibility to use their judgment in treating a patient. Also, some populations and indications would probably never be included in labeling. (See the discussion in Chapter 5.)

If medicines could be used as rigorously in daily practice as they are in clinical trials, perhaps they would be as safe and effective as manufacturers and regulators say they are. However, this would be difficult or at best impractical within the normal arrangements of community and hospital practice. It is increasingly obvious that drug *product* safety is not equivalent to drug *therapy* safety. This distinction is important and far reaching, and a specialized vocabulary is needed to describe it.

Furthermore, once such a distinction is clear, it may become apparent that the risks of drug therapy are not as widely appreciated as the risks of drug products. Few governments, for example, regulate drug therapy, despite strict regulation of drug products. Furthermore, the medication use policies that do exist in hospitals and managed care organizations, and the priorities of many health care professionals and patients, seem inconsistent with a full appreciation either of the problem or of its possible solutions.

Review of Research Data on Adverse Outcomes of Drug Therapy

An expanding literature documents a widespread problem: the legitimate use of governmentally approved drug products often results in adverse effects and treatment failures, and in turn, costly emergency visits, hospital admissions, transfers to intensive care, and deaths. Another related, but less appreciated problem is treatment failure caused by nonuse of needed medicines, because the doctor did not prescribe it, the pharmacist did not dispense it, or the patient did not take it.

Adverse Drug Reactions

According to the World Health Organization (WHO), an adverse drug reaction (ADR) is

> a response to a drug which is noxious and unintended and which occurs in man at doses normally used for prophylaxis, diagnosis or therapy of disease, or for modification of physiological function.

There are literally hundreds of published studies on the prevalence of ADRs. Lazarou et al. reviewed 39 studies, conducted among 62,480 patients over a 32-year period, estimating the risks of adverse drug reactions in hospitals. The overall incidence of serious ADRs was 6.7% of hospitalized patients. The incidence of fatal ADRs was 0.32%. They estimated that in 1994, 2,216,000 hospitalized patients had serious ADRs, including 106,000 fatal ADRs, making these reactions between the fourth and sixth leading cause of death in the United States.[3]

Lazarou et al., among others, assert that ADRs are not preventable by definition. They argue that ADRs (by definition) are unintended and occur at normal doses.[3–5] However, other investigators have found, on review of specific cases, that some ADRs (or at least their consequences) may be preventable. This issue is discussed further below.

Preventable Adverse Outcomes

An expanding literature documents preventable illness, hospital admissions, transfers to intensive care, and deaths caused by the misuse of drug products that had been approved as safe and effective. Two basic approaches have been used to estimate prevalence: medical record review and application of preventable drug-related morbidity (PDRM) indicators.

Medical Record Review

Medical record review, or medical record audit, is so called because the data sources are the detailed records of the admission and stay. Medical record review by qualified experts is generally considered to be the gold standard for evaluations of processes requiring judgment. Some studies reviewed a data summary abstracted from medical records, while others interviewed patients and added the interview results to the data available from the patients' official medical records.

The investigators were usually among the reviewers, and presumably chose additional qualified reviewers when necessary. Some reports described formal means to increase reliability, e.g., having more than one reviewer for each case and using criteria for interreviewer agreement.

In a typical study of drug-related admissions, the sample would comprise patients admitted to one or more hospital units. The clinician-investigators reviewed those records or an abstract (summary) to evaluate the reason for hospital admission. In the studies reviewed below, the reviewers used more or less implicit definitions of drug relatedness and preventability. The investigators then counted the number of drug-related admissions (DRAs) and further subdivided them according to whether they had been preventable. The prevalence would then be calculated as the ratio of DRAs (or preventable DRAs) to the total number of admissions reviewed.

Winterstein et al.[6] carried out a systematic review of preventable drug-related hospital admissions (PDRAs). They selected 15 studies from 8 nations. These studies are summarized in Table 2.1. Details of sampling and study methods varied widely.

The 15 studies report a median DRA prevalence of 7.1 per 100 hospital admissions (range, 2.5 to 25%). The median prevalence of *preventable* DRAs was 4.3 per 100 hospital admissions (range, 1.4 to 15%). Overall, the median preventability rate (PDRAs/DRAs) was 58.9% (range, 32 to 86%).

The range of PDRAs in studies from the United States was 2.3 to 15.2%, with a calculated median of about 7.9%. Two studies from the U.K. showed

TABLE 2.1

Studies of Preventable Drug-Related Hospital Admissions

Author, Year, Country (reference no.)	Sample Size	DRAs as % of Admissions	PDRAs as % of Admissions	Preventability Rate (%)
Bero et al., 1991, U.S. (4)	224	21.1	15.2	76
Bigby et al., 1987, U.S. (7)	686	10.6	6.3	59
Courtman and Stallings, 1995, Canada (8)	150	14.0	12.0	86
Cunningham et al., 1997, U.K. (9)	1011	5.3	4.3	80
Darchy et al., 1999, France (10)	623	6.6	4.8	73
Dartnell et al., 1996, Australia (11)	965	5.7	3.7	66
Hallas et al., 1992, Denmark (12)	1999	8.0	3.8	47
Lakshmanan et al., 1986, U.S. (13)	834	4.2	2.3	54
Lindley et al., 1992, U.K. (14)	416	6.3	3.1	50
Nelson and Talbert, 1996, U.S. (15)	450	16.2	9.5	59
Ng, et al., 1999, Australia (16)	172	18.0	5.8	32
Nikolaus et al., 1992, Germany (17)	87	25.3	12.6	50
Raschetti et al., 1997, Italy (18)	1833	2.5	1.4	56
Trunet et al., 1980, France (19)	325	7.1	4.3	61
Trunet et al., 1986, France (20)	1651	5.9	2.6	44
Median	623	7.1	4.3	59
Minimum	87	2.5	1.4	32
Maximum	1999	25.3	15.2	86

Source: Winterstein et al., *Ann. Pharmacother.*, 36, 1238, 2002.

that PDRAs account for 3.1 and 4.3% of admissions, with preventability rates of 50 and 80%, about at the median found in studies from other countries.

Table 2.2 summarizes six studies of PDRM among hospitalized inpatients. In these studies, patients already hospitalized would be followed, and patients with possible DRM typically would be identified using screening criteria or voluntary reports from pharmacists or nurses. These patients' medical records would then be evaluated for drug-related morbidity by medical record review. The incidence would then typically be calculated as the ratio of DRM or PDRM to the total number of hospital stays (admissions) during the study.

The incidence of PDRM among inpatients ranges from 0.32 to 3.9%, with a median of about 1.5%. The preventability rate ranges from 20 to 56%, with a calculated median of approximately 41%.

Studies of preventable death caused by drug therapy (contrasted to death from an adverse drug reaction) are difficult to review systematically. Most focus on specific diseases, e.g., asthma. Preventable deaths are rather rare events on a population basis. All studies oversampled for death. That is, in effect, they searched for patients who had died, rather than counting the deaths in a sample drawn sequentially or at random from a general population at risk.[27–34] Examples are described below.

Selected Examples

Hospitalization

Bero et al.,[4] at the University of California, followed 706 elderly patients discharged from a California hospital. Within 6 months of discharge, 247 (35%) reentered the hospital. About one fifth (45) of the readmissions were drug related. The most frequently identified drug-related problems were unexpected adverse drug reactions (10), patient noncompliance (10), overdose (8), lack of a necessary drug therapy (6), and underdose (5). Drug-related factors were a major reason for readmission in half the cases. The majority (76%) of the problems identified were potentially preventable. The authors concluded that specific drug-related problems could become targets for preventive interventions.

Bigby et al.[7] studied 686 emergency admissions of patients from their own hospital-based primary care practice. In their judgment, 59 (9%) of the admissions were potentially preventable. Medical care, including inadequate follow-up and adverse drug reactions, caused 40 admissions; lack of patient compliance caused 12; and both medical care and noncompliance caused 7. Adverse drug reactions were the most common cause of treatment problems, and warfarin was the most common cause of an adverse drug reaction. Inadequate follow-up of abnormal physical findings, symptoms, and laboratory test results was also important.

Wayne Ray and colleagues[49] at Vanderbilt studied 1021 patients with hip fractures in a study design that matched injured patients to normal controls.

TABLE 2.2

Preventable Drug-Related Morbidity in Inpatients

Author, Year, Country (reference no.)	Sampling Type, Sample Size, Setting	Sample Description[h]	Prevalence of DRM	Prevalence of PDRM	Preventability Rate
Outcome: Significant, Serious, Life-Threatening, or Fatal Adverse Drug Events					
Bates et al., 1995, U.S. (21)	Prospective n = 4,031 HAs (21,412 IPDs) 2 tertiary hospitals	SRS of (+) all adults admitted to 11 units of 2 hospitals over 6 months, February to July 1993;[a,b] (–) obstetric Pts.	247/4,031 (6.1%) 6.5% adjusted	70/4031 (1.7%)[c] 1.8% adjusted	70/247 (28%)
Bates et al., 1993, U.S. (22)	Prospective n = 420 HAs (2967 IPDs)	(+) All adults admitted to 7 units (2 medical, 2 surgical, 2 obstetric general care, 1 coronary IC) during 37 days in August and September 1990[a]	27/~420[d] (6.4%)	15/420 (3.6%)	15/27 (56%)
Bates et al., 1995, U.S. (23)	Prospective n = 379 HAs	(+) All adults admitted over 51 days during October and November 1992 to 3 medical units: 2 general medical, 1 ICU[e]	25/379 (6.6%)	5/379 (1.4%)	5/25 (20%)
Outcome: Disability, Death, or Prolonged Hospital Stay					
Wilson et al., 1995, Australia (24)	Retrospective n = 14,179 PRs SRS from 28 hospitals with > 3000 admissions in 2 states	(+) RS of at least 520 HAs from each hospital (–) Hospitals with less than 3000 eligible admissions per annum, day-only admissions, admissions to psychiatric wards mean age = 43.8[f]	233/14,179 (1.6%)	84/14,179 (0.6%)	84/233 (36.1%)
Leape et al., 1991, U.S. (25)	Retrospective n = 30,195 PRs	(+) RS of PRs from an SRS of 51 hospitals (NY)[a,f]	0.72% (adjusted)	0.32% (adjusted)	45.2%

Outcome: Cardiac Arrest					
Bedell et al., 1991, U.S. (26)	Prospective n = 203 Teaching hospital	(+) All inpatients receiving CPR and discharged patients with cardiac arrest within 24 h after discharge[g]	15/203 (7.4%)	8/203 (3.9%)	8/15 (53%)

Note: HA = hospital admission; MRA = medical record audit, or review; Pt. = patient; PR = patient medical record; IPD = inpatient day; RS = random sample; SRS = stratified random sample.

[a]Potential cases were assessed by MRAs using two independent reviewers, and a third when necessary to break a tie.
[b]Oversampled specific patient groups. Definite and probable ADEs.
[c]Number of admissions estimated from patient days.
[d]Potential cases were assessed by medical record review using one reviewer (90%) or two independent reviewers (10%).
[e]Records assessed by medical record review using two independent reviewers, and a third when necessary to break a tie.
[f]Two independent reviewers.
[g]Internist reviewed hospital medical charts within 24 h after CPR and interviewed staff for clarification; assessment by three internists.
[h](+) = inclusion criteria; (–) = exclusion criteria.

The risk of hip fracture was approximately doubled for patients taking long-acting psychoactive agents, tricyclic antidepressants, and antipsychotics. The risk went up as dosages went up. "These data support the hypothesis that the ... effects of psychotropic drugs increase the risk of falling and fractures in elderly persons."[49]

Lindley et al.[14] studied 416 successive admissions of elderly patients to a teaching hospital. Twenty-six (6.3%) were attributed to ADRs, including 13 (50%) that were due to inappropriate prescribing. Forty-eight patients (11.5%) had a total of 51 drugs with absolute contraindications, amounting to 3.8% of the prescriptions reviewed in the study. A total of 175 unnecessary drugs were discontinued at admission in 113 (27%) patients. About half of all of the ADRs in the study were due to unnecessary drugs or drugs that were absolutely contraindicated in the patient. This ADR rate was significantly higher than that observed for all prescriptions. The authors concluded that "much drug-related morbidity in the elderly population may be avoidable, as it is due to inappropriate prescribing."

Emergency Department Visits

Three studies of drug-related emergency department (ED) visits are available. Hanlon et al.[35] studied a cohort of 167 high-risk ambulatory older veterans who participated in a 1-year health service intervention trial in a VA General Medicine Clinic. All patients were taking five or more scheduled medications. During exit interviews, the investigators asked patients to describe any potential side effects, unwanted reactions, or other problems from medication during the past year. All reported adverse experiences were assessed for plausibility and categorized by predictability, therapeutic class, and organ system. Eighty self-reported adverse drug events (ADEs) involving 72 medications taken by 58 (35%) of 167 patients were confirmed as plausible. Seventy-six of 80 (95%) ADEs were classified as predictable.

Dennehy et al.[36] retrospectively evaluated a random sample of 1260 patients visiting an ED during October 1994. They excluded cases involving intoxication, suicide attempts, drug abuse, and alcoholism. The proportion of drug-related ED visits to all ED visits was 49/1260 (3.9%) overall, or 49/565 (8.6%) of patients receiving medications. The published abstract does not provide the preventability rate. However, using the typical value from Table 2.1, this study might have included about a 2% prevalence rate of preventable ED visits.

In their review of ED visits in Slamanca, Spain, Otero et al. found that 332 (1%) of 33,975 ED visits resulted from preventable, verified adverse drug events. Of these, 119 resulted in hospitalization. The average cost for each preventable drug-related ED visit was $1707.[37]

Inpatient Studies

Bedell et al. studied cardiac arrest among patients hospitalized during 1981 in a university teaching hospital. They found 203 arrests in which resuscitation was attempted during this 1-year study. Of these, 28 (14%) followed an iatrogenic complication. Seventeen (61%) of the 28 patients died. Patients with iatrogenic arrest were more likely to be taking digoxin or antiarrhythmic medication prior to arrest. The most common causes of potentially preventable arrest were medication errors and toxic effects (44%) as well as suboptimal response by physicians to clinical signs and symptoms (28%), most frequently dyspnea and tachypnea. Among the 28 cases of iatrogenic cardiac arrest, 18 (9% of all arrests) might have been prevented. The authors noted a lack of attention and rapid response to patients' history, findings on physical examination, and laboratory data. They specifically mentioned abnormal drug levels, signs of adverse drug effects, digoxin toxicity, and congestive heart failure.[26]

Brennan and associates at Harvard reviewed 30,121 randomly selected records from 51 randomly selected acute care, nonpsychiatric hospitals in New York State in 1984.[25,38] Adverse events (AEs) were defined as patient injuries caused by medical management. They occurred during 3.7% of the hospitalizations. The authors judged 28% of the AEs to be due to negligence or substandard care.

Seventy percent of the AEs caused disability lasting less than 6 months, but about 3% caused permanently disabling injuries, and 13.6% led to death. Patients with preventable AEs had a significantly higher risk of death than patients with nonpreventable AEs (27 vs. 19%).[39] Drug complications were the most common type of adverse event (19%), followed by wound infections (14%) and technical complications (13%). The authors recognized that prevention of many adverse events must await improvements in medical knowledge; however, they found that many others are potentially preventable now. They recommended identifying the causes or error and developing methods to prevent error or reduce its effects.

When the authors studied interhospital variation in AEs, they found substantial variation in both AE rates (0.2 to 7.9%; mean, 3.2%) and the percentage of AEs due to negligence (1 to 60%; mean, 24.9%) among hospitals. They concluded that AEs and negligence are not randomly distributed. In other words, AE and negligence rates depend on the care system in place. Certain types of hospitals have significantly higher rates of injuries due to substandard care.

Drug-Related Deaths

Dubois and Brook studied preventable deaths in 12 hospitals selected on the basis of having higher-than-average death rates.[29] Although the investigators do not specifically describe drug-related preventable deaths, some of the causes they cite are strongly suggestive of mismanaged drug therapy. According to a majority of their medical reviewers, half of 17 preventable deaths in patients with pneumonia were due to inadequate fluid management or improper antibiotics. Reviewers found that inadequate fluid management or inadequate management of infection explained two of nine preventable deaths in patients with cerebrovascular accidents. Of 23 preventable deaths in patients with myocardial infarction, reviewers attributed 3 to inadequate fluid management, 2 to inadequate control of arrhythmias, and 12 to inadequate management of infection.

Fletcher et al.[32] followed up 35 asthma deaths in children aged 1 to 16 years. Twenty-four of these children had previously received care from a specialist (hospital consultant). There were seven inpatient deaths. Twenty-nine (83%) of the children had a history of severe asthma, 17 of whom had previously experienced a life-threatening attack. Six children (17%) had preceding mild asthma. Potentially preventable factors in management were found in 28 cases (80%). The major factor in 20 deaths (57%) was suboptimal management of the final attack owing to delay in seeking medical attention, inadequate medical response, or both. Only two children had received systemic corticosteroid in appropriate amounts during the final illness. Eighteen of the children (51%) had been chronically undertreated. The authors concluded that families of asthmatic children should be educated to recognize severe symptoms and should have an appropriate response plan.

Indicator (Large Sample) Studies

The studies using medical record review (Tables 2.1 and 2.2) typically established one or more general, conceptual definitions of PDRM, which reviewers then applied to specific cases during review. Although some studies used explicit ADR algorithms to establish the relationship of an outcome to drug therapy, none of those studies provided operational definitions of preventability.

An alternative method for identifying instances of PDRM is to develop explicit descriptions (indicators) of specific examples of PDRM. These descriptions can then be applied to specific cases. PDRM indicators will be discussed in Chapters 7 and 11.

Two studies in the United States have used this method (two others are in progress in the U.K.). Both of these studies first carried out a review of research-based literature describing drug-related patient injury or severe side effects. For example, original articles and research-based textbooks describe the risks of adverse events during therapy with oral anticoagulants. Scenarios were then developed that described a process of drug therapy that might lead to that an adverse outcome, for example,

> Major or minor hemorrhagic event in a patient taking warfarin when a prothrombin time (INR) had not been done before therapy started or had not been done at least every month during therapy.[40]

All such scenarios were then reviewed by an expert panel according to specific criteria for preventability. (See Chapters 3 and 7 for further information.) The scenarios that were accepted by the expert panel were then translated into computer search language (logical expressions in terms of diagnostic and drug codes).

MacKinnon applied 52 PDRM indicators (accepted by 5 or more of 7 panelists) to a data set containing records of 3365 patients enrolled in a Medicare managed care health plan operated by a hospital in central Florida. He used a combination of automated and manual methods to identify patient records that matched an indicator. He identified outcome codes automatically and then searched manually for the processes of care included in the indicators. He found 158 indicator positives, i.e., events that corresponded to both the outcome and process descriptions, involving 97 patients — an overall PDRM prevalence rate of 2.9%. Twenty-three indicators had no positives. The top five indicators accounted for approximately half of all positives.[41]

Forty-nine indicators were accepted by a majority (four or more) of seven panelists in Faris's study. He applied the 49 indicators to a data set containing 11,711 patients enrolled in a health insurance-based Medicare managed care plan in Florida. His search procedure was fully automated, using statements such as those in the following example (diagnostic, procedure, and drug codes, rather than natural language, were used in the actual searches):[40]

> (Physician office visit or emergency department visit or hospitalization) AND (diagnosis or procedure during visit consistent with hemorrhage) AND (drug code for oral anticoagulant) AND (date of visit later than first date of anticoagulant)

Faris found 966 indicator positives, yielding an overall PDRM prevalence rate of 8.2%. A total of 685 patients (5.8%) had one PDRM, while 281 (2.4%) had two or more. Because patients were enrolled an average of 1.32 years, the PDRM rate per year was 6.25%. The two most commonly occurring adverse outcomes (nearly 34% of positives) involved ED visits or hospitalizations following cardiac decompensation due to inadequate drug therapy. The third most common event (9.5% of positives) was gastrointestinal bleeding from nonsteroidal anti-inflammatory drugs. The five most frequently occurring indicators accounted for about 60% of all PDRM; the top ten accounted for 80%. Twenty indicators had no positives.[40]

Studies using indicators of PDRM complement studies based on medical record reviews. They use explicit definitions and are replicable. They include a wider range of consequences than studies of hospital admissions. This method is limited, however, by its specificity. Both Delphi panels were asked to think about circumstances of therapy or definitions of PDRM that were missing from the list of proposed definitions. Some were indeed proposed, but no new definitions were accepted by a majority of panelists. Nonetheless, there may have been types of PDRM that were not included in the indicator set. Some types of PDRM may not even be measurable by the method. For the time being, prevalence estimates based on PDRM indicators should be considered as a lower bound to the true PDRM prevalence in a population. Both of these issues can be addressed by validating the definitions against implicit medical record audit. (See Chapters 3, 7, and 11 for further discussion of this method.)

Possible Significance of PDRM

The true prevalence and cost of PDRM are not known for any defined population. The 15 studies in Table 2.1 were carried out from 1986 to 1999 in eight countries on three continents. However, to appreciate the possible practical significance of PDRA, suppose that the overall median PDRA prevalence (4.3%) represented the United States in 1997. (The median of the three U.S. studies was actually 9.5%, but we chose the median of the larger sample of 15 studies.)

In 1997, in the United States, there were about 114 hospital admissions (comprising about 582 hospital days) per 1000 population.[42] Now, if the median of the 15 reviewed studies was typical of the United States in 1997, then about 5 hospital admissions per 1000 population would have been caused wholly or partially by PDRM.

This would have placed PDRM, as a cause of hospital admission, on a par with cancer (4.9/1000) and higher than myocardial infarctions (2.8/1000), diabetes mellitus (1.9/1000), and asthma (1.8/1000). Comparisons to diabetes and asthma are, ironically, awkward to make because drug therapy is such an important part of their management, and we know that mismanagement of drug therapy is a cause of hospital admission for some patients with these diseases.

Cost of PDRM

Based on expert opinion and a cost-of-illness model, Ernst and Grizzle estimated that the total cost of drug-related morbidity and mortality exceeded $177.4 billion in the year 2000. Hospital admissions accounted for nearly 70% of total costs, followed by long-term-care admissions. The estimated mean cost for a treatment failure was $977. For a new medical problem, the mean cost was $1105. The combined cost of a treatment failure and new medical problem was $1488.[43] To put this in perspective, according to the National Ambulatory Medical Care Survey, $99.6 billion was spent on prescription drugs in 1999.[44]

Assuming that the U.S. population in the year 2000 was $275 million, the average expenditure to correct DRM would be about $644 per capita per year. A typical preventability rate from Tables 2.1 and 2.2 is about 50%. Therefore, the average annual per capita cost of *preventable* DRM would be about $322. This is close to the average prescription expenditure, which was about $390. This is shocking, seemingly incredible. This estimate is based on expert opinion about the frequency and types of care required for DRM, and hard data on the costs of that care. The estimate can be compared with other independent data on the cost of PDRA, preventable ED visits, and inpatient PDRM.

Cost of PDRA

Based on the 15 reviewed PDRA studies in Table 2.1, the number of hospital days in 1997 associated with PDRA would be approximately 4.3% of 582, or 25 hospital days per 1000 population. Assuming that patients admitted because of PDRM have "typical" lengths of stay, at $1000 per day that is $25 per capital per year spent on preventable drug-related hospital admissions.

Looking at this another way, in 1997 there were about three medical office visits per capita (3003 per 1000 population, excluding emergency room visits). The average number of prescriptions written per office visit in 1997 was 1.3.[45] So, the equivalent of $25 annually per capita for U.S. residents is an average cost of roughly $6.50 for every outpatient prescription.

These estimates do not include the costs of ED visits, additional physician visits, and other types of health care expenditures that result from PDRM. They refer to ambulatory care and do not include costs resulting from inpatient PDRM.

Cost of Emergency Department Visits

The cost of ED visits caused by DRM was estimated to be $696 per event by Dennehy et al.[36] and $1444 per event by Tafreshi et al.[46] These studies did not estimate cost per unit population.

The study by Faris was done in a defined population. He found greatly increased health care expenditures in the patients who had a positive PDRM indicator, but he could not attribute the cost to the PDRM. His study found that about 6% of Medicare patients annually may have significant, preventable problems with medications use. The most common outcome in the Faris study was an ED visit or hospitalization due to cardiac decompensation in congestive heart failure. The second most common event was an ED visit or hospitalization because of gastrointestinal bleeding.

If we assume that all of the PDRM in the Faris study resulted in ED visits (i.e., ignore office visits and hospitalizations), we can combine the data in these three studies to roughly estimate the cost of preventable drug-caused ED visits. The average per capita cost is from $42 to $86, based on the two ED studies cited above.

Cost of Inpatient DRM

Bates et al. estimated that in-hospital ADEs increased length of stay by an average of 2.2 days and increased costs of care by $3244 per admission. For preventable ADEs, the associated increase in length of stay (LOS) was 4.6 days at an increased cost of $5857.[47] Given 114 hospital admissions per 1000 population, if 2.6% of inpatient stays have a preventable DRM, there are about 3 inpatient PDRM per 1000 population. If each inpatient PDRM costs an additional $5859, the cost of inpatient PDRM is about $17 per capita.

Summing Up

The total of the three cost estimates (admissions, ED visits, and inpatient PDRM) is about $100 to $150 per capita. There are admittedly some flaws in the logic of making these three estimates and then adding them.* The total does not confirm the $322 estimate based on the Ernst and Grizzle total, but perhaps it adds a lower boundary to the estimate. Hundreds of dollars per capita population would be a staggering economic burden. Even with the lower estimate, the cost of PDRM would be one quarter of the per capita expenditure on prescriptions. This must receive further attention. We should learn more about the true cost and how much could be spent to improve medications use systems.

The studies reviewed in Tables 2.1 and 2.2 were heterogeneous with respect to their definitions of drug-related and preventable sampling and assessment methods. Differences in populations and research methods would affect the precision of prevalence and cost estimates. The range of PDRA prevalence estimates is wide. Some populations may have higher or lower prevalence rates, perhaps depending on patient characteristics and quality of care. Therefore, these cost estimates have debatable validity for the purpose of estimating population prevalence rates and costs (national averages).

These limitations, however, should not obscure the potential significance of these data. The problem of PDRM is significant from economic as well as humane perspectives. It may be possible to improve the outcomes of medication use without adding to the cost of medical care.

PDRM may also involve collateral costs. For example, Bates et al. cite a study by the National Association of Insurance Commissioners showing that treatment with drugs was the most frequent type of procedure-related injury leading to a malpractice claim from 1975 to 1978, accounting for 11% of total indemnity payments.[22]

Summary

Four points seem obvious from these data. First, the prevalence of PDRA may be comparable to diseases such as cancer, heart attacks, diabetes, and asthma. Public and professional awareness of this problem, funding for research into causes and preventives, and preventive programs should also be comparable, but clearly are not.

Second, the research evidence in this field is far from conclusive; however, the possible severity of the problem should motivate more studies, with

* The three are rough estimates at best, as is their total. We do not know for certain how closely the estimates apply to the whole population. The total may be conservative because (a) it used a median PDRA prevalence lower than the median of U.S. studies; (b) it adds averages, ignoring the possibility of a patient having a PDRM at more than one level; (c) it ignores additional prescriptions and physician office visits caused by PDRM, which the Ernst and Grizzle estimate included; and (d) it uses data from various years prior to 2000 but does not correct for inflation.

more uniform and valid research methods, and more reliable and precise population estimates.

Third, preventable hospital admissions, transfers to intensive care, and deaths represent needless human suffering and unnecessary expenditures to correct them. PDRMs represent a form of random waste somewhat analogous to other endemic diseases. Evidently, PDRMs are so expensive that many health care systems could reduce this type of suffering without increasing total health care costs. Some studies (reviewed in Chapter 9) suggest that improving the outcomes of drug therapy may significantly *reduce* total costs, probably by avoiding the expensive consequences of adverse outcomes. To some point, improving the quality of medication use may be free.

Fourth, the wide range of occurrence rate estimates in both ambulatory care and hospitals may be only partially explained by differences in research methods. The wide ranges may also reflect true differences among systems. For example, Brennan et al. found substantial variation among hospitals in both injury rates and the percentage due to negligence. They concluded that rates of injuries due to substandard care and negligence are not randomly distributed.[48] In other words, the incidence of both DRM and PDRM depends on how care is provided. The possibility that PDRM occurrence may be system-dependent suggests that efficient methods of system performance appraisal are urgently needed, both to identify ineffective and unsafe systems and to guide systems development and redesign.

References

1. Hepler, C.D., Pharmacy as a clinical profession, *Am. J. Hosp. Pharm.*, 42, 1298, 1985.
2. Hepler, C.D. and Strand, L.M., Opportunities and responsibilities in pharmaceutical care, *Am. J. Hosp. Pharm.*, 47, 533, 1990.
3. Lazarou, J., Pomeranz, B.H., and Corey, P.N., Incidence of adverse drug reactions in hospitalized patients, *JAMA*, 279, 1200, 1998.
4. Bero, L.A., Lipton, H.L., and Bird, J.A., Characterization of geriatric drug-related hospital readmissions, *Med. Care*, 29, 989, 1991.
5. Bates, D.W., Drugs and adverse drug reactions: how worried should we be? *JAMA*, 279, 1216, 1998.
6. Winterstein, A. et al., Preventable drug-related hospital admissions and morbidity in hospitalized patients: a meta-analysis of prevalence reports, *Ann. Pharmacother.*, 36, 1238, 2002.
7. Bigby, J. et al., Assessing the preventability of emergency hospital admissions: a method for evaluating the quality of medical care in a primary care facility, *Am. J. Med.*, 83, 1031, 1987.
8. Courtman, B.J. and Stallings, S.B., Characterization of drug-related problems in elderly patients on admission to a medical ward, *Can. J. Hosp. Pharm.*, 48, 161, 1995.

9. Cunningham, G. et al., Drug-related problems in elderly patients admitted to Tayside hospitals, methods for prevention and subsequent reassessment, *Age Ageing*, 26, 375, 1997.
10. Darchy, B. et al., Iatrogenic diseases as a reason for admission to the intensive care unit, *Arch. Intern. Med.*, 159, 71, 1999.
11. Dartnell, J.G.A. et al., Hospitalisation for adverse events related to drug therapy: incidence, avoidability, and costs, *Med. J. Aust.*, 164, 659, 1996.
12. Hallas, J. et al., Drug related admissions to medical wards: a population based survey, *Br. J. Clin. Pharmacol.*, 33, 61, 1992.
13. Lakshmanan, M.C., Hershey, C.O., and Breslau, D., Hospital admissions caused by iatrogenic disease, *Arch. Intern. Med.*, 146, 1931, 1986.
14. Lindley, C.M. et al., Inappropriate medication is a major cause of adverse drug reactions in elderly patients, *Age Ageing*, 21, 294, 1992.
15. Nelson, K.M. and Talbert, R.L., Drug-related hospital admissions, *Pharmacotherapy*, 16, 701, 1996.
16. Ng, D. et al., Unplanned medication-related admissions to an acute care general teaching hospital, *Aust. J. Hosp. Pharm.*, 29, 84, 1999.
17. Nikolaus, T. et al., [The early rehospitalization of elderly patients: causes and prevention] Fruhe Rehospitalisierung hochbetagter Patienten: Ursachen und Pravention, *Dtsch. Med. Wochenschr.*, 117, 403, 1992.
18. Raschetti, R. et al., Adverse drug events in hospitalized patients: 1. *JAMA*, 277, 1351, 1997.
19. Trunet, P. et al., The role of iatrogenic disease in admissions to intensive care, *JAMA*, 244, 2617, 1980.
20. Trunet, P. et al., The role of drug-induced illness in admissions to an intensive care unit, *Intensive Care Med.*, 12, 43, 1986.
21. Bates, D.W. et al., Incidence of adverse drug events and potential adverse drug events: implications for prevention, *JAMA*, 274, 29, 1995.
22. Bates, D.W., Leape, L.L., and Petrycki, S., Incidence and preventability of adverse drug events in hospitalized adults, *J. Gen. Intern. Med.*, 8, 289, 1993 [see comments].
23. Bates, D.W. et al., Relationship between medication errors and adverse drug events, *J. Gen. Intern. Med.*, 10, 199, 1995.
24. Wilson, R.M. et al., The quality in Australian health care study, *Med. J. Aust.*, 163, 6 Nov, 1995.
25. Leape, L.L. et al., The nature of adverse events in hospitalized patients: results of the Harvard Medical Practice Study II, *N. Engl. J. Med.*, 324, 377, 1991.
26. Bedell, S.E. et al., Incidence and characteristics of preventable iatrogenic cardiac arrests, *JAMA*, 265, 2815, 1991 [see comments].
27. Bottiger, L.E., Furhoff, A.K., and Holmberg, L., Fatal reactions to drugs, *Acta Med. Scand.*, 205, 451, 1979.
28. Caranasos, G.J. et al., Drug-associated deaths of medical inpatients, *Arch. Intern. Med.*, 136, 872, 1976.
29. Dubois, R.W. and Brook, R.H., Preventable deaths: who, how often, and why? *Ann. Intern. Med.*, 109, 582, 1988.
30. Ernst, P. et al., Risk of fatal and near-fatal asthma in relation to inhaled corticosteroid use, *JAMA*, 268, 3462, 1992.
31. Ferner, R.E. and Whittington, R.M., Coroner's case of death due to errors in prescribing or giving medicines or to adverse drug reactions: Birmingham 1986–1991, *J. R. Soc. Med.*, 87, Mar, 1994.

32. Fletcher, H.J., Ibrahim, S.A., and Speight, N., Survey of asthma deaths in the Northern region, 1970–85, *Arch. Dis. Child*, 65, 163, 1990 [see comments].
33. Spitzer, W.O. et al., The use of beta-agonists and the risk of death and near death from asthma, *N. Engl. J. Med.*, 326, 501, 1992.
34. Waldhoz, M., Improper hospital care caused deaths in up to 27% of cases, Rand Study finds, *Wall Street Journal*, 1988, p. B5.
35. Hanlon, J.T. et al., Adverse drug events in high risk older outpatients, *J. Am. Geriatr. Soc.*, 45, 945, 1997 [see comments].
36. Dennehy, C.E., Kishi, D.T., and Louie, C., Drug related illness in emergency department patients, *Am. J. Health Syst. Pharm.*, 53, 1996.
37. Otero, M.J., Bajo, A., Moran, D., and Dominguez-Gil, A., Economic study of preventable adverse drug events in an emergency department, unpublished manuscript, 1999.
38. Brennan, T.A. et al., Incidence of adverse events and negligence in hospitalized patients: results of the Harvard Medical Practice Study I, *N. Engl. J. Med.*, 324, 370, 1991.
39. Leape, L.L. et al., Preventing medical injury, *Qual. Rev. Bull.*, 19, 144, 1993.
40. Faris, R.J., Explicit Definitions to Identify Preventable Drug-Related Morbidity in an Elderly Population and Their Use as an Indicator of Quality in the Medication Use System, unpublished doctoral dissertation, University of Florida, 2001.DAI, 62, no. 10B, 2001, p. 4448.
41. MacKinnon, N.J., Risk Assessment of Preventable Drug-Related Morbidity in Older Persons (Elderly), unpublished doctoral dissertation, University of Florida, 1999.DAI, 60, no. 06B, 1999, p. 2633.
42. Kozak, L.J.L.L., National hospital discharge survey: annual summary, 1997, *Vital Health Stat.*, 13, Issue 144, 1999.
43. Ernst, F.R. and Grizzle, A.J., Drug related morbidity and mortality: updating the cost of illness model, *J. Am. Pharm. Assoc.*, 41, Mar–Apr, 2001.
44. Eberhardt, M.S. et al., *Urban and Rural Health Chartbook: Health United States 2001*, National Center for Health Statistics, Hyattsville, MD, 2001.
45. Woodwell, D.A., National Ambulatory Medical Care Survey: 1997 summary, *Vital Health Stat. Adv. Data*, Issue 305, 1999.
46. Tafreshi, M.J. et al., Medicine-related visits to the emergency department: a prospective study, *Ann. Pharmacother.*, 33, 1252, 1999.
47. Bates, D.W. et al., The costs of adverse drug events in hospitalized patients, *JAMA*, 277, 307, 1997.
48. Brennan, T.A. et al., Hospital characteristics associated with adverse events and substandard care, *JAMA*, 265, 3265, 1991.
49. Ray, W.A. et al., Psychotropic drug use and the risk of hip fracture, *N. Engl. J. Med.*, 316, 363, 1987.

3

Understanding Adverse Drug Therapy Outcomes

Thought is parent of the deed.

Carlyle

Chapter 2 summarized published data about the preventable drug-related morbidity (PDRM) problem — the prevalence of preventable adverse outcomes of drug therapy. This problem causes significant human suffering and economic waste, perhaps throughout the industrialized world. Its severity may vary, however, among specific populations. Customary approaches to improving medications use have tended (a) to focus on an arbitrary part of the medicines use process such as prescribing or compliance, (b) to be based on general models of error prevention, or (c) to be based on common sense and conventional wisdom rather than a theory of medications use. Another approach, however, is developing. Some leaders, notably including the Institute of Medicine (IOM), have called for a systems view of health care.[1–3]

This chapter will offer a definition of the PDRM problem. It will present a qualitative review of the literature on PDRM (a) to identify and clarify concepts that appear in the literature, (b) to develop a consistent vocabulary, and (c) to construct a model to describe how PDRM happens. This model of medicines use will be used in subsequent chapters to identify and describe safer and more effective medicines use systems.

Changing Attitudes toward Adverse Outcomes of Drug Therapy

Attitudes and assumptions powerfully influence thinking and action, sometimes without regard to their basis in fact and theories. Because they influence the direction of research, education, and system change, attitudes and assumptions regarding patient injury from pharmacotherapy should be critically examined. Attitudes have changed in recent years, at least among thought leaders, but necessary change has not gone far enough among health practitioners and policy analysts.

Many influential professionals were "brought up" in an era when attitudes toward adverse drug therapy outcomes were very different than they are today. Published evidence and public discourse seems to, quite properly, debate details of research methods or findings. Private discourse, however, sometimes seems to distort scientific criticism into denial strategies, consistent with obsolete attitudes.[4–6] The behavior of major health care organizations and informal comments by professionals suggest that new information about the magnitude of the problem and the preventability of drug-related injury are still not accepted widely enough.

The older literature on adverse drug outcomes includes the idea that adverse drug events (ADEs) are an unavoidable hazard of medication use. For example, in 1955 Barr described "hazards of modern diagnosis and therapy" as "the price that we, as responsible physicians, must pay for the inestimable benefits of modern diagnosis and therapy."[7] This speaks volumes about a view that, we hope, is rapidly disappearing. First, the patient and society pay the price for adverse outcomes. The "responsible physician" may pay with regret, but also be paid to correct the problem as best he can. Second, since about half of adverse outcomes from drug therapy can be prevented, we should not be resigned to paying this price.

In 1956 Moser described a series of "diseases of medical progress" with the defining characteristic that they occur only when care followed "sound therapeutic procedure."[8] However, both his and Barr's articles described examples of adverse effects that clearly were preventable even at that time, e.g., digitalis intoxication from physician's "dogmatic insistence on oversimplification of dosage."[8] This is an interesting statement. It recognizes the phenomenon of substandard care justified by physician autonomy: either some doctors were inevitably dogmatic or digitalis intoxication would be avoidable by improving the prescribing or management of digitalis.

In 1971 Melmon wrote an editorial that marked a turning point in medical opinion, away from the older view:

> If most drug reactions resulted from hypersensitivity, idiosyncrasy or the inevitable risk assumed when toxic drugs are used, ... one could lament the facts, being powerless to change them. However ... 70 to 80 percent are predictable. Most of these are preventable without compromise of the therapeutic benefits of the drug.[9]

Two studies of drug-related deaths in hospitalized patients done about 10 years apart may symbolize a fundamental difference in the ability to recognize — and willingness to publicly discuss — the problem. Porter and Jick[10] reviewed adverse drug reaction (ADR) studies published between 1971 and 1976 from seven countries. Overall, this study reported six possibly preventable deaths in 26,462 admissions (0.02%): the authors attributed five of the six deaths to fluid overload and one to hyperkalemia. The fact that the authors recognized only two drug-related causes of death is remarkable. It seems to reflect a very narrow concept of preventability (or very limited data).

In contrast, in their 1985 study of preventable deaths in 12 hospitals selected on the basis of death rates, Dubois and Brook reported that half of 17 preventable deaths in patients with pneumonia were due to inadequate fluid management or improper antibiotics. They found that inadequate fluid management or inadequate management of sepsis explained two of nine preventable deaths in patients with cerebrovascular accidents. Of 23 preventable deaths in patients with myocardial infarction, reviewers attributed 3 to inadequate fluid management, 2 to inadequate control of arrhythmias, and 12 to inadequate management of sepsis.[11]

More recently, reports from the Harvard Medical Practice Study[12–14] and the Institute of Medicine[15] make it clear that some medical researchers are more willing today to recognize and report problems with drug therapy.

Preventable drug death in hospitals has become well known to the general public through newspaper and television. To cite one infamous example, Betsy Lehman, a 39-year-old science writer for the *Boston Globe*, was given a massive Cytoxan overdose while receiving chemotherapy for breast cancer at the Dana-Farber Cancer Institute in Boston. In the journalistic aftermath of her death, a *Boston Globe* story listed ten drug deaths attributed to overdosage of anticancer drugs alone.* Also, in contrast to Barr's parochial view, by 1996 it had become clear that the highest price for drug injury was paid not by physicians but by patients and their families.

The two IOM reports represent a further step in changing attitudes, significant not only for what was said, but also for who said it. The members of the Committee on the Quality of Health Care in America are blue-ribbon members of the health care establishment. Yet the thrust of their reports is unmistakable. Even if it did not cause the quality chasm, the old, physician-centered basic medical science paradigm will not find the bridges across it. We need to understand health care as an integrated, multilevel system.[16]

Causal Attributions of DRM: From the Four Bads to System Failure

H.L. Menken once wrote, "For every complex problem there is always a simple solution. And it is wrong." In the field of medicines use, the simple explanations do appear to be wrong. The literature shows that adverse outcomes result from many stages in the medications use process, and that the most useful

* Knox, R.A. and Mooney, B.C., Hospital Dosage Mistakes Not Rare: Past Cases Reveal Medication Errors, *Boston Globe*, Sunday, April 16, 1996.

explanations for adverse outcomes involve *system failure*, that is, recurring failures in one or more process steps or the coordination of those steps.

The simple explanations for DRM are the "four bads": bad drugs, bad doctors, bad patients, and bad luck. For example:

- Unsafe drug products (this is the original idea of adverse drug reaction).
- Failure of a patient, a professional, or a lay caregiver. This is the idea of error and negligence.
- Bad luck (the idea that DRMs are random events or the result of random events such as errors).
- Attribution of DRM to simple causes may be associated with blame and punishment, such as
  - Withdrawing a drug's marketing approval or removing it from a formulary of approved drugs.
  - Finding professional negligence; discipline or defrocking.
  - Malpractice damages if a professional is blamed.
  - Reduction of damages if a patient is blamed.

Some DRMs may have simple causes and simple solutions, for example, human error. However, the argument for blaming a professional or patient often comes down to their proximity to the event in place or time. If the person lacked the means to avoid error, to detect or to resolve the problem, blame may be scapegoating. Scapegoating is not merely unjust to the scapegoat. If it substitutes for finding and correcting real problems, scapegoating may leave the basic problem unchanged and the door open to future accidents. For example, patient noncompliance was mentioned in nearly every reviewed study of preventable hospital admissions. However, noncompliance is rarely simple or a root cause. For example, if a physician or pharmacist were following a patient carefully, he or she sometimes could have detected the noncompliance and corrected the cause before patient injury had occurred. This idea will be developed further below.

Similarly, when a drug product is blamed for patient injury, there may be a demand to remove it from the market. However, it is not clear how more stringent drug safety laws would prevent the common types of DRM reported in the research literature. Three points are noteworthy: First, PDRMs involve many drugs, therapeutic classes, or mechanisms of action.[17] Second, the drugs that are most often associated with preventable patient injury are "old standbys" like warfarin and digoxin. Third, most research describing preventable injury due to drugs comes from nations with stringent drug product safety and efficacy requirements for drug marketing.*

* Safety and effectiveness exist in a political as well as a scientific equilibrium. Some American patients have demanded that drug products available in other countries be made available in the United States, arguing in effect that drug unavailability prevents desirable outcomes.

Improving or correcting isolated parts of the medications use process may not prevent DRM or improve patient outcomes. For example, prescribing improvement programs such as formularies and physician education often demonstrate changes in the targeted process (e.g., prescribing), but very rarely show improvements in patient outcomes. (See Chapter 6.)

Lucien Leape was quoted as follows in the *Boston Globe* (April 16, 1995):

> Sometimes failures are so terrible that individuals should be punished, but that's not usually the case. We've got to look at these things as system problems rather than as individual failings. Doctors and nurses don't tend to look at them that way. Most people in our society don't look at them that way.

The Medicines Use Process Causes Adverse Outcomes

We need more valid models that describe how adverse outcomes of drug therapy arise and how they can be prevented. Understanding the real causes and preventives of DRM requires an analysis of the *medicines use process*, i.e., the sequence of actions and decisions traditionally used to provide drug therapy. The data have been accumulating, and some authors have begun to organize them into a model.

In their study of avoidable toxicity from theophylline, Schiff et al. wrote:

> A set of recurring management errors was identified as contributing to inpatient theophylline toxicity. Effective preventive mechanisms could have prevented most toxicity and associated morbidity. Theophylline's overall risk-benefit ratio in the inpatient setting may be less than that measured in well-controlled studies of the drug's efficacy because of … management errors.[18]

In their analysis of early readmission of elderly persons to a hospital, Bero et al. found recurring management problems. They concluded:

> The study identifies specific drug-related problems that could become targets for preventive interventions. The majority (76%) of the problems identified were potentially preventable.[19]

Bero et al. found the following recurring categories of causes of preventable early readmission: unexpected adverse drug reactions, patient noncompliance, and inappropriate prescribing (overdose, underdose, and lack of a necessary drug therapy).[19]

Lindley et al. emphasized the kinds of inappropriate prescribing that seemed to result in preventable patient injury: inappropriate choice of drug and inappropriate regimens (dose, route, duration).[20]

Inadequate follow-up — where a test should have been done but was not — and lack of response to abnormal symptoms or clinical findings are also frequently mentioned as causes of PDRM.[18,21–23]

To summarize, most of the PDRMs in the studies reviewed were associated with one or more instances of:

- Inappropriate prescribing
- Unrecognized adverse drug reactions
- Patient noncompliance (including taking too much or too little of a prescribed drug)
- Overdose or underdose, either in general or for a specific patient
- Lack of a necessary drug therapy
- Failure to recognize symptoms, delay in response, inadequate follow-up of clinical signs and symptoms
- Medication administration errors

This list will reappear in Chapter 8 as a partial basis for five principles of pharmaceutical care systems.

Leape et al. have taken the analysis of ADEs well beyond the level of simply identifying where a problem or error may have occurred in the medicines use process. They defined a system as "an interdependent group of items, people or processes with a common purpose"[69] and recognized that a medicines use system would involve external systems, e.g., professional education and information dissemination, and would include subsystems of various complexities.[3]

They first classified errors into 15 types and cross-tabulated them by the stage in order processing where they had occurred. Then they searched for

TABLE 3.1

Process Locations of Errors in Inpatient Studies

Author	Prescribing (Choice of Drug, Dose, Route)[32]	Drug Distribution (Transcription, Dispensing, and Administration)[31]	Follow-up, Monitoring[21]
Bates 1995[a]	68%	29%	2%
Bates 1995[a]	49%	51%	0%
Bedell 1991			Inadequate follow-up
Leape[b] 1991	49%	9%	29%

[a] Includes 264 actual and potential ADEs.

[b] Denominator is 227 drug treatment errors. One error could be classified into more than one error type. Excludes two additional error types: professional practicing outside his expertise (4%) and other (8%).

Note: For literature citations, see Table 2.2 and References to Chapter 2. Two of the six studies included in Table 2.2 are not included in this table. In their 1993 study, Bates et al. did not discuss drug therapy problems as potential causes of inpatient DRM or where in the medicines use process underlying causes may have occurred.[30] Wilson et al.[47] did not discuss causes of DRM specifically.

proximal causes, defined as the apparent reason the error was made.[3] They found 13 proximal causes. Finally, they asked why the proximal cause had occurred and how it could be prevented in the future. They called this third-level explanation a *system failure.*

They identified 16 system (or subsystem) failures. The usefulness of the system view was demonstrated powerfully by the fact that there was not a one-to-one relationship between proximal causes and errors. That is, proximal causes were not just another more basic way of naming an error. Some proximal causes contributed to many error types. Likewise, an error could result from more than one proximal cause. The identification of system failures led the investigators to recommend four specific system changes: computerized order entry, adding a clinical pharmacist to the patient care team, providing electronic drug information, and standardizing doses and administration times.

To summarize, understanding how to improve the outcomes of drug therapy depends in large part on one's perspective on drug therapy and medications use systems. The research literature clearly argues that PDRMs are often the result of errors, unresolved drug therapy problems, and other failures in the medicines use process. Furthermore, some PDRMs result from failure of more than one component.[3] These studies find correctable patterns leading to injury. Such patterns can simplify the task of prevention.

Errors and drug therapy problems are essential components of an understanding of DRM. However, an adequate understanding of the causes and preventives of DRM requires a model — an intellectual framework — composed of clear and consistent terminology, including error, drug therapy problem, system failure, and preventability.

A Model of the Medications Use Process

This section will present a model of the medications use process, and later sections will fill in the details. Figure 3.1 shows a greatly simplified diagram of a typical drug therapy process in ambulatory care. (The model for institutional care would be fundamentally the same, but would account for inpatient drug distribution and nurse administration.)

The process begins with a patient's decision to visit a health practitioner, let's say a physician. The practitioner would then assess the patient's problem, come to a clinical impression, and develop a therapeutic plan. The therapeutic plan may be simple or complex and may include drug therapy. If it does, normally a pharmacist receives the prescription. Or if the patient has brought his complaint to the pharmacist, the pharmacist may refer the patient to a physician or recommend a nonprescription — over-the-counter (OTC) — therapy. The pharmacist dispenses the medicine,

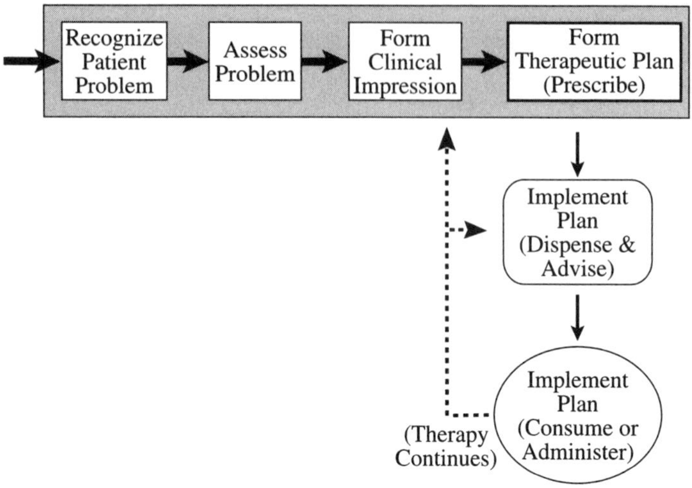

FIGURE 3.1
Diagram of the medications use process.

and the patient or caregiver consumes or administers it (at home or in an institution).*

Figure 3.2 shows the "shadow" of the medications use process depicted in Figure 3.1. During medications use, one or more errors may occur at each step. (Figure 3.2 ignores innocuous errors.) The physician may not recognize or not respond to an indication for drug therapy, may assess the patient incorrectly, form an incorrect impression (diagnosis), or misprescribe (wrong drug, dosage form, dose, directions, duration). The pharmacist may make a dispensing error (wrong drug, dosage form, dose, directions, amount) or provide inadequate advice to the patient about how to use the prescription. The nurse may administer (or the patient may take) an unprescribed drug or too little or too much of the prescription.

In addition, sometimes an event occurs that does not meet any reasonable definition of error. An example is an unknown (unknowable) drug hypersensitivity, or a symptom, not recognized as significant by a patient and not reported to a prescriber during an interview. Technically, the interview could have been more detailed, or the patient could have been more cooperative; but a finding of error might nonetheless be unrealistic. (Hindsight bias, for example, stating that if an injury occurred then an error must have caused it, and then looking for the error is discussed below.)

* Diagnosis (clinical impression, etc.) is included in this description of a medications use process because appropriate medications use clearly depends upon prompt recognition and a correct assessment of a patient's problem.[9] Unrecognized and untreated indications are important causes of DRM. The right drug for the wrong disease is unlikely to improve quality of life. Also, symptoms of some DRMs may be interpreted as new, unrelated medical problems and may be treated with more drugs.

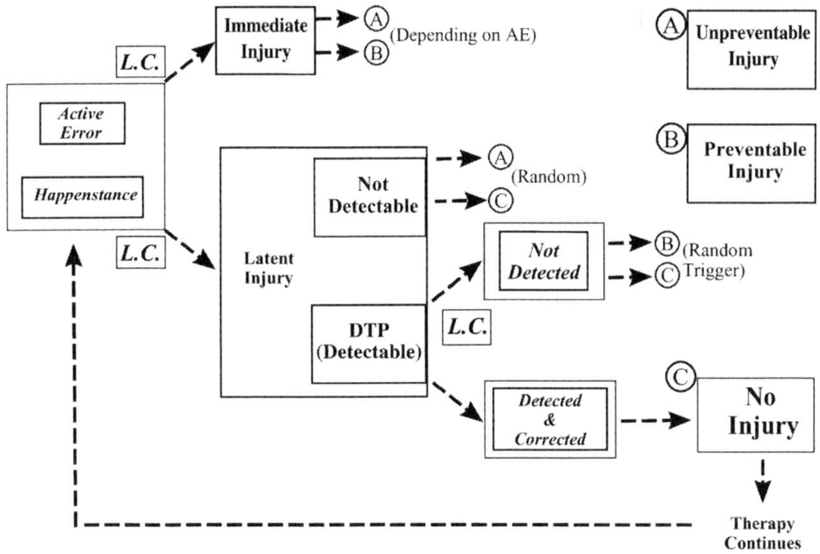

FIGURE 3.2
Model of how DRMs occur in the medications use process. L.C. = latent condition (failure).

Some errors or happenstances do not cause injury, although they may be near misses or important in other respects within the care of the patient. In contrast, others may be sufficient to cause the injury and may cause it almost immediately. James Reason, a psychologist and prominent scholar in the field of human error, has termed such errors (committed or omitted by caregivers or the patient himself) *active failures* (AFs) or *active errors*.

If a significant error (or happenstance) is not sufficient to injure a patient, then it causes a latent injury. A *latent injury* or *latent outcome* is a propensity or predisposition for injury that occurs during the processes of care. Latent injury is an attribute of a patient at a particular time. (A latent failure, condition, or error is a system attribute and is discussed further below.) Some latent injuries may be recognizable and correctable at a subsequent time during therapy.

Some latent injuries follow errors in prescribing, dispensing, or administration. Others may follow happenstance events that do not fit most people's idea of error. For example, a patient may begin to develop an unusual ADR, perhaps mild at first, say a fall in white blood cell count. Some patients may be unforeseeably overdosed on a usual dosage of a drug. A patient may begin to take another drug or eat a food that is incompatible with existing therapy. Grapefruit juice, for example, notoriously interferes with the metabolism of cisapride, some benzodiazepines, and many other drugs, causing toxic reactions at otherwise normal doses. Although this interaction is understood now, for a while patients taking those drugs could not be warned to avoid grapefruit juice because the interaction was not recognized. A patient taking anticoagulants may change his diet and thereby change his intake of vitamin K.

A previously controlled diabetic patient may hurt his ankle, causing him to suspend his daily exercise routine and either undercompensate or overcompensate with adjustments in diet. In order for this model to be useful for understanding DRM and for guiding design of safer systems, it is important to avoid hindsight bias. Patient injury can occur without error.*

A *drug therapy problem* (DTP) is a detectable (recognizable) latent injury. A latent injury may become recognizable as a DTP long before it actually causes DRM, while it is correctable. Other latent injuries may never appear as a DTP. Some latent injuries, including some DTPs, do not become severe enough to be considered DRM. For example, a patient may go for years with an unrecognized side effect. Likewise, a DTP such as somewhat undertreated asthma may go on for years. However, some other event — called a *trigger event* — may occur during the treatment of the patient that causes the latent injury to become an actual manifest injury.

A trigger event can be another error or happenstance, usually one that would not be expected to cause injury by itself. The death of Katherine LaStima (see Preface and Chapter 1) illustrates latent injury, a trigger event, and DRM. Her asthma had evidently been out of control for some time. Probably a number of errors had produced and sustained her latent injury, but she seems to have lived an almost normal life despite her undertreated and barely controlled asthma. Her latent injury was manifest as a DTP. Her pharmacist or physician could have recognized it through her pattern of medications use: overuse of "rescue" medicines and underuse of "preventer" medicines. It could have been recognized medically (by taking a detailed recent history or by examination), by herself or by her parents, had they appreciated the significance of her decision to stop taking her "preventer" steroid medications. This latent injury (DTP) existed for some time because of latent failures in the system and might have continued, except that she went to an agricultural fair where she presumably encountered allergens. The allergens triggered her latent injury (in other words, exacerbated her poorly controlled asthma) to the point that her life could not be saved.

Sometimes a trigger event is not clearly discernible. A patient on nonsteroidal anti-inflammatory drugs (NSAIDs) may develop an oozing gastric lesion and may shed a small, but detectable, amount of blood into his stools. The lesion may gradually enlarge until a larger blood vessel is opened, and the patient may hemorrhage "suddenly." A patient may be slowly accumulating a drug like digoxin or a drug with a sedative side effect. Examples are far too numerous to list here. The description of PDRM indicators in Chapter 7 provides more examples.

---

* For example, if a formerly controlled patient on anticoagulants had a severe bleeding event, hindsight bias would say, "Hemorrhage in an otherwise healthy, formerly controlled patient rarely happens without an error. Since it occurred, there may have been an error. Let's figure out who committed the error." The distinction between a significant and insignificant error admittedly depends on whether a patient was injured. This distinction, however, is necessary to teach the model, but not to apply it for system design.

Now, according to James Reason, systems allow latent injuries to occur through *latent failures*, also called latent conditions or latent errors. Despite the similarity in their names, latent injuries and latent failures are fundamentally different because a latent failure is an attribute of a system, and a latent injury is an attribute of a patient. They are related because latent failures allow latent injuries to continue.

To summarize, this model distinguishes two types of precursors to an adverse effect of drug therapy:

1. "Active" errors and violations that led to injury before they could be detected and corrected.
2. Unresolved latent injuries caused by happenstance and "upstream" errors (errors from earlier in the system). Some latent injuries are detectable drug therapy problems; some are not detectable.

The Adverse Outcome

The main issue involved in defining an adverse outcome is the scope of the definition. The event being defined may denote consequences of (a) drug products per se; (b) drug therapy, which is the use of a drug product to achieve a therapeutic objective; (c) ineffective drug therapy; or (d) lack of drug therapy when it had been indicated. The scope then logically influences both causality and preventability.

Adverse Drug Reactions

By far, the most widely recognized adverse outcome from drug therapy is an adverse drug reaction (ADR). According to the World Health Organization (WHO), an adverse drug reaction is

> a response to a drug which is noxious and unintended and which occurs in man at doses normally used for prophylaxis, diagnosis or therapy of disease, or for modification of physiological function.[24]

This definition refers to the drug product itself. It excludes inappropriate therapeutic intent, inappropriate dose, and injuries caused by undertreatment or nontreatment. Some ADR researchers also would exclude inappropriate route of administration, frequency, and duration. This leads some scholars to conclude that ADRs result from drug products themselves. It has led some authors, for example, Bero et al.[19] and Lazarou et al.,[24] to conclude that ADRs are not preventable, by definition, except by withholding the drug. (Preventability is discussed further below.)

The WHO and related definitions do not consider the severity of an outcome. According to this definition, a nosebleed would be as much an ADR as a hemorrhage. Reidenberg required that an event in his study, to qualify as an ADR, be severe enough to be commented on in progress notes.[25] Seidl et al. required that an event result in further treatment, reduction, or discontinuation of therapy with the causative agent, or that it be seen to increase the potential risk of future use of the agent.[26]

Drug-Related Morbidity and Adverse Drug Event

Table 3.2 lists some examples of terminology from studies of drug-related admissions and emergency department (ED) visits. After ADRs, perhaps the two most familiar terms are drug-related problem (DRP) and adverse drug event.

The most commonly found term for an adverse outcome of drug therapy in outpatient studies (hospital admissions and ED visits) is *drug-related problem.* In inpatient studies, the most commonly found term is *adverse drug event*. The Harvard Medical Practice Study (MPS) identified adverse events as "unintended injury that was caused by medical management and that resulted in measurable disability." The glossary to the IOM report defines an adverse event as "an injury resulting from medical intervention."[15]

Papers from the members of the Adverse Drug Event Prevention Study (ADEPS) have defined an adverse drug event variously as "an injury resulting from the administration of a drug,"[30] "an injury resulting from a medical intervention related to a drug"[31–34] and "injury related to the use of a drug."[36]

The concepts of ADE and ADR differ in two important respects: (1) ADEs do not require that a patient received a drug in "doses normally used," and (2) ADEs require patient injury rather than a "noxious result." Therefore, ADEs extend the scope of definition beyond ADR to include consequences of some important aspects of drug use — specifically *error* (and, by extension, other kinds of inappropriate drug *use*). The definition also excludes noxious responses that do not constitute patient injury. However, these definitions of ADE include toxicities and side effects caused by drug therapy, but exclude consequences such as treatment failure, attributable to ineffective drug therapy, or nontreatment of a valid indication for drug therapy.

Some injuries that are attributable to the disease itself are avoidable by proper diagnosis and therapy, for example, asthmatic crisis where the patient did not receive indicated steroids or was otherwise undertreated.[22] This is very often the purpose of medical care. Nontreatment or undertreatment, including but not limited to patient noncompliance, is reported as a cause of drug-related hospital admissions in many published studies. Examples are patient noncompliance, lack of necessary drug therapy,[19] treatment failure,[37] dose-related therapeutic failure,[28] long term undertreatment and suboptimal management,[22] failure to accomplish intended purpose of the treatment,[38,39] and "success or failure of the medical system as a whole."[23]

TABLE 3.2

Events Leading to Hospital Admissions and ED Visits

Author[a]	Event	Definition, Description, Examples
Bero	DRP	An adverse event related to drug administration or to the lack of a necessary drug therapy; 14 DRP types defined
Bigby		Success or failure of the medical system as a whole, as well as possible success or failure of individual providers and patients: failure to follow up an abnormal symptom, sign, or laboratory test result; adverse drug reaction; complication from a procedure; misdiagnosis; NC
Courtman et al.	DRP	ID, ADR, DI, NC, UI; from Strand et al. (27)
Cunningham	DRP	ADR, UD, UI, IP, OD, WI, DP, DI; based on Strand et al. (27)
Dartnell	Adverse events related to drug therapy	OD, UD, CI, IF, IP, inadequate counseling
Hallas et al. (28)	Drug events	ADR, dose-related TF
Lakshmanan et al.	Adverse effects	OD, SE, DI, IMR, drug-disease interaction (CI?), idiosyncratic reactions
Lindley		IP, CI, WI, DI, ADR
Nelson et al.	Drug-related event	ADR, dose-related TF[28]
Ng	Adverse medication-related event (AMRE)	UI, WD, UD, OD, ADR, DI, NC (not receiving prescribed drug), WI; based on Bero et al. (19), Wilson et al. (47)
Raschetti	ADE	ADR, dose-related TF, DI, interactions of a drug and alcohol
Tafreshi	DRP	UI, IP, UD, OD, NC and FP, ADR, DI, WI[29]
Trunet	Iatrogenic disease, specifically drug-induced illness	Disease that is independent of underlying disease and results from drug administration [or] therapy; ADR, therapeutic errors: OD, CI, therapeutic antagonism or inappropriate route of administration

[a] See also Table 2.1 and the references for Chapter 2.

Note: In most cases the original term used in the individual studies was retained. Consistent abbreviations were used, as follows: DI = drug interaction; DP = duplicate prescription (therapeutic duplication); DSE = side effect of drug; FP = failure to receive prescribed drug; ID = inappropriate dose; IF = inadequate follow-up; IMR = immunological reaction; IP = inappropriate prescribing (including wrong directions); NC = patient noncompliance or nonadherence; OD = excessive drug dosage; TF = treatment failure; UI = untreated indication; UD = underdosage; WD = wrong drug taken; WI = drug use without indication.

A term is needed to encompass all of the adverse outcomes of drug therapy described in the literature, including serious undesirable drug effects and the outcomes of nontherapy and ineffective therapy. DRP could be used, but it has, confusingly, been used to refer both to the medications use process and to the outcome of that process. The definition of an ADE could be extended to include treatment failure and nontreatment. Such cases, however, may not have been included in previous ADE studies.

This book uses the term *drug-related morbidity* (DRM). A DRM is an unintended patient injury* with a scientifically plausible relationship either to (a) drug therapy or (b) an untreated indication for drug therapy. *Plausible* means a valid theoretical relationship and chronology. A DRM is, essentially, an adverse drug event, as defined above, *plus* injury caused by nontreatment or undertreatment.

Broadly, a DRM is the malfunction or miscarriage of drug therapy. DRMs include (a) significant adverse or toxic effects (ADR and ADE), as defined above; (b) treatment failures, i.e., occasions when drug therapy was attempted but did not achieve a realistic, intended outcome in a reasonable time; and (c) occasions when a patient did not receive an indicated or necessary drug therapy.

The concept of DRM is related to usages of drug-related problems to denote outcomes and to *drug-related adverse patient events* (DRAPEs).[37] It reframes definitions that require that an injury not be due to the disease itself.

Finally, a patient can feel ill from drug therapy and may seek additional professional care or stop therapy, regardless of whether the cause of the illness is professionally recognized. DRMs encompass both drug-related illness and drug-related disease. In its clinical (objective) manifestation, e.g., when there is sufficient evidence that symptoms are caused by drug therapy, DRM may be called a drug-related disease. When a DRM is primarily in terms of patient experience, it should properly be called a drug-related illness. The distinction may be especially useful in studies of hospital admissions and other ambulatory care studies.

Errors, Drug Therapy Problems, and System Failures

Researchers frequently use three terms to describe the genesis of DRM. These are *error*, *drug-related problem*, and *system failure*. The three terms as commonly used denote different components of a DRM model.

Errors

The Harvard Medical Practice Study and the IOM report have "emphasized the serious problem of human error in medicine."[40] The MPS investigators looked for explanations of adverse events in terms of errors and negligence. Error was defined as "a mistake in performance or thought." Negligence was "a failure to meet the standard of care reasonably expected of an average physician qualified to take care of the patient in question."

The Adverse Drug Event Prevention Study, a successor to the MPS, has continued to use *error* to explain DRM. In their 1993 study, Bates et al. identified ADEs and then looked for explanations involving error.[30] This paradigm connects *error* to *preventability*, for example, in the phrase "[drug-

---

* That is, a severe, dangerous, injurious, or disabling clinical outcome that was not correctable or required significant additional medical care to correct, e.g., emergency treatment or hospitalization.

related injuries] that might be due to errors and therefore potentially preventable."[3] Error is an explicit part of the definition of a *potential* ADE, but not of the definition of an ADE itself.

In their 1995 study, Bates et al. identified medication errors primarily, and then traced them to their possible conclusion as an ADE.[32] This study defined medication error as "errors occurring at any stage in the process of ordering or delivering [dispensing or administering] a medication." (The word *error* itself is not defined.)

Error refers to process — in this instance the medications use process. According to dictionary definitions, an act would be most easily judged to be an error if it were a deviation from a process standard. Pertinent dictionary definitions of *error* include

> **a:** an act or condition of ignorant or imprudent deviation from a code; **b:** an act involving unintentional deviation from truth or accuracy; **c:** an act that through ignorance, deficiency or accident departs from or fails to achieve what should be done ... Error suggests the existence of a standard or guide and the straying from the right course through failure to make use of this.[41]

James Reason defines error in terms of an *act* in the context of *intention* and *outcome*. The glossary of the IOM report defines error similarly:

> [Error is] a generic term to encompass all those occasions in which a planned sequence of mental or physical activities fails to achieve its intended outcome, and when these failures cannot be attributed to the intervention of some chance agency.[15]

Reason identifies three primary error types: *mistakes*, *slips*, and *lapses*. He defines *mistakes* as errors in judgment while planning an action. He further classifies mistakes as due to failure of expertise, when a preexisting rule or formula is misapplied, or lack of expertise, where the actor had no preexisting response and had to invent one. *Slips* are errors of execution. *Lapses* are storage (memory) errors between planning and execution.

Actions (and errors) can be further classified as *skill-based* (SB), *rule-based* (RB), or *knowledge-based* (KB). SB actions are "highly routinized activities in familiar circumstances."[51] In colloquial terms, one might say that SB actions are habitual responses to familiar situations. SB actions are not the focus of the actor's attention while being performed, and are controlled automatically by means of a learned pattern. Think, for example, of a regular commuter driving an automobile under usual conditions of traffic and weather.

In contrast, RB and KB acts are nonroutine problem-solving activities. They are the focus of the actor's attention. RB acts are controlled by rules, somewhat more automatically than KB acts. RB acts are controlled consciously, for example, by feedback (trial and error, feeling one's way).

An example of SB problem solving relevant to medications use might be a prescriber's apparently habitual use of a particular drug regimen for a specific patient presentation. For example, suppose a prescriber routinely recommends acetaminophen (Tylenol®) or aspirin for initial pain management for osteoarthritis (OA). If this were truly SB, the recommendation would require no reflection and no hesitation. Usually the prescriber could make the recommendation correctly, but a *slip* would be possible if, for example, he were thinking of another problem, and instead of saying "try Tylenol," he told the patient to "try Tylox®." (Tylox is a combination of acetaminophen with a narcotic, and not available without a prescription.)

Now suppose that the patient returned complaining that the acetaminophen did not suffice. The prescriber had not recorded the earlier recommendation and did not remember it. If the prescriber again recommended acetaminophen, as if it were a new recommendation, that would be a *lapse*.

Faced with a treatment failure from his first choice, the prescriber may consult his mental rules, such as "when acetaminophen or aspirin fails as initial therapy for OA pain, try using both together or try another nonsteroid." (His rules may also include a simple question for the patient before actually making a recommendation.) Given the RB output, to use an NSAID, the prescriber may then return to the SB level and automatically recommend or prescribe his usual NSAID regimen (drug, dose, frequency).

Continuing the example, suppose that the patient returns again, with a report indicating that the NSAID was not acceptable, for example, because of gastric discomfort or lack of pain control. If this were a relatively rare occurrence for this prescriber, it might provoke him to reevaluate not only the drug regimen but also the clinical impression of OA. In other words, it may provoke a knowledge-based response. He might find a *mistake* in his earlier impression about the cause of the patient's discomfort.

According to Reason's general error model (GEM), "human beings are furious pattern matchers."[51] That is, people recognize familiar patterns and prefer to respond to them automatically. Reason sees most problem solvers as reluctant to think through a problem and as strongly preferring SB over RB responses.

If the problem solver sees that preexisting, automatic actions are not having the expected effect (or senses that they would not reach the objective), he or she would next attempt to apply rules. If the application of rules has the desired effect, the person may switch back to SB behavior again. Alternatively, "the problem solver realizes that none of his or her RB solutions is adequate to cope with the problem"[51] and switches into KB mode. Only when the problem solver has no useful rules will he or she actually try to think through the problem.

Reason's analysis and modeling lead to the identification and classification of the causes of error, e.g., perceptual confusion and inattention (SB level); misapplication of a good rule or application of a wrong or inadvisable rule (RB level); bounded rationality (i.e., the limitations of rational abilities vs. problem complexity) and an incomplete or inadequate mental model (KB level).

The concept of error is a necessary building block for a systematic model of medication use outcomes. However, it is not sufficient. According to Reason,[51] "error does not capture all the ways in which human beings contribute to major accidents." He observes that people do not behave in isolation, but within "a regulated social milieu."

> While errors may be defined in relation to the cognitive processes of the individual, violations can only be described with regard to a social context in which behavior is governed by operating procedures, codes of practice, rules, and the like. For our purposes, *violations* can be defined as deliberate — but not necessarily reprehensible — deviations from those ... practices deemed necessary ... to maintain the safe operation of a potentially hazardous system (p. 195).[51]

Violations may be unintentional (where they overlap with errors), well-intentioned shortcuts, or intentional sabotage (which is outside the scope of this analysis). Routine violations seemingly result from a natural human tendency to find the path of least resistance. If these shortcuts or work-arounds occur in an environment that does not somehow punish them (or reward compliance), violations can become routine. Some violations are, in effect errors. They may cause overt or latent injury. Other violations connect the concept of error to the concept of a system if they cause a latent failure or manifest system failure.

Critique of Error

Error and violation are necessary concepts in this model of medications use but have significant limitations. The dictionary suggests that an error can be found when an action departs from a standard. Reason stresses that *error* depends on intention. In a like manner, *violations* depend on social norms and rules. In short, error presupposes a structure of standards and intentions that may not exist in many health care situations.

Professionals claim the right to be autonomous and value autonomy. Some autonomy may be essential for proper practice because of variations in the needs and problems of specific patients. Some autonomy, however, may simply seek to rationalize random variations in decision making. Evidence of irrational practice pattern variation seems to undercut some of the argument for professional autonomy. In any event, there are few specific guidelines covering necessary details of common therapies.

Explicit standards covering circumstances that are known to cause injury are few. For example, standards of practice rarely require (a) documentation of therapeutic intention or other necessary details of what a physician, pharmacist, or nurse was thinking when he made a decision; (b) monitoring and documentation of progress toward therapeutic objectives; and (c) prompt response to drug therapy problems. Therefore, many instances of PDRM involve decisions or actions for which standards are implicit or do not exist at all.

This may come as a surprise, because we seem to have many standards for appropriate prescribing, accurate dispensing, and correct administration. These are standards to prevent active errors, however. We lack standards to define latent error. If an asthmatic patient begins to slip out of control and compensates with overuse of his "rescue" inhaler, who is to say whether an error was committed? Much of drug therapy involves professional judgment, and it can be difficult to call a judgment erroneous. Documentation of therapeutic objective is rare, especially in community practice, but even in teaching hospitals.

When both the performance standard and the intention of a specific instance of medications use are merely implicit, a finding of error can be, at best, debatable. Likewise, violations can be difficult to detect when the rules are vague or nonexistent. For practical reasons, these are severe limitations which may sometimes complicate or disable the application of error and violation.

Its kinship with negligence taints error with a pejorative connotation that cannot be removed for some observers. Some writers use the concept of error and then argue against blame. This may be a distinction that is beyond the psychological flexibility of many people. In this view, errors are committed by individuals, and the question often becomes one of blaming or excusing the individual.

For example, some researchers have excluded some DRMs from the preventable category apparently because they were reluctant to find an error. For example, Hallas et al.[52] excluded injuries such as gastrointestinal hemorrhage associated by NSAIDs, because some NSAID use was from over-the-counter medicines or otherwise beyond the control of a physician. The logic seems straightforward, for the physician could not be blamed (or held accountable) for a patient's actions. The problem is not with the researchers' logic. The problem is with their premise that preventability requires an error by an individual. Likewise, if the stakes are seen to be high (as they usually are), a professional involved in a DRM might defend against the idea that it was caused by an error, unless there was a clear mistake, slip, lapse, or violation of an explicit standard.

The second limitation in applying error and violation to medications use is that DRMs are too prevalent to investigate individually. Many DRMs are misattributed or pass unremarked. Aircraft disasters, nuclear reactor meltdowns, and the like are more public, even though fewer people may be injured in these disasters than by DRMs. Disasters involve danger or personal injury to more people per event than do DRMs. Because they are infrequent and injure many people at once, they receive attention and can be followed up at length.

Few DRMs result in formal inquiries like those that followed disasters such as Chernobyl, Tenerife, Three-Mile Island, or Bhopal. The two limitations compound each other. The practical outcome is that few DRMs, treated as errors, result in structural assessments or changes. Even when DRMs have prompted public inquiries, they often have been in the form of lawsuits, usually for negligence, but sometimes with another objective, e.g., to rescind a drug's marketing approval. (Drug withdrawals are discussed in Chapter 5.) Such proceedings are blame oriented rather than system oriented, and are retrospective rather than directed at preventing future injuries. Negligence suits are frequently settled out of court, in confidential (secret) agreements.

Finally, using error to explain preventable DRM can just beg the question of whether the error was avoidable.

Drug Therapy Problems

Another necessary building block for a model of medications use is the concept of a drug therapy problem.* A *drug therapy problem* is any circumstance that a competent professional would judge to be inconsistent with achieving the objective of drug therapy. A DTP is overt, i.e., potentially detectable by a patient, caregiver, or professional, and is specific to a patient and time. In other words, DTPs are detectable in principle, although many may be undetected in fact.

A DTP is part of the *process* of care, in contrast to ADR, ADE, and DRM, which are *outcomes* of medications use. In systems terminology, a DTP is a state of an individual in a medications use system, an intermediate result of therapy.

A DTP is a possible precursor to a drug-related morbidity. The difference between a DRM and a DTP seems subtle at first, but maintaining a clear distinction between process and outcome is very important to understanding the model.

The notion of a DTP complements error and violation in three ways. First, DTPs are important and common latent injuries that can lead to DRM. Latent precursors include both latent injuries (a state of a patient in therapy) and latent failures (a state of a system's process or outcome) that result from human errors and violations, but which do not constitute or cause injury by themselves.** Latent injuries may continue indefinitely without causing injury until they are triggered, e.g., combined with other precursors. Reason called a latent error a *resident pathogen.* In this metaphor, a resident pathogen in a system is like a bacterial pathogen that can exist for a time in the body without causing disease. A latent injury, then, is like an impairment in a patient's immune system. The patient is susceptible to the pathogen. Then,

---

* The original term was *drug-related problem.*[27,29] The term originally referred to the process of care. Unfortunately, some studies used DRP to denote an outcome, that is, as a kind of DRM. For example, suppose a patient were admitted to a hospital because of overdosage — too much of the correct drug. That confuses process with outcome. Drug overdose is a part of the process of care. Some people who receive excessive dosages show a toxic manifestation, and some do not. In all but exceptional cases, the toxic manifestation, the outcome, would have been the reason for admission, not the overdose. The distinction is important, so a new term was needed.

** Out of respect for clear terminology (and for James Reason), the original definition of latent precursor included only what we are calling latent failure. My usage somewhat expands the original. Understanding medications use requires a term for deficiencies (in the patient, so to speak) that were caused by the system, i.e., what I call latent injury.

when the pathogen finds the compromised host, the patient shows manifest infection, i.e., injury.

Second, DTP is useful in circumstances where error or violation would be ambiguous, as described in the preceding section. DTPs include events or states (circumstances in the process of therapy) that may not clearly result from a deviation; a slip, lapse, or mistake; or the violation of a social norm. This may avoid the tendency toward finger pointing and defensiveness that often result from ambiguous allegations of error. Some DTPs have unknown etiology. They may result from unrecognizable, possibly chance, events or from the intersection of multiple causes that would be innocuous in isolation but deleterious in combination.

To return to an earlier example, consider a patient who experiences gastric hemorrhage. Endoscopy reveals a number of oozing gastrointestinal lesions and one large one, which is the apparent source of the hemorrhage. A medication history reveals that the patient has been taking prescribed NSAID medicine for more than 2 years. Also, he (unwittingly) takes a proprietary over-the-counter medicine for heartburn, an effervescent powder containing aspirin. He denies black, tarry stools until 2 days before admission. His record does not include evidence that his physician monitors hematocrit or performs tests for occult blood. One could debate (endlessly) whether the prescriber or the patient had committed an error or violation. While voluntary guidelines for the use of NSAIDs certainly do exist, there is no official requirement for monitoring NSAID use. If there was an error, there is room for debate about whether it was inappropriate prescribing, inadequate patient information, patient nonadherence, the fault of the OTC manufacturer, etc. Or one could say that there are two DTPs — two potentially recognizable circumstances that are inconsistent with the therapeutic objective — duplicate therapy and long-term therapy with NSAIDs without monitoring.

In the story of Katherine LaStima, it is not necessary to find an error in order to understand what happened. Was her overuse of her rescue medication and underuse of her preventer medication an error? Perhaps it was her decision to go to the fair. The pharmacist in this case actually committed a clear violation of the insurance company's policy regarding frequency of refills. The absence of a medication use standard, and his failure to appreciate the clinical significance of the early refill, however, was a latent failure. The violation did not kill her, but the latent failure contributed to her death. Perhaps she or her parents were not well informed about the management of asthma or distracted by other concerns. Error does not help us to understand the system that killed her (or allowed her death). The pattern of prescription refills certainly indicates a DTP to be investigated further. DTP does move us closer to an understanding. The failure to recognize and resolve Katherine's DTP was the proximate cause of her death.

The third way that DTPs complement error is that DTP changes the focus from the *details* of process (who did what, when) to the *management* of process — anticipation of likely outcome (what is likely to result).

Classification of DTP

Despite the complexity of terms used in the literature and in Tables 3.2 and 3.3, there are relatively few types of DTPs. Bero et al. defined 14 types.[19] Cipolle et al. have developed an exhaustive categorization of potential DTPs into eight types that are useful for practice and research.[42] This will be described in more detail in Chapter 10. For purposes of modeling medications use and the genesis of DRM, we can think of DTPs as falling into three basic types. During the process of therapy, the patient, caregiver, or health professional could have observed one or more problems with:

1. *Access*: that the patient was not receiving necessary therapy for a valid indication
2. *Effectiveness*: that therapy was not having the intended effect within a reasonable time
3. *Safety*: that therapy was producing an undesired effect

System Failures

We can define a *system* as "a set of interdependent elements interacting to achieve a common aim." System elements may include people, equipment, and techniques.[15] Reason's definition of error (above) refers to the actions of an individual. It also provides a ready template for a definition of system failure, which refers to the actions of many individuals (and, perhaps, of one individual over many discrete episodes):

> System failure is an occasion in which a planned sequence of discrete interdependent decisions and actions, carried out by many individuals and directed at a common objective, fails to achieve its intended outcome, when the outcome had been achievable.

In this definition, *achievable* simply requires the objective to be possible. It excludes (a) unpredictable and undetectable errors, (b) unpredictable idiosyncratic circumstances such as allergic reactions that develop so suddenly that they could not be interrupted, and (c) uncorrectable random interference, such as, for example, a treatment that does not succeed because a patient was injured by an agency entirely outside of the medications use process (e.g., an accident unrelated to medications use).

System failure, by this definition, refers more to outcome and less to process than does error. In contrast to a finding of error, a finding of therapeutic system failure depends on the clarity of an objective, but depends little on process standards. A therapeutic objective may be — should be — the purpose of every occasion of medications use, so a finding of therapeutic system failure should be less ambiguous and more accurate than a finding of error. If an explicit therapeutic objective were absent, the implicit objective might be much more obvious (easier to establish) than would be an implicit process standard needed to establish error.

TABLE 3.3

Abbreviated Descriptions or Criteria for Preventability

Author (reference no.)[a]	Preventability Term Used	Criteria for DRM Preventability
Bedell	Preventable	None
	Not preventable	A known complication
Bero	Potentially preventable	None; some examples in discussion
Courtman et al.	Avoidable	(1) Therapy was obviously inappropriate or contraindicated drug treatment; (2) no measures to counteract known effects of the drug; (3) or the patient was noncompliant or insufficiently educated about his or her medications
	Possibly avoidable	Drug therapy was not altered in response to changes in patient's disease state
Cunningham	Definitely preventable	Drug therapy was inconsistent with present-day knowledge or clearly unrealistic in the circumstances (see entry for Hallas et al. below)
	Possibly preventable	[Therapy] not erroneous, but [DRM] could have been avoided by appropriate measures beyond obligatory requirements
	Not preventable	[DRM} could not have been avoided by any reasonable means or was an unpredictable consequence of appropriate therapy
Dartnell	Avoidable	The likelihood that the admission could have been avoided if appropriate measures had been taken by health workers
Hallas et al. (28)	Definitely avoidable	Drug event was due to a drug treatment procedure inconsistent with present-day knowledge of good medical practice or was clearly unrealistic, taking the known circumstances into account
	Possibly avoidable	[Therapy] not erroneous, but drug event could have been avoided by an effort exceeding obligatory demands
Lakshmanan et al.		(1) Drug toxicity where levels could have been checked or were available but ignored; (2) use of CI drugs; (3) failure to detect adverse effects that were present long before admission; excluded: immunologic or idiosyncratic reactions; predictable but unavoidable side effects, e.g., chemotherapy-induced neutropenia; rapidly developing effects
Lindley	Avoidable	Inappropriate prescribing (as defined)
Nelson et al.	Definitely avoidable	(1) Patient did not take a drug known to reduce/prevent symptoms according to prescribed directions; (2) patient had known allergy to a prescribed drug; (3) patient had a disease for which the drug was contraindicated; (4) patient took a drug that was not indicated

TABLE 3.3 (CONTINUED)

Abbreviated Descriptions or Criteria for Preventability

Author (reference no.)[a]	Preventability Term Used	Criteria for DRM Preventability
	Possibly avoidable	Therapy was not monitored by physician at reasonable time intervals, including patient inability to see a physician (e.g., financial difficulties)
Ng	Preventable	No definition
Raschetti	Avoidable	See entry for Hallas et al. above
Tafreshi	Preventable	History of allergy, previous reaction to drug, DI, NC, IP, OD, UD, IF, prescribing, dispensing, and administration errors
Trunet (50)	Preventability	Not defined; some preventable events involved therapeutic error
ADEPS (31, 36)	Preventability	Preventability usually equated to error; for example, "[Some ADE] are due to error and are therefore by definition preventable"[36]; one study refers to "preventable by any means currently available"[31]
Kohn et al. (15)	Preventable adverse event	An adverse event attributable to error is a "preventable adverse event" (p. 28)

[a] See also Tables 2.1 and 2.2, and the references for Chapter 2.

Note: In most cases, the original term used in the individual studies was retained. Consistent abbreviations were used, as follows: DI = drug interaction; DP = duplicate prescription (therapeutic duplication), DSE = side effect of drug; FP = failure to receive prescribed drug; ID = inappropriate dose; IF = inadequate follow-up; IMR = immunological reaction; IP = inappropriate prescribing (including wrong directions); NC = patient noncompliance or nonadherence; OD = excessive drug dosage; TF = treatment failure; TI = untreated indication; UD = underdosage; WD = wrong drug taken; WI = drug use without indication.

Consider, for example, the evidence and reasoning required for a finding of system failure in the case of Katherine LaStima, compared to the evidence and logic required for a finding of error. Some observers could decide that no specific error had led to her death. No reasonable observer could deny that there was a system failure — specifically treatment failure. Many people and institutions failed, but any one of them may have been able to prevent her death.

Errors are often random events. However, as Leape and others have pointed out, a well-functioning system can detect errors and avoid a system failure.[3] In fact, that is a major reason for understanding and constructing systems. Although it is common for an inquiry to find a human error as the proximate cause of system failure, this may reflect a cultural bias. As a causal theory, error proneness does not withstand careful reflection. In most functioning systems, it is rare to find an error-prone person and even rarer to find a profile that reliably identifies error-prone people in advance.

System failures are *not* random events. Rather, they are the result of weaknesses in system design or performance, especially what Reason calls latent failures. Well-designed systems make people less likely to commit errors and make the errors easier to correct in time to prevent injury. In contrast, poorly designed systems continuously rely on people to compensate for design weaknesses. Some "errors" may be little more than an individual's failure to compensate for a poor system. System failure need not lead to blame, but may lead to problem solving and system improvement.

Two major types of latent failures are operational failures and design failures. Operational failures can be violations of procedure. They are described below, under "Preventability," as failures to detect and resolve a DTP. Design failures are the holes in the system that cause unintended consequences. By analogy to a computer program, they are the bugs that cause the program to crash.

Pure examples of DRM from design defects are rare, but design defects often combine with operational failures. For example, a patient presented to a Florida hospital with a coronary heart attack. The admitting physician ordered an appropriate drug, TPA, to dissolve the clot. To prevent permanent myocardial damage, the clot dissolver should be given within 30 min. TPA, however, was not in the hospital formulary. The hospital had streptokinase on hand (another clot-dissolving drug), and it had a procedure for responding to nonformulary drug requests, but the procedure made no exception for emergency drugs.

The patient received neither drug and claimed permanent myocardial damage. Technically, this was also operational failure because a DTP was manifest (untreated indication for a drug.) However, the nurse and pharmacist involved would have had to violate hospital policy to obtain treatment within the window of opportunity. They were blamed for not doing so, and maybe they should have. This is nonetheless an example of a design defect.

The death of Donald Ashwell, described in Chapter 5, is an example of a system failure caused in part by a design defect. Mr. Ashwell's Medicaid program would pay for up to five prescriptions. Mr. Ashwell was chronically mentally ill and had five prescriptions to control his mental illness. His sixth prescription was for an antibiotic to treat pneumonia. The Medicaid program presumably had an appeal process for when the sixth prescription was necessary, but Mr. Ashwell did not use it, probably because he did not know about the loophole. A pharmacist refused to fill the prescription because Mr. Ashwell was over his limit and had no money to pay. The untreated pneumonia was obviously a DTP caused by a system design defect. However, the pharmacist did not correct the DTP. Mr. Ashwell did not get his prescription and later died of pneumonia. The design defect, DTP, and process failure are obvious in both examples, but whether injury was caused by error was hotly debated by those accused.

A useful test of whether human error (vs. system failure) was truly the cause of system failure would be to ask if another person would have been equally likely to have committed the alleged error, or whether removing the person would probably have reduced the likelihood of the alleged error. For example, according to the facts reported in the news coverage, Mr. Ashwell's pharmacist apparently recognized the DTP but did not correct it or refer it to someone else. Perhaps another pharmacist would have behaved differently, but the system surely failed to provide backup (redundancy). In the case of Katherine LaStima, it may be tempting to blame the pharmacist, especially, or the physician, but the standards upon which one would blame them are not clear. It seems clear that even revoking the licenses of *both* the doctor and pharmacist would not change the likelihood of the same outcome occurring, by the same mechanisms, in other people.

Preventability

The remaining piece of the DRM model is the question of which adverse effects are preventable and how they can be prevented, in theory. Prevention arguably is the payload of a theory of medications use. The rest of the book will build on this foundation as it addresses practical issues in the design and operation of medications use systems.

Despite its importance, preventability is perhaps the least well defined concept. The motivation for a precise definition is both scientific and practical. The scientific motivation is to provide a foundation for research that can be compared and compiled. Some studies of preventable DRM did not publish even a description of preventability (or avoidability). Studies that did publish a description or definition show little agreement, as shown by Table 3.3.

Published studies may also have applied preventability definitions to specific cases inconsistently. No study provided explicit criteria, a reliability measure for preventability judgments, or formal validation of their definitions or judgments. These greatly limit the replicability and generalizability of study findings. Other investigators cannot apply identical methods (including definitions) to new samples for purposes of replication. The lack of replicate studies in different populations made the meta-analysis in Chapter 2 difficult to summarize toward a population prevalence estimate.

The second motivation is practical and political impact (credibility). A critical reader cannot decide whether he or she agrees with the classification of some cases of DRM as preventable, or even which cases would be included or excluded from the definition.

Preventability in Medical Record Reviews

Most studies of preventable DRM classify cases as preventable or not preventable using medical record review. Medical record review by qualified experts is generally considered to be the gold standard for evaluation of processes requiring judgment. Some studies reviewed a data summary abstracted from medical records, while others interviewed patients and added the interview results to the data available from the patients' official medical records.

The investigators were usually among the reviewers, and presumably chose additional qualified reviewers when necessary. Some reports described formal means to increase reliability, e.g., having more than one reviewer for each case and using criteria for interreviewer agreement.

Hallas et al. described a good example, one of the more careful medical record review procedures to be found in the literature. After an initial case finding, the review team interviewed patients and family members to obtain a detailed drug history covering the 14 days prior to admission. Interviews were carried out by a clinical pharmacology trainee, usually within 2 days of admission. The typical case review team comprised the senior investigator (Dr. Hallas), the chief of the relevant clinical service, and a clinical pharmacologist. They contacted the patient's general practitioner (GP) for additional information in all definite or probable drug events and reevaluated cases with a fourth member of the team (a GP).[28]

Hallas et al. defined *avoidable* in two categories as follows (see Table 3.3):[28]

> *Definitely avoidable*: "Drug event was due to a drug treatment procedure inconsistent with present-day knowledge of good medical practice, or was clearly unrealistic, taking the known circumstances into account."
>
> *Possibly avoidable*: "[Therapy] not erroneous but drug event could have been avoided by an effort exceeding obligatory demands."

During the process of review, the team would have used this definition and judged whether a therapeutic procedure was inconsistent with present-day knowledge of good medical practice or whether it was clearly unrealistic for the circumstances. Assuming that the three or four people on the review team carried out independent reviews, the *reliability* of those judgments may have been reasonably high. That is, it would be likely that the same team would make the same judgment about a very similar case. That might not have been so in studies that obtained less data or used fewer reviewers.

However, the *validity* of such judgments is difficult to assess. The definition contains important terms that are not defined and about which reasonable people might disagree: *inconsistent*, *knowledge*, and *unrealistic*. The definition of possibly avoidable refers to "effort exceeding obligatory demands." The context suggests to me that this refers to obligatory demands on a physician, but perhaps should have included others. What assumptions are implicit in obligatory demands?

DRM that seem not to be preventable in one system might seem preventable in another. Once the medical community has learned the number and types of avoidable hospital admissions, it should change its notion of obligatory demands.

Definitions of preventability in terms of error may be similarly ambiguous. The studies from the ADEPS are prominent examples. Some of the ADEPS papers catalog errors extensively. Although this reduces ambiguity somewhat, as I argued above, *error* is an incomplete basis for defining preventability.

Proposed Definition of Preventability

The following definition of preventability combines the major elements from the definitions summarized in Table 3.3, in the context of the DRM model given in Figure 3.1. A preventable DRM is defined as one with the following four attributes:

- The DRM was preceded by a *recognizable* DTP.
- The DRM was reasonably *foreseeable* under the circumstances.
- The cause of the DTP and resulting DRM was *identifiable*.
- The identified cause of the DTP (and resulting DRM) was *controllable* within the context of therapy (i.e., without sacrificing essential therapeutic objectives).

Some examples are given in the next section. According to the model, some DRMs, whether caused by error or happenstance, first manifest as recognizable DTPs, while some do not. (See Figure 3.1.) The former meet the four-part definition of preventability; the latter do not.

Some DRMs that follow recognizable DTPs may not have been reasonably foreseeable, for example, if a common and usually self-limiting side effect unexpectedly (unaccountably) developed into a DRM. The cause of a recognizable DTP may not be identifiable or it may not be controllable within therapeutic priorities. For example, a patient receiving cancer chemotherapy might experience disabling nausea, bone marrow suppression, etc., that would meet the definition of a DRM. It would not meet the definition of preventability if preventing the DRM would compromise the cancer therapy.

System failure and preventability are partially reciprocal concepts. In Figure 3.1, an important type of system failure is failure to detect and resolve a DTP. A preventable DRM is the manifestation of system failure.

This general four-part definition seems to encompass all of the specific types of events that were included under the definitions in Table 3.3, with one possible exception. It is not clear whether definitions of preventability in terms of error would include slips, lapses, and violations that had not become visible before the DRM. A slip or lapse might not become visible if the erroneous sequence was carried out in a brief time period by a single actor, for example, a drug administration error at the bedside. DRM from such causes would not be judged as preventable according to the four-part definition. However, DRM caused by slips, lapses, and violations would be considered preventable if they had become recognizable as DTPs before the appearance of the DRM.

The four-part definition does not require a finding of error as a prerequisite to preventability, substituting system failure as the prerequisite. Therefore, the definition includes cases where no error was committed, for example, when an observable ADR, initially mild, was allowed to develop into a patient injury (a DRM). This definition would not eliminate all reliability and validity problems, but it is a step in that direction. The theory is applied through the use of PDRM indicators, described in the next section.

PDRM Indicators

The four-part definition of preventability was validated by using it to construct specific definitions (indicators) of PDRM. In three separate studies, MacKinnon,[44] Faris,[45] and Morris et al.[46] developed proposed indicators, each in the format of outcome + process. Each was based on clinical literature connecting an adverse outcome with a pattern of care, e.g., excessive use of NSAIDs, lack of monitoring, and gastrointestinal bleeding. Each indicator was specific with regard to an adverse outcome and a process of care that was known sometimes to lead to the outcome. Each outcome appeared to be potentially preventable, according to the four-part definition, when it followed the specific process of care, for example, for gastritis (or upper GI bleeding or GI perforation or GI ulcer) and anemia

a. following the use of two or more NSAIDs concurrently for at least 2 weeks or
b. in a patient with a history or diagnosis of ulcers or GI bleeding, and NSAID use for at least 1 month

Proposed indicators were submitted in writing to a Delphi panel, a select group of physicians and pharmacists. MacKinnon[44] asked his panel to vote on each of the four components for each proposed indicator:

- Given the outcome and pattern of care, was a DTP recognizable? If so,
- Was the DRM reasonably foreseeable?
- Was the cause of the DTP and DRM recognizable?
- Would that cause be controllable within the scope of usual therapeutic objectives?
- Overall, does this indicator describe a PDRM as defined (recognizable, foreseeable, identifiable, controllable) and on the overall scenario, for each proposed definition?

The panelists reviewed the proposed indicators and voted to agree or disagree, using a two-choice scale (MacKinnon, Faris) or a five-choice scale (Morris et al.). Panelists could also propose modifications of existing definitions and propose additional definitions. The investigator compiled each panelist's written votes and critical comments anonymously. The investigator then deleted proposed definitions that lacked consensus and repeated the process. The compiled results of each Delphi round were then submitted to the panel in the next round, and the process continued until consensus had been reached either to keep or delete each proposed indicator.

Two or three rounds normally were required to obtain consensus (e.g., five or more votes of seven panelists). In the example, a Delphi panel agreed that there were recognizable DTPs in each hypothetical instance: (a) concurrent use of two or more NSAIDs, and (b) long-term use of an NSAID in a patient with a history of bleeding. They agreed that the possibility of an adverse outcome would be foreseeable. In this case, the cause is given and the panel agreed that it was controllable, e.g., by changing therapy or by careful monitoring.

The indicators accepted by the Delphi panels (usually about 50) were then applied to medical information in a patient database or other records. MacKinnon[44] and Faris[45] used databases from two Medicare managed care populations, and Morris et al.[46] used computerized records from a GP group practice in the U.K. Both MacKinnon and Morris et al. used a combination of manual and computerized searches to identify cases of PDRM. Faris coded the definitions completely and used computer searches of a U.S. health insurance database to identify cases of PDRM. The results were described in Chapter 2.

MacKinnon[44] submitted two of his indicators to criterion validation by medical record review. (Only two indicators — myocardial reinfarction and hospitalization due to hyperglycemia — had enough cases for reliable estimates of their individual specificity and sensitivity). A blinded panel of five clinical pharmacists reviewed medical record abstracts of all indicator positives and a random sample of matched indicator negatives for the two indicators (21 and 24).

(21.) An ER visit or hospitalization due to hyperglycemia has occurred after the following pattern of care:
  1. Use of an oral hypoglycemic agent (e.g., chlorpropamide, etc.)
  2. Hemoglobin A1c level not done at least every 6 months

(24.) A patient has had a second myocardial infarction after the following pattern of care:
  1. History or diagnosis of myocardial infarction
  2. No use of ASA or a beta-blocker

Overall, the indicator positives and negatives tended to be highly predictive of a patient having or not having the adverse outcome. By chart review, the two indicators had a sensitivity of 87.5% and a specificity of 73.5%. The sensitivity of indicator 21 (hyperglycemia) was 93.3% (95% confidence interval from 68 to nearly 100%), and the specificity was 81.3% (95% confidence interval from 54 to 96%).* For indicator 24 (second myocardial infarction), the sensitivity was 82.4% (95% confidence interval from 57 to 96%), and the specificity was 66.7% (95% confidence interval from 41 to 87%).

Summary (Preventability Definition)

Three independent panels of physicians and pharmacists have face- and content-validated specific PDRM indicators. Each indicator was based on the four-

* Specificity and sensitivity express measurement validity. Validity is discussed in Chapters 7 and 11. Interestingly, the Faris panel rejected MacKinnon's indicator 21 because they preferred blood glucose level over glycosylated hemoglobin as a more sensitive measure for diabetes control.

part definition. By accepting the specific definitions, the panels also have accepted the underlying four-part definition from which they were derived.

These indicators are explicit; in fact, they have been applied to computer databases. Their specific content is open and available for review. Their reliability and validity can be more easily evaluated. Studies based on them can be replicated.

Evidence-based PDRM indicators that have been accepted by an expert Delphi panel provide a balance between scientific evidence and local best practice. This might increase their applicability as performance indicators, as described in Chapters 7 and 11.

For research purposes, however, local variation may not be as desirable. Some readers of a research report might not concur with the Delphi panel's opinions about the face validity of some indicators. A national or international blue-ribbon panel could be used to provide a broader scope of medical authority.

The use of explicit definitions, which improve interpretation and potential replication of results, is also its major limitation as a research tool. There may be types of PDRM that were not included in the original indicator set and that were not added by the Delphi panel. Perhaps there are types of PDRM that are not even measurable by the method. Both of these issues can be addressed by a large-scale criterion validation against medical record audit. For the time being, PDRM indicators, as research tools, should be interpreted as providing a lower bound to the true PDRM prevalence in a population.

Preventability Depends on Assumptions and Paradigm

Decisions about preventability also depend on assumptions (sometimes implicit) about the nature of professional practice and the medications use process. For example, Hallas et al. consider some adverse outcomes to be only possibly avoidable if preventing them would exceed obligatory demands of medical practice.[28] Wilson et al. define a standard of preventability in terms of "the current level of expected performance for the average practitioner."[47] Both of these reflect a *descriptive* rather than a *prescriptive* approach to standards, and rest to some extent on unstated assumptions about current practice.

In contrast, DRMs that are not considered to be preventable in a process view might become preventable in a systems view. We can adopt a somewhat more active (interventionist) perspective, similar to that of a system's engineer. We can imagine and design systems in which more DTPs will be recognized and corrected. Two especially instructive examples involve the alternative interpretations of DRM caused by patient medication-taking behavior (e.g., noncompliance) and by ADRs.

Patient Medication Use

One the one hand, some investigators would argue that DRM resulting from patient medication-taking behavior is not preventable. For example, they may explain that a patient's taking the "wrong" amount of a prescribed medicine is beyond professional control. In the case of OTC drugs, neither what is taken nor how it is taken would be subject to professional control. Also, OTC drugs are often not recorded in medicine databases. However, a patient may experience a DRM from a combination of OTC and prescribed medicines, for example, hemorrhage from a combination of OTC and prescribed NSAIDs.

On the other hand, while professionals cannot *control* patient behavior, they can *influence* patient behavior, which might affect the incidence of adverse outcomes. Furthermore, if a patient is in a physician's care, or even if he buys OTC medicines in a pharmacy, problems resulting from patient medication-taking behavior could often be detected as a DTP, e.g., from early signs of treatment failure or toxicity, from pharmacy records. This would be an opportunity for a professional to discuss the patient's medication-taking beliefs and behaviors and to recruit the patient's cooperation in his own care.

Adverse Drug Reactions

Because of the documented prevalence of ADRs, the question of preventability of ADRs is potentially quite significant, for example, as it would encourage or discourage appropriate efforts to improve outcomes. Lazarou et al., among others, assert that adverse drug reactions are not preventable, by definition, because they are unintended and occur at normal doses.[16,19,24] However, 4 of the 15 PDRA studies reviewed in Chapter 2 found that hospital admissions or transfers caused by ADRs may be preventable.[23,48–50]

Some ADRs begin to manifest themselves with reversible symptoms that fit the definition of DTP but not DRM. For example, patients taking warfarin may experience bleeding. Any episode of bleeding from warfarin at "normal" doses would be noxious and unintended, and therefore would meet the WHO definition of an ADR. However, because of the mechanism of action of warfarin, severe over-anticoagulation usually develops over time, with manifestations that proceed from minor (bruising, nosebleeds, bleeding gums) to major (hemorrhage).

Before significant hemorrhage can occur, increases in prothrombin time can be observed (if we look for them). Furthermore, many patients may experience bleeding gums, nosebleeds, increased tendency to bruise, and occult blood in stools or urine. Perhaps such technical ADRs as nosebleeds, etc., from warfarin can be prevented, perhaps not. However, the clinically important point is clear: if excessive anticoagulation is recognized as a DTP — while it is relatively minor — then serious blood loss (the DRM) can be avoided. Therefore, DRMs caused by ADRs, i.e., serious *consequences* of ADRs, may be preventable.[20,21,23,31]

Lindley et al. also recognized that an ADR caused by an unnecessary drug is also a preventable ADR. The assumption that "ADR[s] are not preventable, by definition," while perhaps technically correct, is seriously misleading.[20]

Active Errors and Theoretically Perfect Systems

The preceding discussion of preventability concerns latent injuries. Improving the system's performance would require elimination of latent failures. So far, I have said little about active errors, i.e., errors that are sufficient to cause immediate injury, e.g., injection of a drug into an artery instead of a vein, or all at once (intravenous push) instead of by slow drip. Figure 3.2 (at the top) diagrams active errors. The figure suggests that deciding whether an immediate injury was preventable depends on the preventability of the error itself. The preventability of such injuries may be much more difficult to decide than latent injuries that become manifest.

The preventability of an injury from an active error surely depends in part on the error itself. Should the operator have known better, thought more, been more careful? Was his slip, lapse, mistake, or violation one that never should have happened, or can it be prevented from happening again? In this instance, perhaps, happenstance would include unforeseeable and unique contributing circumstances. Some misapplication of rules or errors of judgment seem inevitable under some circumstances. Therefore, some immediate injuries might be considered preventable, some not, depending on the nature and circumstances of the active error itself. This is a different matter than the preventability of DRMs that depend on the nature of the latent injury.

This is emphatically not meant to suggest that we can tolerate errors in the operation of a system in the mistaken belief that they will be detected later on. It is axiomatic that safer and more effective systems "do it right the first time" more often than other systems. On the contrary, some errors cannot be detected and resolved before injury has occurred. Preventing them in the first place is the only way to prevent the injuries they cause. How many *can* be prevented, however?

Some experts would argue that an injury caused by active error should have been prevented by the system, just as with latent injuries. But perhaps the difference between active injury and latent injury is fundamental. Perhaps designing systems to prevent injury from active error is self-defeating. (The issue here is the preventability of the error and the performance of the system. Accountability for the injury and culpability for the error are separate issues.)

The box labeled "L.F.?" between error and injury at the top of Figure 3.2 represents the idea that active errors injure people through latent failures, i.e., system deficiencies that do not stop or neutralize the errors. The question mark represents controversy about how many active errors system design should be able to intercept.

According to the view of high reliability theory (HRT), all errors can be prevented or caught before they injure a patient. Advocates of high reliability theory would argue that a system can be designed to operate without adverse outcome. According to this theory, the question mark should be small or absent. Any error that proceeds to injury indicates a system failure.

According to normal accident theory (NAT), however, there is a point at which error prevention and detection efforts become self-defeating because the efforts themselves begin to cause errors or worsen their effect on outcomes. To oversimplify, would a fail-safe system be too complex and tightly linked to operate safely? Advocates of NAT might insist that injury does not necessarily indicate system failure because systems cannot be perfected. They also argue that some complex systems are a form of Russian roulette. They can appear to be operating safely for a while, but only as long as luck holds out. That is, they have inherent and irremediable latent failures that sooner or later will be triggered into disaster.

The performance of most medications use systems is probably so far short of perfection that the issue of HRT vs. NAT seems academic, even for a theoretical discussion. In some ways, operation of a health care system, with millions of unprogrammable decisions made in tight time constraints, is quite different from the operation of, say, a nuclear power plant, a dam, or an airplane. The immediate practical issue is which end we should start with: active errors or latent errors?

Two important points come from this discussion. First, my preference would be to build and improve medications use systems that are designed to detect and reverse latent injuries. Then we can apply what we have learned to detecting and stopping active errors. Second, simplicity in drug therapy may be a greatly underappreciated value. Perhaps there are patients with so many problems that some of those problems cannot be treated as aggressively with drugs as they would in a patient with fewer problems. Perhaps some regimens, although not theoretically the best, are more manageable.

Summary of the Preventable DRM Model

The model developed in this chapter proposes a medications use process of patient assessment, prescribing, dispensing, consuming, and monitoring (Figure 3.1).

1. The medications use process can have three outcomes: the therapeutic objective, a new medical problem created by therapy, or treatment failure. The three names for adverse outcomes are:

   Adverse drug reactions (ADRs) — any noxious and unintended effect caused by the drug itself.

   Adverse drug events (ADEs) — patient injury caused by the drug itself or by an error in how a drug is used.

   Drug-related morbidities (DRMs) — patient injury caused by a drug or nontreatment of a valid indication. DRMs include ADEs and patient injury when no error was obviously present, usually the result of latent causes.

2. Errors may occur in the process of medications use. An error is most broadly defined as an occasion when a planned sequence of activities fails to achieve its intended outcome, and these failures cannot be attributed to the intervention of chance. In popular use, however, an error is an ignorant or imprudent and unintentional inaccuracy or deviation from a code. Error suggests the existence of a standard or guide and the straying from the right course through failure to make use of it. There are four kinds of errors:

   Mistake — an error when planning an activity

   Lapse — failure of memory

   Slip — failure of execution

   Violation — intentional deviation from a rule or procedure
3. Furthermore, events may occur that do not meet the definition of an error. Some errors and other events may begin to injure the patient immediately, some may be recognizable drug therapy problems, and others may remain undetectable as latent injuries. Unresolved drug therapy problems, latent injuries, are immune deficiencies. Latent errors and latent failures are resident pathogens. They do not harm the patient but may combine with each other to cause injury, often suddenly.
4. A drug therapy problem is a circumstance that is inconsistent with achieving a therapeutic objective, but which is not particularly injurious in itself or difficult to correct. Some drug therapy problems are errors or are caused by errors that happened earlier in the process. Others, however, result from chance events or interactions of errors and chance events.
5. A *preventable* ADE or DRM follows a recognizable, correctable drug therapy problem when the possibility of injury was reasonably foreseeable.
6. A latent failure is a system defect in operation or design that permits latent injury to persist. A system failure is the possible culmination or manifestation of latent failure. It is similar to an error, i.e., an occasion when a planned sequence of activities fails to achieve its intended outcome, except that a system failure, by definition, involves more than one event and focuses on the result rather than what went wrong in the process.
7. The distinction between system failure and error is important. It is reasonable to say that an error caused an injury if and only if the error caused injury before it could be recognized as a drug therapy problem. If an error could have been detected as a DTP before it injured the patient, then the failure of the system to detect the error is the proximate cause of injury. This point is fundamental to constructing and operating medications use systems that are reliable and in which accountability can be shared.

Where Do Medications Use Systems Fail?

All of the preventable drug-related hospital admission (PDRA) studies included in Table 2.1 identified DTPs that had been associated with DRAs. Four of the six inpatient studies (Table 2.2) mentioned errors or DTPs and the stage in the medications use process where they may have occurred.

Hospital Admissions Studies

Table 3.4 classifies DTPs according to their likely place in the medications use process shown in Figure 3.1. This approach is analogous to the one used by Leape et al. to classify adverse drug events occurring in a hospital: physician ordering, transcription and verification, pharmacist dispensing, and nurse administration.[3]

The main categories are prescribing (Rx) drug choice, Rx dosage, drug distribution (dispensing, administration, consumption), and therapeutic effect. Main categories are further subdivided to retain, as much as possible, the terminology used in the report. So, for example, the paper by Lakshmanan[53] reported that 3% of patients with drug-related hospital admissions had a prescription for a contraindicated drug (CI).

Table 3.4 contains many blank cells because different authors used different terms. For example, the Dartnell et al.[48] study did not report any patients with CIs prescribed, but reported that 26% of patients had inappropriate prescribing (IP). Some investigators used fewer terms than others; consequently, those terms may have included a variety of specific DTPs. For example, Hallas et al.[52] used only ADRs (but including drug toxicity) and dose-related therapeutic failure (including noncompliance, inadequate monitoring, and low dosage). Hallas et al. surely observed other DTPs, e.g., inappropriate prescribing, but reported them in just two groups.[28]

The summary row in Table 3.4 labeled "NStudies" shows the number of studies that mentioned percentages for DTPs under each of the four categories. The row labeled "Avg. % of Patients" reports average proportions for each of the four categories, based on these ten studies.

Percentages add across and down. For example, Trunet[54] reported that 25% of patients admitted to intensive care had a DTP involving drug choice. Five of the 10 studies reported problems with drug choice, and the overall percentage of patients with drug choice DTPs was 6.3%. (Note that the denominator is the sum of all ten studies' reporting percentages.) The summary percentages are not, however, valid estimates of population data. The bottom section of the table summarizes the five studies that only mentioned DTPs, but did not give percentages.

The studies in Table 3.4 tended to clearly state the nature of the DTP, which was implicated as a cause of a DRM. This information should help to identify the problems that should be addressed to improve drug therapy. The studies

TABLE 3.4
DTPs Mentioned in PDRA Reports

	Rx Drug Choice						Rx Dosage				Drug Distribution			Therapeutic Effect						
Author[a]	**CI**	**WD**	**IP**	**UI**	**WI, DP**	**Total**	**UD**	**OD**	**ID**	**Total**	**NC**	**FP**	**Total**	**ADR**	**TF**	**IF**	**DSE**	**IMR**	**DI**	**Total**
Studies with Quantitative Data (%)																				
Bigby											36		36	64		X				64
Dartnell			26			26					27		27	47						47
Hallas														73	27					100
Lakshmanan	3					3		23		23							54	20	0	74
Nelson								12		12				33	55					88
Ng		0		3	3	6	3	16		19		16	16	58					0	58
Niklaus											55		55	45						45
Raschetti														32	56				11	99
Trunet	3					3		29		29				56					12	68
Trunet	8		17			25		17		17				58						58
NStudies						5				5			7							10
Avg. % of Patients	1.4	0	4.3	0.3	0.3	6.3	0.3	9.7		10.0	11.8	1.6	13.4	46.6	13.8		5.4	2.0	2.3	70.1

Studies with Qualitative Data Only (Mention)

Bero			X	X		X	X	X		X	X		X	X					X	X
Courtman				X		X			X	X	X		X	X						X
Cunningham			X	X	X	X	X	X		X		X	X	X					X	X
Darchy			X	X		X			X	X						X				X
Lindley	X		X		X	X								X						X
NStudies						5				4			3							5

[a] See also Tables 2.1 and 2.2 and the references for Chapter 2.

Note: Numbers are percent of admissions as reported. X = qualitative mention in report; NStudies = number of studies that mentioned a DTP in the group; Avg. % of Patients = sum of percent mentions divided by 10. The original terms used in the individual studies were retained in most cases, abbreviated as follows: DI = drug interaction; DP = duplicate prescription (therapeutic duplication); DSE = side effect of drug; FP = failure to receive prescribed drug; ID = inappropriate dose; IF = inadequate follow-up; IMR = immunological reaction; IP = inappropriate prescribing (including wrong directions); NC = patient noncompliance or nonadherence; OD = excessive drug dosage; TF = treatment failure; UI = untreated indication; UD = underdosage; WD = wrong drug taken; WI = drug use without indication. Some terms may be synonymous, while others may have overlapping meanings. For example, various investigators have named an inappropriate drug order as inappropriate prescribing, contraindicated drug, wrong drug, duplication of therapy, and untreated indication.

often did not state as clearly the step in the medications use process where the DTP had occurred. Some DTPs could have involved more than one step. For example, Bero et al.'s "lack of a necessary drug therapy"[19] clearly belongs to "prescribing," but it includes failure to recognize a valid drug indication, failure to prescribe for the indication, and a patient's general lack of access to medical attention. Overdosage and underdosage seem to refer to the prescribing step, but for a few reports, they could have referred to drug administration or consumption.

Despite such ambiguities, however, Table 3.4 suggests, in broad terms, which parts of the process are most in need of improvement.

Therapeutic effect was the most frequently occurring group of DTPs associated with DRAs. It was first on the basis of both number of studies (10/15) and average proportions of admissions (70%). The group includes admissions related to ADRs, treatment failures, inadequate follow-up, drug side effects, immunological reactions, and drug interactions.

The most frequent DTP subgroups, in descending order, were ADRs (46.6%), treatment failure (13.8%), patient noncompliance (11.8%), overdose (9.7%), and inappropriate drug (4.3%, or 5.7% if we include the CI category). Some of these drug-related admissions obviously were preventable. Others, in particular admissions caused by ADR, will be discussed further below.

Table 3.4 provides valuable information to guide approaches to prevention. It suggests two important points for reducing the prevalence of drug-related hospital admissions. First, DRMs arise from problems that occur at each step in medications use, and prevention should address all steps, not just one. Simple preventives, even if highly successful, could affect only a minority of cases. Second, the step in medications use accounting for the largest proportion of DRM is drug consumption — especially unmanaged adverse drug reactions and treatment failures. This group was more prevalent than the usual suspects of inappropriate prescribing and noncompliance. *If only one aspect of the medications use process were to be targeted, however, the greatest impact might result from improved monitoring and follow-up.*

Inpatient Studies

Table 3.1 summarized the four studies from Table 2.2 that provided information about the stage in the medications use process where DTP may have occurred. Two studies suggest that lack of follow-up is a significant problem, while two do not.

Comparing the inpatient and ambulatory care results is a bit dangerous because the inpatient data are much more homogeneous with respect to investigators, methodology, setting (country and region), and time interval represented. If the inpatient data do represent a wider group of hospitals, prescribing improvement would seem somewhat more justified in the inpatient setting than in ambulatory care.

Although the studies might explain why medical and pharmacy school academics tend to emphasize problems with prescribing, they also show that extending such a preoccupation into the ambulatory care arena would be unjustified. The drug-related problems of ambulatory care may be quite different than those in a hospital.

Chapter Summary

1. Attitudes about drug-related morbidity are changing from a physician-centered perspective to a patient-centered perspective. They are changing from a view that DRMs are rare, caused by bad drugs, bad prescribing, bad patients, or bad luck, to a view that they are common and caused by system failures.
2. A model explaining how preventable DRMs come into existence was developed. Some DRMs have simple causes; some preventable DRMs involve an error, i.e., a failure by an individual. Most, however, appear to have complex causes involving failure in systems design, operation, or both. Each person operating a system should appropriately share responsibility for detecting and resolving drug therapy problems and should be potentially accountable for injury, along with the person committing the original error.
3. The majority of patient injuries from inpatient medications use systems involve prescribing problems. However, prescribing is the least common type of problem leading to hospital admissions, after ADRs, inadequate follow-up, and noncompliance.

Conclusion: Looking Forward to Systematic Medications Use Management

The analysis leads us away from simple cause-and-effect explanations. It leads toward a systems model of drug therapy that includes organized patient monitoring and cooperative actions by patients, caregivers, physicians, nurses, pharmacists, and others.

According to this model, the key to prevention is recognizing and correcting latent precursors of system failure called drug therapy problems. A well-constructed medicines management system would have a low likelihood of creating DTPs, a high likelihood of detecting and resolving DTPs, and a means of monitoring, evaluating, and improving its structure and performance with respect to DTPs.

From this perspective, many health care systems seem to have tremendous scope for systems improvement. For example, consider the typical ambulatory care system described above and illustrated in Figure 3.1. There are six major points to make about the usual medications use process shown in Figure 3.1:

1. Many patients take OTC medicines and prescribed medicines from many concurrent and past providers, dispensed by more than one pharmacy. The possibilities for latent errors and interactions involving latent errors may be far greater than the figure implies.
2. Furthermore, the process is infinitely recursive (in practical terms), especially for chronic disease. The patient's medical condition and other circumstances change with time. The process spirals along the time dimension as therapy progresses. Therapy must be monitored.
3. This structure does not adequately promote communication and cooperation. Information flows poorly through it, from patient to physician to pharmacist to patient, despite all good intentions to the contrary. The physician may focus on medical problems but be unaware of some important details of the patient's medications use. The pharmacist may be unaware of the therapeutic objective and of other information about the patient necessary for properly advising the patient and for monitoring. The patient may leave the pharmacy without knowing how to interpret the effects of the medicine and when to seek professional advice.
4. This process often attempts to educate the patient or caregiver at psychologically the worst moment — when he or she may be tired and ill — at the end of an episode of care.
5. From the time outpatients or family caregivers receive the prescription, they are in charge of their drug therapy. This authority may actually begin when they leave the physician's office, because patients can decide whether to obtain the medicine. For many patients, following doctor's orders may not withstand the first subjective experience of a side effect, regardless of whether actually caused by the medicine.
6. This process lacks an effective *feedback* loop for patient outcomes. It may isolate the patient's or caregiver's opportunity to *observe* the immediate consequences of therapy from the professional's ability to *interpret* them properly. In theory, the patient or caregiver can notice potentially significant therapeutic outcomes and seek professional advice to interpret them. The literature suggests, however, that this frequently does not occur.

These weaknesses may exacerbate each other. They can add up to an unmanageable (at least, unmanaged) medications use process. The prevention of DRM depends on the management of drug therapy, which depends in part on how systems are designed and operated, which in turn depends on how designers and professionals think about drug therapy and medications use.

Many different medications use systems coexist in most populations, so it is difficult to provide detailed criticisms or solutions that would apply to all medications use systems. Later chapters will describe system problem-solving approaches and tools that can be applied to a variety of circumstances. However, few system tools are robust enough to be used without some theoretical understanding of medications use systems.

References

1. Institute of Medicine, *Crossing the Quality Chasm: A New Health System for the 21st Century*, National Academy Press, Washington, D.C., 2001.
2. Berwick, D.M., A user's manual for the IOM's Quality Chasm Report, *Health Aff.*, 21, 80, 2002.
3. Leape, L.L. et al., Systems analysis of adverse drug events: ADE Prevention Study Group, *JAMA*, 274, 35, 1995.
4. McDonald, C.J., Weiner, M., and Hui, S.L., Deaths due to medical errors are exaggerated in Institute of Medicine report, *JAMA*, 284, 93, 2000.
5. Dunn, J.D., Patient safety in America: comparison and analysis of national and Texas patient safety research, *Tex. Med.*, 96, 66, 2000.
6. Brennan, T.A., The Institute of Medicine report on medical errors: could it do harm? *N. Engl. J. Med.*, 342, 1123, 2000.
7. Barr, D.P., Hazards of modern diagnosis and therapy: the price we pay, *JAMA*, 159, 1452, 1955.
8. Moser, R.H., Diseases of medical progress, *N. Engl. J. Med.*, 255, 606, 1956.
9. Melmon, K.L., Preventable drug reactions: causes and cures, *N. Engl. J. Med.*, 284, 1361, 1971.
10. Porter, J. and Jick, H., Drug-related deaths among medical inpatients, *JAMA*, 237, 879, 1977.
11. Dubois, R.W. and Brook, R.H., Preventable deaths: who, how often, and why? *Ann. Intern. Med.*, 109, 582, 1988.
12. Brennan, T.A. et al., Incidence of adverse events and negligence in hospitalized patients: results of the Harvard Medical Practice Study I, *N. Engl. J. Med.*, 324, 370, 1991.
13. Leape, L.L. et al., The nature of adverse events in hospitalized patients: results of the Harvard Medical Practice Study II, *N. Engl. J. Med.*, 324, 377, 1991.
14. Localio, A.R. et al., Relation between malpractice claims and adverse events due to negligence: results of the Harvard Medical Practice Study III, *N. Engl. J. Med.*, 325, 245, 1991.
15. Kohn, L.T., Corrigan, J.M., and Donaldson, M.S., *To Err Is Human: Building a Safer Health System*, National Academy Press, Washington, D.C., 2000.
16. Bates, D.W., Drugs and adverse drug reactions: how worried should we be? *JAMA*, 279, 1216, 1998.
17. Hallas, J. et al., Drug related events and drug utilization in patients admitted to a geriatric hospital department, *Dan. Med. Bull.*, 38, 417, 1991.

18. Schiff, G.D. et al., Inpatient theophylline toxicity: preventable factors, *Ann. Intern. Med.*, 114, 748, 1991.
19. Bero, L.A., Lipton, H.L., and Bird, J.A., Characterization of geriatric drug-related hospital readmissions, *Med. Care*, 29, 989, 1991.
20. Lindley, C.M. et al., Inappropriate medication is a major cause of adverse drug reactions in elderly patients, *Age Ageing*, 21, 294, 1992.
21. Bedell, S.E. et al., Incidence and characteristics of preventable iatrogenic cardiac arrests, *JAMA*, 265, 2815, 1991.
22. Fletcher, H.J., Ibrahim, S.A., and Speight, N., Survey of asthma deaths in the Northern region, 1970–85, *Arch. Dis. Child*, 65, 163, 1990.
23. Bigby, J. et al., Assessing the preventability of emergency hospital admissions: a method for evaluating the quality of medical care in a primary care facility, *Am. J. Med.*, 83, 1031, 1987.
24. Lazarou, J., Pomeranz, B.H., and Corey, P.N., Incidence of adverse drug reactions in hospitalized patients, *JAMA*, 279, 1200, 1998.
25. Reidenberg, M.M., Registry of adverse drug reactions, *JAMA*, 203, 85, 1968.
26. Seidl, L.G., Thornton, G.F., and Cluff, L.E., Epidemiological studies of adverse drug reactions, *Am. J. Public Health*, 55, 1170, 1965.
27. Strand, L.M. et al., Drug related problems: their structure and function, *Ann. Pharmacother.*, 24, 1093, 1990.
28. Hallas, J. et al., Drug related hospital admissions: the role of definitions and intensity of data collection, and the possibility of prevention, *J. Intern. Med.*, 228, 83, 1990.
29. Hepler, C.D. and Strand, L.M., Opportunities and responsibilities in pharmaceutical care, *Am. J. Pharm. Educ.*, 53 (Suppl.), 7s, 1989.
30. Bates, D.W., Leape, L.L., and Petrycki, S., Incidence and preventability of adverse drug events in hospitalized adults, *J. Gen. Intern. Med.*, 8, 289, 1993.
31. Bates, D.W. et al., Incidence of adverse drug events and potential adverse drug events: implications for prevention, *JAMA*, 274, 29, 1995.
32. Bates, D.W. et al., Relationship between medication errors and adverse drug events, *J. Gen. Intern. Med.*, 10, 199, 1995.
33. Bates, D.W. et al., The costs of adverse drug events in hospitalized patients, *JAMA*, 277, 307, 1997.
34. Bates, D.W. et al., Patient risk factors for adverse drug events in hospitalized patients: ADE Prevention Study Group, *Arch. Intern. Med.*, 159, 2553, 1999.
35. Cunningham, G. et al., Drug-related problems in elderly patients admitted to Tayside hospitals, methods for prevention and subsequent reassessment, *Age and Ageing*, 26, 375, 1997.
36. Leape, L.L., Preventing adverse drug events, *Am. J. Hosp. Pharm.*, 52, 379, 1995.
37. Grymonpre, R.E. et al., Drug-associated hospital admissions in older medical patients, *J. Am. Geriatr. Soc.*, 36, 1092, 1988.
38. Bergman, U. and Wiholm, B.-E., Patient medication on admission to a medical clinic, *Eur. J. Clin. Pharmacol.*, 20, 185, 1981.
39. Bergman, U. and Wiholm, B.-E., Drug-related problems causing admission to a medical clinic, *Eur. J. Clin. Pharmacol.*, 20, 193, 1981.
40. Cullen, D.J. et al., Prevention of adverse drug events: a decade of progress in patient safety, *J. Clin. Anesth.*, 12, 600, 2000.
41. *Webster's Ninth New Collegiate Dictionary*, Merriam-Webster, Springfield, MA, 1986.

42. Cipolle, R.J., Strand, L.M., and Morley, P.C., *Pharmaceutical Care Practice*, McGraw-Hill, New York, 1998, p. 1.
43. Gurwitz, J.H. et al., Thiazide diuretics and the initiation of anti-gout therapy, *J. Clin. Epidemiol.*, 50, 953, 1997.
44. MacKinnon, N.J., Risk Assessment of Preventable Drug-Related Morbidity in Older Persons (Elderly), unpublished doctoral dissertation, University of Florida, 1999. DAI, 60, no. 06B, 1999, p. 2633.
45. Faris, R.J., Explicit definitions to identify preventable drug-related morbidity in an elderly population and their use as an indicator of quality in the medication use system, unpublished doctoral dissertation, University of Florida, 2001, DAI, 62, no. 10B, 2001, p. 4448.
46. Morris, C.J. et al., Preventing drug-related morbidity-determining valid indicators, *Int. Soc. Qual. Health Care Oxford Univ. Press*, 14, 183, 2002.
47. Wilson, R.M. et al., The quality in Australian health care study, *Med. J. Aust.*, 163, 458, 1995.
48. Dartnell, J.G.A. et al., Hospitalisation for adverse events related to drug therapy: incidence, avoidability, and costs, *Med. J. Aust.*, 164, 659, 1996.
49. Courtman, B.J. and Stallings, S.B., Characterization of drug-related problems in elderly patients on admission to a medical ward, *Can. J. Hosp. Pharm.*, 48, 161, 1995.
50. Trunet, P. et al., The role of iatrogenic disease in admissions to intensive care, *JAMA*, 244, 2617, 1980.
51. Reason, J., *Human Error*, Cambridge University Press, Cambridge England, 1990.
52. Hallas, J. et al., Drug-related admissions to a department of medical gastroenterology: The role of self-medicated and prescribed drugs, *Scand. J. Gastroenterol.*, 26, 174, 1991.
53. Lakshmanan, M.C., Hershey, C.O., and Breslau, D., Hospital admissions caused by iatrogenic disease, *Arch. Intern. Med.*, 146, 1931, 1986.
54. Trunet, P. et al., The role of drug-induced illness in admissions to an intensive care unit, *Intensive Care Med.*, 12, 43, 1986.

4

People and Purpose in Medication Use

Power consists in one's capacity to link his will with the purpose of others, to lead by reason and a gift of cooperation.

Woodrow Wilson

Sasha Diehl is a 50-year-old lawyer. He belongs to the local yacht club and is a weekend boater and tennis player. He was diagnosed with hypertension last year. His physician, Dr. Jones, initially tried a low-salt diet and aerobic exercise, but when Mr. Diehl's blood pressure did not fall, he moved on to diuretics and then to nadolol, a nonspecific beta-blocker. Mr. Diehl visited Dr. Jones yesterday. When the nurse took his blood pressure, it was 150/110. Dr. Jones told him that if the hypertension was not lower in 4 weeks, he would increase the dose of medication.

Mr. Diehl telephoned his pharmacist to request a refill of his blood pressure medication. The prescription is for

Nadolol, 40 mg #60

Sig: 1 q.d. for blood pressure

The last refill was a little more than 10 weeks ago.

The pharmacist, Ms. Piazza, makes it a point to speak with Mr. Diehl when he comes in, and after a small discussion about boats, she takes his blood pressure. It is 140/90, standing. Mr. Diehl told her that it is usually about 130/90, sometimes a little higher, when he takes it himself at home.

Mr. Diehl confides that he is reluctant to take any medication. He says that friends have taken medicine for their hypertension and "never get off the stuff, like they get hooked or something." He is especially reluctant to increase the dose. On the contrary, he is thinking of stopping the medicine altogether. When Ms. Piazza asked why, he explained, in effect, that he never really agreed with Dr. Jones's decision to initiate therapy or to increase the dosage of the medicine.

He comments that he has no symptoms of hypertension and had been surprised when the doctor told him he had it, because he's not the nervous type. He admits that he has not been taking the medicine as prescribed, but adds that he has sufficient reason not to. He took the medicine as prescribed for a while, but feels much better when he is not taking the prescribed dosage. When he was taking it, he experienced fatigue and dizziness, which he attributes to the nadolol. He has experienced some occasional impotence, and he thinks the nadolol is the cause.

He did not tell this to Dr. Jones. Dr. Jones has explained that hypertension is a serious disease, and Mr. Diehl has not told him that he is skipping doses, especially on the weekend. Mr. Diehl says, "You gotta live while you're alive. You can't keep hoping to live forever." But, at Mrs. Diehl's insistence, he has agreed to try the medicine again until his next physician visit.

Introduction

People use medications for specific purposes, but those purposes differ from person to person. The case of Mr. Diehl raises a number of important questions. How many purposes are there for using medicines, and who should be involved in deciding what those purposes should be? What is the possible range of relationships, and who should be in charge? Does patient-centered care relieve caregivers of some responsibility for bad outcomes?

The vignette shows that Mr. Diehl has taken charge of his medication use (at least in the negative sense), regardless of whether his doctor and pharmacist agree. Therefore, the most important issue in the care of Mr. Diehl is how he experiences his care in the context of the quality of his life, how he feels and thinks about it. However, a sovereign consumer has to be able to make informed decisions.

Mr. Diehl may have treatable hypertension. He may have the phenomenon known as "white-coat hypertension," when a patient's blood pressure is high in the doctor's office but normal (or nearly so) at other times. White-coat hypertension may mean that a patient's blood pressure is unstable and needs to be treated. Whatever sort of hypertension he has, it is asymptomatic. He is the expert on how he feels on any given day. If Mr. Diehl has severe hypertension, however, he may not be able to make an informed decision about his long-term interest. Of course, that's what Dr. Jones is for, but how do Mr. Diehl and Dr. Jones work together?

This chapter will address three important issues: (1) what is meant by health-related quality of life, (2) how patients' and professionals' perspectives may differ, and (3) how professional relationships may influence resolution of differing perspectives and values. That discussion will establish two conclusions.

First, an effective therapeutic relationship usually requires *negotiation*. The participants in drug therapy differ in what they know, what they value, and possibly how they think. Each brings necessary elements to the relationship. Their specific decisions and actions may depend greatly on those differing perspectives. Second, active *cooperation* by all direct participants may be necessary to achieve the multiple, possibly conflicting objectives of therapy. An organized understanding of these different viewpoints might help one to understand how they fit together into a medication use system.

The People in Medication Use

Many people and institutions have a stake in medications use. The simple stereotype is a triangle of physician, patient, and pharmacist. This is, however, an oversimplification in modern society, so it is more useful to discuss these in terms of basic functions instead of occupations.

Effective drug therapy requires three overlapping functions: *prescribing*, which is the initiation of therapy based on medical problem assessment; professional *supervision* or *management* of therapy by the prescriber or a co-therapist (e.g., pharmacist, nurse, or physician's assistant); and *facilitation* or actual administration of therapy, e.g., by the patient, a family caregiver, nurse, etc. These *three primary functions of drug therapy* are drawn inside the dotted line in Figure 4.1, each connected to the other by a two-headed arrow denoting communications in both directions.

Today, dentists, clinical nurse practitioners, physician's assistants, pharmacists, and others have the authority to initiate therapy by prescribing prescription-only medicines, and patients and caregivers can initiate therapy with

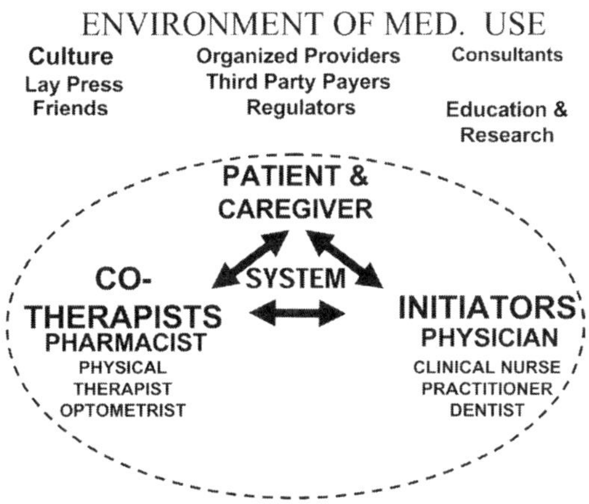

FIGURE 4.1
Participants in drug therapy.

nonprescription medicines, alternative medicines like food supplements, or even with prescription medicines that were prescribed for someone else.

Likewise, a variety of occupations may act as co-therapists, providing professional knowledge and skill to help manage the use of medicines. Finally, most people administer their own medicines, while others, such as the very young and the very old, need assistance from family members or other caregivers. Patients and lay caregivers administer the medications as prescribed, maintain administration equipment, and otherwise facilitate therapy.

These three primary functions are more distinct in ambulatory care than in institutional care. Most hospitals and nursing homes have standard procedures for medication administration that combine the co-therapist and facilitator functions, but sometimes medications are administered by a nursing assistant who follows orders with little professional judgment.

Environment of Medication Use

Medication use takes place in an environment that includes the medical care system, cultures (which communicate shared assumptions, beliefs, and values), laws, regulations, voluntary accreditation programs, professional and biomedical research and education, pharmaceutical manufacturers, and third-party payers. (These are drawn outside the dotted line in Figure 4.1.)

Each part of the environment may influence medication use in both overt and subtle ways. State and federal governments influence access to drug products and the information provided about them by their manufacturers. Hospitals and managed care organizations may further control access through lists of approved medicines. Professional and popular media (journals, magazines, Internet) influence knowledge and beliefs about drugs. They are protected by the first amendment, and not regulated by the Food and Drug Administration (FDA).

Consider, for example, the interconnections among (a) published research in a professional journal about nonsedating antihistamines, (b) an article about them in a popular magazine, (c) direct-to-consumer advertising of the same drug product (which is regulated by the FDA), (d) consumer demand for a prescription for the product, and (e) consumer expectations, e.g., that an insurance company will pay for it and about the effects of the medicine.

Objectives of Medication Use

Common objectives of drug therapy are summarized in Table 4.1. They are usually interrelated. Professionals typically use medicines to obtain a clinical

TABLE 4.1

Objectives of Medicines Use

Professional Objectives
Cure or control of disease
Amelioration or control of symptoms
Diagnosis
Providing valuable product or service
Expression of concern, legitimization
Personal Objectives
Improved (or protected) health-related quality of life
Comprehension (interpretation and understanding) of illness
Legitimization and self-expression
Compliance with authority (following instructions)
Economy, useability, compatibility with style, convenience

outcome, which they and their patients, especially, expect will improve or protect the quality of their lives in the short or long term.

Professional Objectives

The traditional and most familiar purposes of medication use are professional objectives. The most obvious professional objectives are clinical objectives: (1) to cure, arrest, slow, or prevent disease; (2) to eliminate or reduce a patient's symptoms; or (3) to assist in diagnosis or monitoring, e.g., as with radioactive pharmaceuticals.[1–3]

This is not to suggest that patients do not share professional objectives. Certainly control of symptoms may immediately improve quality of life, and clinical objectives may trump all others for life-threatening or highly symptomatic diseases. But clinical objectives may be abstract or vague to some patients — Mr. Diehl, for example. When possible, clinical objectives should be *explicit* and connected to a personal outcome.

Radioactive drugs and contrast media are pharmaceutical products that are used to diagnose disease. They have all of the properties of medicines except that their usual purpose may be diagnostic rather than therapeutic. In addition, some therapeutic drugs are used to diagnose disease or, perhaps, to circumvent diagnosis. For example, attention deficit hyperactivity disorder (ADHD) should be diagnosed by careful attention to a person's patterns of behavior, i.e., as described in the *American Psychiatric Association's Diagnostic and Statistical Manual of Mental Disorders* (DSM-IV).[4]

However, some doctors combine the diagnosis and treatment of ADHD in children by simply giving the child a medication like methyphenidate (Ritalin®). If the behavior improves, the "diagnosis" is in effect made by the treatment. A related example is "empiric" use of antibiotics (treating the symptoms of an infection before tests have identified the causative organism and determined what antibiotics are actually effective). In that case, a true diagnosis may never be made.

In addition to the obvious clinical purposes of medicines, doctors use drug therapy as a means of providing professional services to satisfy patient demand, to symbolize care or power, and to legitimize a patient's illness. Pharmaceutical manufacturers sell drug products as articles of commerce, as a kind of highly regulated fine chemical. Pharmacists seem to have both motives — sometimes dispensing drug products as an article to sell, part of the manufacturers' channel of distribution, and sometimes using drug products as an instrument of professional pharmaceutical service.

Personal Objectives

When a disease is rapidly life threatening or markedly reduces quality of life, the distinction between professional and personal outcomes is often neglected. However, personal outcomes obviously should be addressed for many relatively asymptomatic ("silent") diseases, especially those with a slow course and diseases in which symptomatic treatment may conceal a worsening of the underlying disease, such as asthma. Furthermore, even patients with extremely symptomatic or life-threatening diseases may choose not to treat them if they decide that the treatment would be worse than the disease, or even worse than dying, for them or their loved ones.

In the vignette that opens this chapter, Mr. Diehl is concerned about his ability to enjoy life. He does not experience symptoms from his hypertension. In fact, he doubts that he has hypertension, while he attributes symptoms that he does experience, e.g., impotence, to his medication. Trying to trump his quality-of-life concerns with clinical objectives may not succeed, especially if this is attempted by means of professional authority. He admits that he is not cooperating in his care as well as he could. His cooperation may well be necessary to obtain the professional objective of disease control.

In addition to producing clinical effects that are visible to patients, medicines may help patients to understand, interpret, or accept an illness. Drug therapy for depression is an example. People sometimes say, in effect, "I'm not crazy, I have a biochemical imbalance that can be corrected with medicine." This is also an example of a medicine being used to make legitimate an otherwise vague illness.

Some people take medicines mainly to follow doctor's orders. This applies not only to a patient in a paternalistic relationship, in which the patient may take his medicines regularly regardless of their desirable or undesirable effects, but also to some caregivers, nurses, and pharmacists who carry out doctors' orders without questioning the effect of the medicine on a patient.

Finally, from a negative perspective, patients may choose *not* to take medicines or may use them incorrectly because they cannot afford them, because they do not know (or accept) the correct method of use, because the medicine is incompatible with diet or other aspects of their lives, or because using them is inconvenient. There are many examples. "Three times a day after meals" does not mean the same thing to a middle-class matron as it does to a homeless person. The dietary needs of a diabetic may not fit well with budget or with menus planned by another. A schoolchild's need to use an asthma inhaler may be incompatible with his desire not to appear different, especially if school rules restrict his access, e.g., by requiring that medicines be left with the school nurse.

Employers may in turn value people's wellness and quality of life, because people with a higher quality of life tend to be more effective. Governments may value quality of life because it satisfies the electorate, and because populations with higher quality of life may be more effective citizens. The significance of health professions to a society may be greater than just keeping its population disease-free.

Medicines as Instruments

The foregoing discussion illustrates that drug products and drug therapy have little value in themselves, even though they sometimes may be priceless as instruments or means to a valued objective. This idea may seem obvious when written down. However, it is apparently ignored in at least two important ways by some stakeholders.

First, if professionals and patients respect the usefulness of a medicine, it is amazing that they often do not think it necessary to discuss the goals of drug therapy, let alone agree and communicate these goals to other direct participants. When the goals are not clear, therapy may simply be allowed to happen without active management. Then professionals can only rely on the patient's willingness to follow instructions obediently, instead of harnessing the patient's motivation to achieve a mutually agreed-upon and valued outcome.

Second, pharmaceutical manufacturers, many insurance programs, and some pharmacists seem to be preoccupied with buying or selling drug products as articles of commerce. For example, the predominant approach to influencing drug therapy (the formulary or list of approved drugs) tries to influence only part of prescribing — choice of therapeutic agent — without reference to the objectives of therapy or any other specific circumstances. Insurance programs often will pay only for such favored formulary drugs. Some hospitals delay providing nonformulary drugs to patients. Likewise, the predominant approach to evaluating the appropriateness of drug therapy is drug use evaluation (DUE). DUE considers how often approved and unapproved drug products are prescribed, but ignores the objectives of care in individual patients. This will be described further in Chapters 5 and 6. For now, I am pointing out the popularity of DUE merely as an example of an emphasis on drug products that ignores the objectives of their use in patients.

Quality of Life

During recent public debate about whether insurance companies should pay for drugs that improve sexual performance, some financial analysts and insurance company executives dismissed sexual function as a "quality of life issue," as distinguished from a "medical necessity."* This use of quality of life to denote recreation or enrichment shows confusion — and perhaps *sows* confusion. The analyst's implication was that quality of life is a luxury that health insurance need not cover. He has it backwards. Feeling well and being able to meet one's social obligations, including work, child rearing, and so forth, is a necessity, not a luxury. For many people, it is a sufficient reason to take or not take medicines. Sexual functioning is part of quality of life, and its importance depends on the patient. Whether improving sexual functioning is worth the potential expense to the insurance company and its members is a fair question, but it is a separate question from quality of life.

Quality of life (QOL) is the generalization of a person's ability to live his life, including its physical, mental, and spiritual dimensions. This includes somatic (bodily) sensations and psychological state as they are reflected in ability to carry out occupational and other social functions. Quality of life depends on a person's state of health, in addition to many other psychological, social, economic, and political factors.

According to the World Health Organization, a state of *health* refers to complete physical, mental, and social well-being and not merely the absence of disease. A somewhat more straightforward definition is *the proper functioning of the whole organism*. So QOL is a part of these definitions of health.

Health-related quality of life (HQOL) is an attempt to narrow the concept to the effects of wellness or illness and its therapy on quality of life.[5] HQOL is partially subjective and depends in part on a person's expectations. However, some parts of HQOL are objective. A person who cannot stand up without getting dizzy from postural hypotension (a temporary drop in blood pressure), or a person with untreated severe pain, is experiencing a physiological phenomenon that is just as definite as many diseases. It is subjective in the sense that the patient feels it, but objective in the sense that it can cause the patient to avoid some work or recreational activities, and can have sequelae such as injury from a fall. The importance of each dimension varies from person to person and from time to time. However, it seems that there is a cross-cultural agreement about certain domains of health-related quality of life. These domains are:

- Physical (symptoms, physical limitation, days in bed, pain, physical well-being, energy, vitality)
- Mental (cognitive function, concentration)
- Emotional and psychological (fear, depression, psychological well-being, emotional control)
- Social (personal relationships)

* Ginsberg, T., N.J. to Pay for Viagra® on Limited Temporary Basis, Philadelphia Inquirer, June 5, 1998, p. B2.

TABLE 4.2

Dimensions of the SF-36

Dimension	Examples
Vitality	Feeling full of pep, tired
General health perception	Sense of getting sick a little easier than other people; sense of excellent health; expectation that health will worsen
Physical role	Reduction in the amount of time spent on work or other activities; difficulty performing work or other activities (for example, it took extra effort)
Bodily pain	Bodily pain during the past weeks; pain interfering with normal work (including both work outside the home and housework)
Physical functioning	Ability to engage in activities, e.g., bathing or dressing oneself; bending, kneeling, or stooping; carrying groceries; moving a table, pushing a vacuum cleaner, bowling, or playing golf; walking a block, several blocks, a mile; running, lifting heavy objects, participating in strenuous sports
Mental health	Being a very nervous person; feeling down in the dumps, downhearted, blue; feeling calm and peaceful; being a happy person
Emotional role	Less time spent on work or other activities; accomplished less than you would like; didn't work as carefully as usual
Social functioning	Physical health or emotional problems interfered with normal social activities

Source: Medical Outcomes Trust: How to Score the SF-36 Health Survey, 1994.

- Role (ability to perform daily work)
- General health perception (current perception about health, expectations)

HQOL measurements are well established in outcomes research. They may also be useful in clinical practice, although this use is still very much in development. In outcomes research, scientifically valid and reliable questionnaires have been developed to measure HQOL in groups of people. One of the best-established general HQOL instruments is the Medical Outcome Study Short-Form 36, usually abbreviated MOS SF-36 or just SF-36. The SF-36 measures eight underlying dimensions of HQOL, as shown in Table 4.2.

Different diseases and treatments seem to affect quality of life in different, specific ways. For example, some of the questions useful to evaluate the effect of arthritis and arthritis therapy on HQOL should be different from the questions that would be useful for a person with asthma. However, the basic dimensions are essentially the same. An example of a disease-specific HQOL instrument is Hyland's Living with Asthma Questionnaire (LWAQ). The underlying dimensions of this are shown in Table 4.3.

Health care programs can use HQOL questionnaires to evaluate their overall impact and the state of well-being of their patients or members. Clinicians can use HQOL questionnaires to assess an individual's quality of life. This use is not as well established as their use with populations. An

TABLE 4.3

Dimensions of the Living with Asthma Questionnaire

Dimension	Examples
Seriousness	Would it make any difference if I forgot my inhaler? Does asthma makes a difference in the way I work? Not bothered by asthma. My asthma is not a serious health problem.
Drugs	Having to use an inhaler is a nuisance. I worry about the long-term effects of asthma drugs.
Leisure	Asthma limits the type of vacation I can take. I miss out because there are some sporting activities that I cannot join.
Consequences	I sometimes let people down because asthma stops me from doing something I agreed to do. There are times when I have difficulty getting around. I sleep badly because of my asthma. I tend to cough a lot at night. I can walk up one flight of stairs without stopping. I sometimes feel frustrated sexually because of my asthma.
Affect (emotions)	I don't feel in control of my asthma. It is difficult to do some activities like simple repairs. My asthma makes me feel so helpless. I feel inadequate because of my asthma. I feel in charge of my life. I feel depressed because of my asthma.

Source: Adapted from a shortened version of LWAQ from Ried, Nau, and Grainger-Rousseau, *Qual. Life Res.*, 8, 491, 1999. The LWAQ was developed by Hyland, Fennis, and Irvine (see Appendix 2).

individual's interpretation of a specific question could be different from the intended interpretation. However, most scales have more than one question. Also, an HQOL instrument can be used with discussion or dialog, as described in Chapter 10. The clinician could follow up certain responses to get a clearer idea about problems, their meaning to the patient, and possible solutions. Furthermore, the underlying dimensions are a useful framework for guiding a clinical dialog and for documentation. For example, Mr. Diehl's comments seem to refer to the vitality and either physical functioning or social functioning dimensions of SF-36.

HQOL problems may represent clinical problems — specifically drug therapy problems (DTP), as described in Chapters 3 and 10. Mr. Diehl seems to be describing an actual DTP — although his comments about lack of energy and concerns about impotence may need clarification. A clinician, say the pharmacist, Ms. Piazza, could connect the patient's illness experience to resolvable DTPs. In this example, Mr. Diehl is mentally connecting his illness experience to drug therapy. However, his interpretations may be incorrect. Although his beta-blocker can cause fatigue and impotence, Mr. Diehl may be attributing symptoms to his drug therapy that actually have another cause, e.g., his hypertension, an undiagnosed intercurrent disease, or even his relationships at home or at work.

Understanding the relationship between drug therapy, clinical effects, and HQOL effects can be difficult. Particular caution would be necessary about whether the problem is known to occur in similar circumstances and whether it has a plausible relationship to the patient's therapy.

Quality-of-life assessment by health care providers is necessary in order for them to understand their patients' needs and provide appropriate care, especially when:

- The burden of therapy (side effects, etc.) could be (or seem to the patient) worse than the benefit.
- A therapy will last a long time, e.g., to control a chronic disease.
- Two regimens would have approximately equivalent clinical effectiveness, but different side effects or other burdens for a patient.
- A regimen is palliative and not curative.

Three Basic Relationships

A major objective of a professional should be to establish and maintain therapeutic relationships. A therapeutic relationship can initiate, direct, and sustain dialog and cooperation in treatment. It is the professional's place to initiate this relationship. "As physician, the task [of establishing a productive relationship with a patient] was mine, not his, and the instrumentality would be dialogue."[6]

Professional relationships involve, among other things, the distribution of power and authority. Therefore, because the stakes are usually high, professional relationships may reflect and amplify human virtue and weakness. The many possible forms of a professional relationship can be simplified into the three general patterns shown in Table 4.4: paternal, consumerist, and therapeutic. Although these are oversimplifications of real relationships, they illustrate the range of possibilities along the three dimensions of perspective: values, beliefs, and decision making.

Paternal Relationship

A paternal relationship is at one extreme in which the balance of power is toward the professional. Here the professional is all-powerful and active while

TABLE 4.4

Three Basic Relationships

	Paternal	Consumerist	Therapeutic
Whose values?	Professional's	Patient's	Patient's
Whose beliefs?	Professional's	Patient's	Professional's
Whose judgment?	Professional's	Patient's or shared	Professional's or shared

the patient is powerless and passive.[7] The professional decides what is best for the patient and acts, if necessary, without the patient's explicit consent.

In some cases, of course, the patient may be unable to participate in his own care, e.g., because of emergency or unconsciousness. A paternalistic relationship can exist, however, between a professional and a mentally competent patient. In this relationship, the patient is expected to adopt, or at least accept, the professional's values, beliefs, and decision-making processes as they concern the purpose of the encounter. Patient participation would consist mainly of responding to questions asked by the professional and following treatment instructions. In the authoritarian extreme, the patient may be expected "neither to question nor to argue or disagree with the orders he receives." In a gentler (less authoritarian) version, the practitioner may explain his thinking to the patient to develop a "guidance-cooperation" relationship.[7]

Consumer Relationship

The medical consumer movement has sought to redefine the passive patient (the origin of the word *patient* is "one who suffers calmly") into an intelligent consumer of medical services. It is an understandable response to professional condescension, unsolicited paternalism, unexplained practice pattern variation, and self-fulfilling professional decisions done in the name of philanthropy or altruism.[8,9] However, consumerism brings with it a business approach to purchasing professional services (including the doctrine of caveat emptor). This ignores the basic issue that consumers of highly valued, very complex, and personally intimate services may be inherently disadvantaged in a marketplace.[10] A time of illness (with attendant distractions) is not a good time to attempt to learn complex knowledge well enough to make informed medical decisions, as a consumer must.

The power relationship is reversed in a consumer relationship. The objective is customer service, much as in a business relationship between a customer and a highly skilled service provider. Patient satisfaction with care would be paramount. A professional in a consumer relationship would tend to accept the customer's values about outcomes, operate within the customer's belief system, and leave many nontechnical decisions to the customer.

For example, a consumerist engineer might not ask why a bridge is needed in a certain time and place. A plastic surgeon might not question whether a patient would really look better with fuller lips created by a collagen injection. A pharmacist or nurse might not ask why a medicine is needed, but just go ahead and provide it. Any nagging questions about propriety would be answered (in this example) in terms of consumer sovereignty.

This need not be quite as extreme as it may first appear. The professional would still be expected to possess the necessary technical skill and to exercise the necessary care and vigilance in providing service, but would interfere the least with the patient's intentions. Advice might emphasize the use of a product or service, but real education would often be seen as unnecessary.

Therapeutic Relationship

William May has proposed that the ideal relationship between professional and client is described as a covenant.[8] As used here, a covenant is a solemn, secular, binding agreement between people (usually two) for the performance of unspecified actions or the exchange of unspecified gifts. There may be a contract contained in a covenant, but a contract is legally enforceable, while a covenant (as defined here) is not. Covenants transform relationships in ways that contracts cannot.

Marriage is a familiar example of a personal covenant: marriage is a solemn, binding agreement between two people to "love, honor, and cherish" one another for life. It is solemnized by a civil or religious ceremony. Marriage may contain legal obligations, e.g., spousal support, but loving, honoring, and cherishing are not legally enforceable. This secular covenant lasts as long as the parties to it continue to exchange those gifts.

A professional covenant is a solemn and binding agreement between a professional and a client in which the professional promises the client competent care and the client promises to yield authority to the professional.[8–11] There is an implied contract for services within most professional covenants, but often the most important aspects of the relationship cannot be legally enforced.

Accordingly, Hepler and Strand state that "the fundamental relationship in pharmaceutical care is a covenant, a mutually beneficial exchange in which a patient promises to grant authority to the provider, and the provider promises competence and commitment to the patient."[12]

Authority

The notion of covenant recognizes people's sovereignty over their own bodies and minds, but recognizes limits to some people's ability to exercise that sovereignty without expert help. In the covenantal ideal, the patient freely grants to the professional authority to influence both the patient's beliefs (e.g., the definition of the problem) and behaviors (e.g., actions necessary to solve the problem).[10] Professional practice is virtually impossible if the patient withholds such authority.[8]

Caring

Care encourages the relationship needed by *both* the professional and the client for the professional to succeed in improving the client's situation, and may itself improve outcomes. Once a professional aims for an outcome, the necessity of client cooperation usually becomes apparent. Once the professional recognizes that need for cooperation, competent caring becomes a necessity. In the view developed here, the motivation to care is related to the motivation to succeed.

Among the usual meanings of *care* used as a noun are "a disquieted state of blended uncertainty, apprehension and responsibility," "watchful attention," "regard coming from … esteem," "maintenance," and "supervision."[13] However, emotional attachment is not required for professional care. Confusion about this point may be quite troublesome. Professionals are obliged to behave as if they care, e.g., provide watchful attention, whether or not they like or even approve of their clients.

Competence

Competence is the ability to use personal and environmental resources to reach one's objectives. Professional competence includes scientific knowledge, skill (e.g., problem-solving and communications), and attitudes of painstaking attention and commitment to the client's interests.[8,11,14,15] It includes teaching patients or caregivers the spectrum of options and consequences, and helping them to make informed choices.

The objective is to direct professional competence toward outcomes that the patient values and can choose when he knows the possibilities and costs (risks). So, a therapeutic relationship falls between the extremes of paternalism and consumerism. In a therapeutic relationship, the patient and provider might negotiate within all three dimensions, but ideally the patient's values would take precedence over the professional's, the professional would attempt to teach his knowledge and beliefs to the patient (or the patient would accept professional knowledge), and decision making would be shared. The patient and professional would apply the professional's scientific knowledge and experience and the patient's personal experience to develop a plan intended to achieve goals valued by the patient.

Sasz and Hollender suggest a number of prerequisites for this model of mutual participation. Each person needs to be able to recognize emotional connections with the other (common humanity), balanced with respect for and ability to tolerate differences. It is crucial that each recognize dependency on the other for the purpose of reaching shared goals.[7]

Example

Consider the use of morning-after pills, i.e., oral contraceptives used in high doses after sexual intercourse to prevent implantation of a zygote. This is a difficult and controversial topic in the ethics of professional relationships that may clarify how perspectives are handled in the three types of professional relationships.

> Sally Fourth has been a patient of Dr. Brown and has been receiving oral contraceptives for some years. She gets her prescription filled at the Grey Pharmacy. Some months ago, she decided to stop taking her

> oral contraceptives because she had become celibate after breaking up with her boyfriend. One morning, she called Dr. Brown to explain that she and her old boyfriend were attempting a reconciliation and had unprotected sex the previous night. She told Dr. Brown that she was afraid she may become pregnant. She asked Dr. Brown if he would prescribe a morning-after pill.

In a paternalistic relationship, Dr. Brown might be much more likely to try to convince Ms. Fourth of his opinion about whether she should use a morning-after pill. His advice might mainly reflect his own opinion of Ms. Fourth's best interest. He might discount her knowledge and disregard her wishes. He might even try to manipulate behavior (this is beyond paternalism into an authoritarian extreme). The motto for this is "doctor knows best."

In a consumerist relationship, Dr. Brown might disregard his own values, beliefs, and judgment. He would discuss the problem carefully with Ms. Fourth, but he would accept her perspective and knowledge within the broadest limits. The motto (and basic argument) might be that it is her body, her life, and her decision.

In a therapeutic relationship, Dr. Brown might help Ms. Fourth to clearly identify her desired outcome but not try to change it. He would try to make sure that she had an accurate, scientifically based understanding of the major physical, social, and psychological consequences and would try to correct misunderstandings. He would help her to develop a realistic sense of her feelings if she used the treatment, and how she could cope with any repercussions, such as regret. Together they would decide what to do.

This example also can illuminate the environment of medication use: the role of culture, research third-party payers, and government. Our culture has some shared values, assumptions, and beliefs about the proper use of medicines, and about childbearing, and some controversies. Pregnancy and abortion have become for many a passionate sociopolitical issue. There may be only a small step from Sally's philosophy that she has sovereign control of her own childbearing to an insistence on a consumerist relationship with Dr. Brown.

Culture is communicated in news broadcasts and magazine articles. It may be reflected in laws about medication use. In the United States, pregnancy tends to be viewed as a medical issue (if not a disease), and legal access to oral contraceptives is limited to a doctor's prescription. In some countries, however, the patient can decide whether to get oral contraceptives without a prescription or from a doctor. However, Ms. Fourth may not need Dr. Brown's cooperation to get the medicine she wants. Information about how to use oral contraceptives as morning-after pills is available from magazine articles or the Internet, or even from a friend. She may already have the oral contraceptive tablets on her kitchen table or be able to get some from a friend.

Control of pregnancy is, for our purpose here, a symbol of people's desire to maintain or improve the quality of their lives as they believe is best.

They may make decisions based on whatever understanding they have, and sometimes regardless of what medical or governmental authorities may intend. A therapeutic relationship is premised in part on respect for this need and a willingness to use scientific knowledge to help people toward this goal.

Two Main Perspectives on Drug Therapy: Illness and Disease

A fundamental distinction is made in the sociology of medicine between how a patient *experiences* illness and how a professional *thinks about* it. The terms *illness* and *wellness* refer to a person's subjective feelings and perceived ability to function. For example, Mr. Green knew that he felt tired and occasionally dizzy. Furthermore, a person may act *sick*, i.e., change his normal activities as a result of illness. Illness experience is the primary reality of health care. That is, people experience illness directly. Illness often comprises the motivation for, and basis of, health care and may powerfully influence a person's other life experiences.

The term *disease* is reserved for a professional interpretation of the person's (patient's) account of illness experience and any additional objective or subjective information the professional obtains, e.g., from physical examination or laboratory tests. A disease is an abnormality or derangement of structure or physiology. Although the derangement must be objectively verifiable, the diagnosis of disease is often an inference about reality rather than reality itself, a theoretical construct based on data. Disease can be thought of as a professional's *secondary* perception of the primary illness experience.

> Mrs. Loring, a 60-year-old white female in apparently good health, went to Dr. George with complaints of vague chest pain. Her cholesterol was slightly elevated, so Dr. George ordered a treadmill stress test with the injection of a radioactive dye that would allow the cardiologist to visualize the overall coronary blood flow. Mrs. Loring showed good coronary blood flow before exercise, some EKG abnormalities before and during exercise, and a "cold spot" after exercise, suggesting that blood flow to part of her heart muscle was less than it should be in response to exercise. The cardiologist recommended a cardiac catheterization, in which dye was injected directly into her coronary blood vessels so that they could be visualized. The result showed 25% blockage in one artery, not enough to explain her chest pain. The cardiologist did, however, diagnose a minor problem with Mrs. Loring's mitral valve, which he said was consistent with her symptoms.

Naming and classifying disease is fundamental to medical practice because once a doctor recognizes a disease or syndrome, he gains access to a wealth of scientific knowledge that may be essential in managing the patient — some as part of the doctor's educational background and even more through clinical experience and current literature. In this example, although the cardiologist may not know a great deal about Mrs. Loring's mitral valve prolapse (MVP), he may know a lot about MVP from scientific studies and clinical experience. He can, with the exercise of clinical judgment, apply his general knowledge to Mrs. Loring's case.

However, MVP is arguably not what is really wrong with Mrs. Loring. The symptoms are real, but the diagnosis is little more than a proposition to explain the symptoms. Despite its great value, general scientific and experiential knowledge of disease is abstract knowledge about people other than the patient. It complements, but does not substitute for, the patient's primary experience.

> During a routine visit, Mr. Green asked his doctor if ibuprofen can make you feel tired and sometimes make you dizzy. Dr. Smith replied that although dizziness and drowsiness are occasionally reported side effects of ibuprofen, they may go away during treatment and usually do not require medical attention. She reviewed his record and noted that he was not taking any other medications. Just to be sure, however, she asked Mr. Green about other medicines that he might have been using and verified that he was not taking any others. His diet and sleep habits were normal. She recommended that he get plenty of sleep and keep well hydrated in hot weather. They chatted briefly, and then Mr. Green left. A week later, Mr. Green's daughter called 911 because his weakness and gray pallor frightened her. In the emergency room, his hematocrit and red blood cell count showed that he was extremely anemic. He required transfusions of whole blood. Tests for occult blood in his stool were positive. Endoscopy showed that Mr. Green had bled from a gastric lesion.

Mr. Green's question unintentionally diverted Dr. Smith's attention to the ibuprofen. Had he asked Dr. Smith about gastrointestinal bleeding from ibuprofen, she surely would have replied that it is quite common and recommended a course of action that might have avoided his collapse. Perhaps Dr. Smith dismissed weakness and dizziness because they are not recognizably symptoms of an adverse reaction to ibuprofen. She answered correctly in the narrow context of direct side effects of ibuprofen, but incorrectly in the broad context of Mr. Green's health.

Despite Mr. Green's question, Dr. Smith should have asked herself, "Why does Mr. Green feel dizzy?" Scientific thinking about drug products instead of patients can mislead a health professional if the patient appears not to have a disease known to have a particular symptom or is not taking a drug known to have a particular side effect. While it is rare for a pharmacist or physician openly to deny a patient's illness experience, it may not be unusual for them to ignore it (in effect) or to decide that nothing can be done. Subjective symptoms (pain, weakness, fatigue) of unknown cause are common examples.

Sickness and Legitimization

As *illness* denotes a person's feeling of not being well, and *HQOL* denotes a person's subjective feeling of capacity to perform normal activities and to meet normal obligations; *sickness* is used to denote behavior consistent with illness or low HQOL. That is, a person may *feel* ill and *act* sick, for example, by not engaging in normal behavior such as recreation, work, or child care. Just as a person with a disease may or may not feel ill, a person who feels ill may or may not act sick. However, since sickness is a behavior, it can be measured, e.g., as days of lost work due to sickness.

Sometimes a person's report of feeling ill is enough to excuse sickness behavior, e.g., being excused from normal duties. Sometimes it must be formalized or legitimized. For example, when a student has missed an examination or an employee has used too many days of sick leave, a note from the doctor may be required in order for the absence to be excused.

This takes medicine out of a personal relationship between a doctor and patient and moves it into a political or even legal arena. Prescription-only medicines are another example. Authority to legitimize sickness and to authorize prescription-only medicines increases the social power of the medical profession. It also leads to the phenomenon of "medicalization," which is the making of normal human experiences into medical events that are treated almost as if they were diseases. Examples include not feeling well enough to work, childbirth, and death. Normal events of everyone's life, however, are not diseases in the usual sense of disordered physiology.

Some social critics claim that this process has made medicine into a modern pseudoscientific priesthood that has expropriated human experience, and that will lead to industrialization of medicine and ultimately to "medical nemesis," the failure of medicine as a helping profession.[16]

Some people's HQOL may be influenced more by their feelings of illness or wellness than by objective disease status. Many people are ill without a (recognized) disease, just as others may have a disease without feeling ill. Therapy may influence a patient's illness (wellness) experience and quality of life through simple or complex mechanisms; for example, a patient may feel that drug therapy is reducing his quality of life (e.g., by causing side effects) or is affecting the lives of family and friends (e.g., by taking up resources that might have been used for something else).

Family and friends' reactions to drug therapy may in turn affect a patient's HQOL. Therefore, it is possible for the treatment of disease to increase feelings of illness or reduce HQOL more than the disease itself. For example, Jachuck et al.[17] reported on the outcome of the treatment of hypertension, as reported by a patient and the patient's physician and family members. Physicians reported that 90% of the patients were doing better. However, only half of the patients reported that they felt better, while 95% of family members felt the patients were doing *worse*. This illustrates the contrasts among the outcomes valued by the clinician, patient, and family member.

Models of Disease and Therapy

Whatever their educational background and culture, people seek to understand the significant experiences of their lives, including illness. Modern medicine represents an attempt to explain illness experience scientifically and to develop rational treatments. This enterprise has been spectacularly successful in many areas, including drug therapy. However, scientific models do not explain some illnesses.

Many of the illnesses seen in office practice are not really diagnosed, just labeled (e.g., respiratory symptoms as "a cold") or treated empirically. The causes of mental illness, cancer, and AIDS were scientifically unknown for years. Some disagreement still exists, for example, about the causes of AIDS.[18] Neither does scientific medicine explain the impact of diseases and their treatments on people's lives as well as it explains the biology of the disease. For example, think of migraine, epilepsy, or insulin-dependent diabetes, or almost any serious disease, especially as it complicates the life of a child and his or her family.

The limits of scientific medicine leave room for alternative interpretations, explanations, and therapies, for example, alternative medicine like chiropractic, homeopathy, acupuncture, aromatherapy, and a multitude of herbs and "natural" folk remedies. Some people are reluctant to use governmentally approved and regulated remedies, regardless of testing, and prefer to use relatively untested and loosely regulated "nutraceuticals" (drugs marketed as foods). (See Chapter 5.)

Some people are reluctant to immunize their children because of concerns that vaccines carry unknown risks of poisoning or exotic animal diseases. Others worry that immunizations are wrongfully withheld. The medical community decided that smallpox had been eradicated, and smallpox immunization had no benefit to offset its risks. In 2002, following fear of biological terrorism, the unimmunized population seemed vulnerable. Some asked how we know that smallpox really has been eradicated. There are no definitive scientific answers to such questions because they require proof of a negative. Statistical evidence simply begs the question.

Some forms of alternative medicine have no theoretical foundation and no empirical support, and seem to be fraudulent attempts to exploit human suffering. However, the history of medicine includes a number of folk remedies that were "discovered" and subsequently absorbed by mainstream medicine, with or without scientific proof. Examples include digitalis, rauwolfia, and smallpox vaccinations. Acupuncture may be moving from illegitimacy to legitimacy.

The point is not to indict scientific medicine, far from it. Scientific medicine, however, has definite limits. People's desire for meaning and action will sometimes move them beyond the limits of medical science to make sense of their experiences and to find solutions to their problems.

When that's the case, common sense dictates that a bit of scientific humility — recognition that science does have narrow limits — could do a lot to maintain a therapeutic relationship.

Clinical Negotiation

Differences in perspective (value, belief, and reasoning processes) challenge mainstream practitioners' respect for scientific medicine on the one hand and patients' beliefs on the other. The patient's active participation in his own care may be necessary to improve his quality of life with drug therapy. It is fair to ask whether Mr. Diehl actually has hypertension that is serious enough to require treatment with a beta-blocker — he might be better off if he would ask that question rather than decide on his own not to take his medicine. Since he believes incorrectly that hypertension is a symptomatic disease, perhaps diet and exercise failed because he did not give them a fair trial.

Assuming for the moment that he does have serious hypertension, Mr. Diehl seems to be asserting his right to refuse care so that he can enjoy his life. In a paternalistic relationship, this is out of bounds. His doctor may feel (and actually say) that Mr. Diehl can either follow medical advice or find another doctor. The polite version of this is to call him noncompliant or nonadherent. In a consumerist relationship, it is his life and he can do as he pleases with it. However, in a therapeutic relationship, a professional would question his beliefs and clarify his unstated assumptions. For one thing, if he really does have serious hypertension, he may assume that he will have an acceptable quality of life, enjoying sex, playing tennis, and sailing his boat until some unspecified time in the distant future when, old and tired, he will die suddenly and painlessly from a heart attack. This is not the typical course of untreated hypertension, and his decision might change if he knew the more probable consequences of untreated hypertension. His unstated assumptions may make him take his disease and its therapy less seriously than he would if he were better informed.

Second, he may be attributing symptoms to his drug therapy that actually have another cause. There are other medicines that would be worth a trial if he would cooperate in evaluating them. As a co-therapist, the pharmacist might show Mr. Diehl how to keep a diary of when he took his medicines, what his blood pressures readings were at various times of the day, and how he felt. This would provide the information needed by Dr. Jones to treat Mr. Diehl effectively and needed by Mr. Diehl to participate actively in his care.

Summary

Patients and professionals may have competing objectives of care and alternative explanations for the experience of illness, its human meaning, and its treatment. Patients seek to improve the quality of their lives. Since they are actually living their lives, the short term is usually more significant to them than to their doctor and pharmacist. ("This may sting a little" has a different meaning to the patient than it does to the doctor.)

In contrast to paternalism, the idea that patients should be in control of their care sounds very attractive. However, patients should never become "consumers" of health care. They need valid explanations of disease (as far as possible), respect for their attempts to understand that which is mysterious, advice about how to care for themselves, and loyalty to their interests. A professional who seeks more than a clinical outcome for his patients will often need active cooperation from patients and family caregivers. Many patients will not easily yield their autonomy to claims of professional authority. However, they may willingly cooperate in a therapeutic relationship in which the common objective is to achieve clinical outcomes that improve quality of life.

References

1. Hepler, C.D. and Strand, L.M., Opportunities and responsibilities in pharmaceutical care, *Am. J. Hosp. Pharm.*, 47, 533, 1990.
2. Strand, L.M. et al., Levels of pharmaceutical care: a needs-based approach, *Am. J. Hosp. Pharm.*, 48, 547, 1991.
3. Strand, L.M., Cipolle, R.J., and Morley, P.C., *Pharmaceutical Care: An Introduction,* The Upjohn Company, Kalamazoo, MI, 1992.
4. American Psychiatric Association, *Diagnostic and Statistical Manual,* 4th ed., American Psychiatric Association, Washington, D.C., 1994.
5. Spilker, B., *Quality of Life and Pharmacoeconomics in Clinical Trials,* 2nd ed., Lippincott-Raven, Philadelphia, 1996.
6. Engel, G.L., How much longer must medicine's science be bound by a seventeenth century world view? in *The Task of Medicine: Dialogue at Wickenburg,* White, K.L., Ed., Henry J. Kaiser Family Foundation, Menlo Park, CA, 1988, p. 113.
7. Sasz, T.S. and Hollender, M.H., The basic models of the doctor-patient relationship, *Arch. Intern. Med.*, 97, 595, 1956.
8. May, W.F., Code and covenant or philanthropy and contract? *Hastings Cent. Rep.*, 5, 29, 1975.
9. Eisenberg, J.M., *Doctors' Decisions and the Cost of Medical Care,* Health Administration Press, Ann Arbor, MI, 1986.
10. Hepler, C.D., Pharmacy as a clinical profession, *Am. J. Hosp. Pharm.*, 42, 1298, 1985.
11. Veatch, R.M., *A Theory of Medical Ethics,* Basic Books, New York, 1981, p. 110.
12. Hepler, C.D. and Strand, L.M., Opportunities and responsibilities in pharmaceutical care, *Am. J. Pharm. Educ.*, 53 (Suppl.), 7s, 1989.
13. *Webster's Ninth New Collegiate Dictionary,* Merriam-Webster, Springfield, MA, 1986.

14. Ramsey, P.G. et al., Use of peer ratings to evaluate physician performance, *JAMA*, 269, 1655, 1993.
15. Petersdorf, R.G., Defining the good doctor, *JAMA*, 269, 1681, 1993.
16. Illich, I., *Medical Nemesis: The Expropriation of Health,* Pantheon Books, New York, 1976.
17. Jachuck, S.J. et al., The effect of hypotensive drugs on the quality of life, *J. R. Coll. Gen. Pract.*, 32, 103, 1982.
18. Cohen, J., The Duesberg phenomenon, *Science*, 266, 1642, 1994.

Appendix 1: How to Get the SF-36 and SF-12

The SF-36, SF-12, and other HQOL measures, with manuals, instructional materials, etc., describing how to use them in research and clinical practice, are available from QualityMetric Inc., a company formed by John E. Ware, Jr., Ph.D., to develop and disseminate the "next generation of outcome assessments and analytic services for improving health care from the patient point-of-view." QualityMetric Inc. and its affiliate, the Health Assessment Lab, have two locations:

QualityMetric Inc.
640 George Washington Highway
Suite 201
Lincoln, RI 02865
Phone: (401) 334-8800 or (888) 947-9800
Fax: (401) 334-8801
E-mail: info@qmetric.com

The Health Assessment Lab
750 Washington Street
Boston, MA 02111
Phone: (617) 636-8098 or (800) 572-9394
Fax: (617) 636-8077

Permission to use the SF-36 and SF-12 is often granted royalty-free for individual research and institutional noncommercial use. Permission to use the SF-36 may be requested on the World Wide Web from http://www.qmetric.com/forms/permission.php3.

Appendix 2: How to Get the Living with Asthma Questionnaire

Write to:

Dr. Michael E. Hyland
Department of Psychology
University of Plymouth
Plymouth PL4 8AA, U.K.
E-mail: mhyland@plymouth.ac.uk

Permission to use the LWAQ is often granted royalty-free for individual research and institutional noncommercial use.

5

Access, Cost, and Quality Issues in Medication Use

> Mere parsimony is not economy ... expense, and great expense, may be an essential part of true economy.
>
> **Edmund Burke**

Introduction

Chapter 2 presented data suggesting that severe problems exist in medications use, especially in ambulatory care. Chapter 3 described a model to explain how preventable drug-related mortality (PDRM) can happen. Chapter 4 discussed the objectives of medications use. Other fundamentals are necessary for a critical understanding of medications use.

This chapter will introduce access, cost, and quality, three basic criteria for evaluating the overall ability of a health care system to deliver services to a population. Some of the PDRMs described in Chapters 2 and 3 resulted in part from problems with one or more of the issues discussed in this chapter. This chapter will also describe some common aspects of medications use in the real world: how people really have access to drug products, how to calculate the real cost of drug products, and how drug product quality is regulated. Chapter 6 will add detail about access to medications: how physicians decide what to prescribe and how managed care (broadly speaking) tries to influence those decisions.

This chapter and Chapter 6, in a sense, describe the frameworks that people have typically used to think about medications use. Some limitations of this paradigm may become clear. The description of an ideal medication use system will then begin with Chapter 7.

Relationship of Access, Cost, and Quality

Some writers assume that improving quality costs more. Some health economists even speak of an "iron triangle" of access, cost, and quality. According to the iron triangle metaphor, quality cannot be increased without corresponding decreases in access to care or increases in cost of care, or both.

The iron triangle metaphor has been used to discourage proposals to improve quality when resources were (or seemed to be) especially limited. For example, "We can't afford quality improvement because (a) our costs are already too high, or (b) we have so many unserved or underserved people." At the time of this writing, an *access* variation on this theme is popular because Congress is once again reconsidering a Medicare prescription benefit, which both political parties promised during the 2000 presidential election. Then the budget appeared to tighten, and the iron triangle metaphor was frequently invoked. Too bad we lack a common vocabulary in this field.

The iron triangle metaphor may be true or false depending on how quality is defined. If quality improvements are defined in terms of structural or procedural changes that have no demonstrated effect on outcomes, costs might have to increase. Examples are the latest, most expensive drug products, more elaborate dosage forms, and more drugs. Many such notions of quality of medications use exist without clear, empirical relationships to improved patient outcomes. Increasing that kind of quality would inevitably cost more, by definition. Then, all other things being equal, access would be reduced.

If quality improvements in structure and process are changed in ways that are known to have the potential to improve outcomes, and if systems are operated to reach that potential, then quality can indeed be free or even reduce cost or increase access. Such quality improvements would increase effectiveness, safety, timeliness, appropriateness, etc. These can be implemented in a system that promotes desired outcomes and reduces adverse outcomes. Given the estimated costs of adverse outcomes from Chapter 2, it is theoretically possible to improve quality of medications use at a lower total cost by changing the way that medications are used to produce outcomes. This can reduce average total costs of care per person.

The iron triangle assumption may persist as a vestige of the historical emphasis on structure and process definitions of quality. It is easy to see that the iron triangle can be broken when structure and process quality standards have been validated in part by demonstrating that they are associated with improved outcomes (see the definitions of quality by the Institute of Medicine (IOM) or the U.S. Office of Technology Assessment (OTA) below). This is illustrated with respect to access later in this chapter.

In principle, if improved quality improves outcomes or efficiency, it may be free or even decrease cost or increase access. That is a basic thesis of this book and of all modern health care quality improvement programs. In particular, improved access and quality of drug therapy can dramatically improve outcomes and lower total costs by avoiding expensive adverse outcomes and treatment failures.

Accessibility of Care

Accessibility of care is about how easily patients can obtain the care they need when they need it. It can be measured by how many people who need services actually receive them or how long they have to wait to receive them. Two main subtopics are physical and financial access. Some access-to-medications issues are controversial, for example, the questions raised by the death of Donald Ashwell (below). As this chapter will illustrate, the various stakeholders in medications use have different perspectives, which can lead to strong differences of opinion about results.

Physical Access

Physical access to care generally involves the geographical distribution of people and providers, including distribution of primary care providers and specialists, health care facilities, and transportation facilities.

Physical access to prescription medications, however, requires an unbroken chain of decisions and actions that are often more important than geographic location. In order for a patient to have physical access to drug therapy for a particular indication, a drug product would have to exist for that indication. This is not quite as obvious or as simple as it may first appear. Drug products (whether natural or synthetic) have to be discovered and developed. An approved manufacturer must have produced and tested a drug product. Before a drug product can be marketed within legitimate channels in the United States, its sponsor (manufacturer) must have received Food and Drug Administration (FDA) approval. Approval is for specific indications, and the manufacturer cannot promote the product for other (off-label) uses. According to the pharmaceutical industry, developing a new drug product requires an average of 15 years and costs an average of $880 million.

No drug therapy has been approved for thousands of rare or "orphan" diseases, even if a potentially safe and effective therapy may exist. (See Appendix 1.) Many approved drugs have unapproved indications, however. A possibly safe and effective therapy would not have been approved for a rare disease or even a common indication without formal sponsorship and testing. Without approval, the drug cannot be promoted for the indication. A physician can prescribe for an unapproved drug or indication if he knows about it and is willing to disregard the apparatus of FDA approval. A pharmacist can dispense it if he can obtain a supply of reliable purity and potency. Some drug products that are not available here are available in other countries. The Internet, especially, has made it easy for a patient to go abroad to get a drug. But that deprives the patient of the protection of U.S. drug standards.

The problem has resulted in a gray market in foreign drugs, including many drugs approved for treating AIDS and its complications. The FDA has allowed some exceptions to its usual drug approval procedures for AIDS drugs, putting them on a fast track. Another example is RU-486, mifepristone, used in combination with misoprostol to produce abortions. The combination was shown to be as effective in ending pregnancy in U.S. women as in women tested previously in France. In July 1996, an FDA advisory committee recommended that mifepristone be approved for pregnancy termination when used in combination with misoprostol. An "approvable" letter was issued September 18, 1996. The drug was not finally approved by the U.S. Food and Drug Administration until September 2000, and U.S. shipments to health care providers began on November 20, 2000. The delay was in part because of political opposition to abortion.* (Federal drug law is briefly outlined below.)

Another necessity for physical access is that the patient be able to actually get and use the therapy, meaning in most instances a prescription from a doctor, a local pharmacy or mail-order service, and a means to pay. The prescription requirement obviously means that a physician or other licensed prescriber must agree that the patient needs the therapy. The pharmacy must stock the medicine or be willing to get it. Some prescribers will not prescribe, and some pharmacies will not dispense, a necessary medicine or amount of medicine. Chronic severe pain and the opiate drugs used for it are common examples of this problem, especially for terminally ill patients who may require unusually high dosages. Another example is ethically or politically controversial treatments, e.g., morning-after contraceptives that are already on the market but which some health professionals will not recommend, prescribe, or dispense because of their personal beliefs or values. Finally, the patient must learn how to use the drug correctly. For example, the patient has to be able to correctly use a metered-dose inhaler, an injectable drug such as insulin, a suppository, or a vaginal tablet. This illustrates the need for access to *information about drugs* as a part of access to the drug products themselves. Of course, physical access also depends on financial access. The patient has to be able to afford the therapy and the associated medical care.

Financial Access

Donald Ashwell of Harrison County, Mississippi, took five drugs every day to control schizophrenia and manic depression. The medicines worked well,

* Kolata, G., Abortion Pill Tests Well in United States, Drug's Sponsor Says, *The New York Times*, April 30, 1998, p. A24 (column 1).

and the 37-year-old man became a frequent and popular volunteer at area health clinics. One day, Mr. Ashwell went to the emergency room at the local hospital. The emergency room doctor diagnosed early stage pneumonia and prescribed an antibiotic. But Mississippi limited how many prescriptions it would purchase each month for Medicaid patients, and someone at the drugstore said that Mr. Ashwell had reached his limit. According to the hospital, Mr. Ashwell could not buy a sixth drug, the antibiotic, "because of financial problems." Unable to pay for the $45 antibiotic, he went home. Three days later, his infection had worsened severely and he was hospitalized. Hospital records describe painful and expensive attempts to save Mr. Ashwell after his untreated pneumonia worsened, but it was too late. He died, and Medicaid had a $4900 hospital bill.*

In the United States, financial access to health care is controlled through a staggering combination of mechanisms and financing schemes:

- Private health insurance, including classic health insurance, preferred provider organizations, and HMO contracts
- Federal and state health financing, e.g., Medicare and Medicaid (each state has its own Medicaid program)
- Direct provision, e.g., through the Veterans Administration and USPHS Indian Health Service
- State, county, and religious hospitals that provide "uncompensated" (charity) care

There are approximately 43 million people in the United States without health insurance, and perhaps an equal number with inadequate coverage, particularly for medications. The larger policy questions of who should have health insurance and how it should be paid for are beyond the scope of this book. Some people who have health insurance, however, may still have major financial access problems. For example, outpatient medications are not covered under Medicare. Although their inclusion was promised by the presidential candidates of both major political parties in 2000, this promise was later reevaluated.

The question of why otherwise insured people do not have adequate coverage of drug therapy should provoke curiosity. Speaking of the Ashwell case, Cynthia Folcarelli of the National Mental Health Association said, "This is a dilemma that thousands … of people across the country face every month." The lack of access to a needed medicine, such as the antibiotic that might have saved the life of Donald Ashwell, is not isolated, is not new, and is not excusable.

William Waldman, a spokesman for the American Public Human Services Association (APHSA), which represents state Medicaid directors, was interviewed for the Associated Press (AP) story about Ashwell. According to the

---

* From Lauran Neergaard, Mississippi Death Raises Questions about Medicaid Prescription Limits, Associated Press, June 30, 1999, 13:18.

AP report, Mr. Waldman explained that medications were the fastest-growing health care cost, so limiting them is logical when budgets are tight. It is important to examine this rationalization because it represents a common, perhaps prevailing, view in managed care.

Arbitrarily limiting access to medications, in order to control costs, could seem logical as a means for shifting necessary costs to people who could and would pay. However, cost shifting would rarely be effective in a Medicaid program, which is for the poor and medically indigent, and which uses strict means tests. Prescription limits in a Medicaid program today ignore the reason that drug therapy is used at all. Drug therapy is not a cost of business, it is a modality of treatment, intended to cure or control diseases and symptoms. This is not mere rhetoric. Arbitrary restrictions on a patient's prescription expenditures, while usually successful for that limited objective, are indiscriminate. They may deter the use of necessary drug therapy. Prescription limits or exclusions have never been shown to decrease total health care costs per patient. (See Chapter 6.) They don't work because prescription limits are frequently associated with increases in other costs of care.

This has been likened to squeezing a balloon, where air just moves from the restricted end to bulge out somewhere else. However, this analogy understates the case, because limiting drug expenditures may not merely redistribute costs. The evidence shows that it often hurts people and significantly increases total costs of care.

The clearest examples of this phenomenon were reported by Steven Soumerai and his group at Harvard. During an 11-month period, New Hampshire established a three-drug limit per Medicaid recipient. Soumerai et al. studied the care given to 268 chronically mentally ill patients in New Hampshire and compared it to the care given to 1959 patients in the New Jersey Medicaid program (which had no prescription limits) at the same time. The investigators reported an immediate and statistically significant reduction (15 to 49%) in use of a variety of psychoactive drugs. So the limit did reduce prescription utilization. However, there was also a coincident increase of 1 or 2 visits per patient per month to community mental health centers (43 to 57% increase), and increases in emergency service utilization and partial hospitalizations (1.2 to 1.4 episodes per patient per month). There was no change in psychiatric hospital admissions. The average increase in mental health care cost per patient was $1530, exceeding drug cost savings by a factor of 17. The authors concluded that limits on Medicaid coverage of prescription drugs increased use of acute mental health services among low-income patients with chronic mental illnesses and increased costs to the Medicaid program. In addition, it decreased their health-related quality of life (HQOL).[1]

Furthermore, Soumerai et al.[2] compared 411 elderly New Hampshire Medicaid recipients to a matched comparison group of 1375 people in New Jersey. In New Hampshire, use of drugs declined by 35% after Medicaid applied the prescription limit. This was associated with a near-doubled rate of admission to nursing homes. Drug use and nursing home admission rates in the comparison group did not change.

The authors considered patients who regularly took three or more study medications before the limit. For these people, the risk of admission to a nursing home during the limit period more than doubled, and the risk of hospitalization increased by 25%.

The authors concluded that limiting reimbursement for effective drugs puts frail, low-income, elderly patients at increased risk of admission to nursing homes and may increase Medicaid costs. Further, and perhaps most costly, few of the institutionalized elderly returned to their communities after discharge from the hospital or nursing home.[2]

These studies explain why the death of Ashwell, and the $4900 additional cost to Mississippi Medicaid, is a predictable consequence of the attempt to save a $45 prescription charge. They discredit the rationale given by the APHSA.

A survey by the Health Care Financing Administration, which oversees Medicare and Medicaid, found that at least 11 states restrict the number of prescription drugs nonhospitalized Medicaid patients can receive per month. Limits vary from 3 in Arkansas to 10 in West Virginia. In the AP news story, Waldman cautioned that there must be safeguards to ensure that critical care is not denied. And in fact, most state Medicaid programs have provisions to waive prescription limits when medically necessary — at least in theory. But even in states that provide waivers for emergencies, the patient must know how to work the system. Many do not. Patricia Vinciguerra, Ashwell's sister, told the AP, "It's mind boggling, all the red tape and things people have to go through. If you don't (know how), you are in trouble."

There is yet another facet to physical access to drug therapy: insured patients with drug coverage who find out that their health insurance will not cover therapy with a particular drug product that their doctor has prescribed. Although this situation clearly involves access, it is more complicated than that. Cost shifting to people who can afford the differences between covered drugs and excluded drugs is also a matter of cost control. Drug coverage may also be an issue of quality. While it is possible that an insurance company or HMO is excluding high-quality, but expensive drug products, it may also be that the company is excluding therapies that offer poor value for money or that are inappropriate. Also, this involves prescribing decisions and prescribing influence. So, we will defer full discussion of this situation until we have discussed cost and quality.

Costs of Drug Therapy

The United States spends a larger share of its gross domestic product (GDP) on health than any other major industrialized country. In 1998, U.S. expenditures on health amounted to 13.0% of the GDP. To put this in perspective, the countries with the next highest shares of GDP spent on health were Switzerland and Germany (10.4 to 10.6% each) and Canada and France (9.5

to 9.6%). The rate of increase in the medical care component of the consumer price index (CPI) increased to 4.1% in 2000 from 3.3% per year during 1995 to 1999. The CPI for hospital and related services showed the greatest price increase in 2000 (5.9%), compared with other components of medical care.

In 1999, prescription drug expenditures totaled $99.6 billion, 8.2% of the total health expenditure of $1211 billion. In the same year, prescription drug expenditures increased 17% higher than the average annual rate of increase of 12% between 1995 and 1998. From 1990 to 2000, the CPI for prescription drugs increased by 3 to 6%. Prescription drugs posted one of the highest rates of CPI increase in 1999, 5.7%, while it dropped to 4.4% in 2000.

In 1999, 43% of prescription drug expenditures were paid by private health insurance (up from 25% in 1990), 35% by out-of-pocket payments (down from 59% in 1990), and 17% by Medicaid.[3]

Are drug prices too high? That turns out to be a topic of endless debate, because of the economics of the pharmaceutical industry — a subject that would fill a separate book. From our perspective, pharmaceutical pricing policy is a part of the environment of medications use and can receive only passing attention.

The pharmaceutical industry is, first of all, global. Second, it is based on very expensive research and development. Over the past decade, companies have gotten larger through mergers and acquisitions to increase the pile of capital available for expensive projects. Often, basic research was paid for by government grants (in the United States or elsewhere). Development cost, however, includes clinical testing and everything else necessary to bring a product to the market. As mentioned earlier, the industry claims that the average drug product costs $880 million and requires 15 years to bring-to-market. Meanwhile, patent protection, which started early in the drug's development, is running out.

It is a high-risk industry. Many products never make it to the market, despite millions of dollars invested. In contrast to development costs, production costs in the pharmaceutical industry tend to be rather low, even with exacting quality standards, expensive record keeping, and so forth. So the pharmaceutical industry prices it products to recover its investment plus profits commensurate with the risk. That means that it routinely charges *dollars* for products that cost *pennies* to produce. It also means that the industry prices according to supply and demand, i.e., what the traffic will bear. Because of federal drug regulations, it is difficult (to say the least) to import products purchased in other countries into the United States. This segments the market and allows the industry to sell a product in South America and Central America for a fraction of what it charges in the United States and Canada. The manufacturer can make money whenever it can sell a product for more than its marginal cost of production (the cost of producing the next tablet, so to speak). So, in effect, wealthier nations subsidize the poorer. Or, if you are so inclined, wealthier nations pay a fool's tax for drug products. Also, from time to time over the years, a relatively few, but highly publicized cases like chloramphenicol, Mer-29®, Pondimin®, and Redux® have shown examples that some manufacturers may put profit way ahead of public interest.[4,5]

This makes the industry vulnerable to criticism of astronomical overpricing and of profiting from the implicit subsidy by wealthy nations. The fact that people need medicines they cannot afford can easily lead to charges of profiting on people's misery. The industry's defense is threefold: new therapies are cost-effective and have revolutionized health care; the industry has a splendid track record of developing new, safe, and effective drugs; and finally, if it cannot remain profitable, it cannot attract capital. Without capital, research and development will dry up. These arguments have plenty of facts to support them, but this does not mean that prices in the United States are as low as they could be.

So, the debate goes on. On the one hand, we get a lot of value for 8% of health care expenditures. On the other hand, much of that $99.6 billion is spent out-of-pocket, so people feel the pain of expensive prescriptions. Medicare does not cover outpatient prescriptions, and many insurance programs force people to pay a significant share of prescription costs. Prescription drug expenditures are rising rapidly. This looks to many people like a budget that could be trimmed.

This is all background. From the perspective of medications use systems, the topic of interest is not to evaluate the industry's pricing structure, but rather to reflect on how patients and providers process information about prices and the relationship between cost, access, and quality, There are two fundamental frameworks for thinking about prescription drug costs: (a) as isolated components, as the discussion above has implied; and (b) as inputs to a health care system whose objective is to achieve therapeutic goals and improve the quality of people's lives.

The interplay is illustrated by the following fictional vignette (any similarity to real drug names is accidental):

> Bill Dowers went to see Dr. Brown because of frequency and urgency of urination and pain when he urinated. Dr. Brown diagnosed Bill's problem as a urinary tract infection (UTI). The symptoms seemed rather severe, and this was Bill's third UTI within the past 24 months. Dr. Brown prescribed a long course of Megaflox. Although Megaflox was expensive, it had many advantages for a patient like Mr. Dowers. Dr. Brown told Bill to return in a week for a follow-up.
>
> Bill Dowers stopped at the pharmacy on his way home to get the prescription filled. He felt lousy, and he was worried about needing to find a bathroom. In fact, that was his first question to the pharmacy clerk. The clerk took the prescription, but in a few minutes the pharmacist, Ms. Dee Spencer, asked Bill to return to the prescription department. She explained that Strongarm Health Plan, Bill's HMO, had a list of drug products that it would pay for, but that Megaflox was not on the list because it was too expensive. She could fill the prescription with Megaflox, but Bill would have to pay the $150 charge, or she could call Dr. Brown to get the prescription changed. Bill asked Ms. Spencer to discuss the problem with Strongarm. She replied that she had already tried, but the HMO would

not authorize Megaflox unless Dr. Brown could justify requesting it for Bill. Bill then accepted the pharmacist's offer to call Dr. Brown.

When Ms. Spencer called, Dr. Brown had left for the day. The on-call physician approved a 5-day supply of SulfoMeth, a drug commonly used for UTI. Ms. Spencer left a message for Dr. Brown to call her back the next day and filled the SulfoMeth prescription. She cautioned Mr. Dowers to take the medicine until it was all gone and to drink lots of water.

Bill took the prescription, and in 3 days all of his symptoms were gone. He felt much better. The SulfoMeth bothered his stomach, and without his urinary symptoms to remind him, he forgot a few doses, and then a few more. The symptoms did not return, and he was free of the heartburn that he usually got after taking SulfoMeth.

Six months later, Bill Dowers returned to Dr. Brown with a backache. Dr. Brown diagnosed a kidney infection. He took a urine sample for culture and sensitivity, but he wanted to get Bill started on a potent antibiotic right away. He wanted to prescribe Megaflox, but his records showed that he had prescribed it for Bill 6 months earlier, so it might not have been effective. He was chagrined when he heard Bill's account of what had really happened at the pharmacy, and that Bill had not finished taking the SulfoMeth. It appeared to him that Bill had not taken his medical problem very seriously. He said that this time Bill might have to go into the hospital if the Megaflox did not work.

Table 5.1 shows two ways of expressing input costs and three ways of expressing effectiveness. The most elementary approach is generically called *cost of illness*. A cost-of-illness study would attempt to measure defined direct and indirect expenditures by people with a defined disease or syndrome. It could also be used to measure the cost of drug therapy per time period or per course of therapy for a disease. For example, a cost-of-illness study would tell us how much it costs per year to treat a patient with AIDS,

TABLE 5.1

Five Types of Cost Study

Type of Study or Analysis	Example Question	Accounts for Outcomes
Cost of illness (cost of therapy)	What does treatment cost? What is the distribution of expenditures?	Ignores outcomes
Cost minimization	Which treatment has the lowest drug cost?	Assumes outcomes of all treatments are equivalent
Cost-benefit analysis	Which treatment is most efficient?	Converts outcomes to "present" dollars
Cost effectiveness	What is the lowest cost per unit result or of result per dollar?	Retains "natural" units for outcomes, e.g., cure
Cost utility	What is the lowest cost per unit of patient satisfaction (subjective utility)?	Outcomes converted to patient satisfaction or other value measures

including how much the drug bill was. The approach has also been used to measure the cost of a drug-induced disease.

Eisenberg et al. measured the cost of nephrotoxicity (kidney damage) associated with the use of an aminoglycoside antibiotic.[6] They reviewed the records of 1756 patients who received aminoglycosides and compared them to those of a sample of patients without nephrotoxicity. Of the 1756 patients, 129 (7.3%) developed nephrotoxicity. The mean total additional cost of this nephrotoxicity was $2501. The average additional cost per patient receiving aminoglycosides was $183.

Cost minimization is in a similar vein. It asks the question, "How can we carry out a defined process (e.g., provide drug therapy) as cheaply as possible?" Questions of cost minimization sometimes ignore differences in outcome, which is another way of saying that they may assume that all outcomes are equivalent.

This approach appeals to some hospitals and managed care organizations, especially when they are paid by a fixed formula instead of a markup. The implicit assumption of cost minimization applied to drug therapy seems to be that all of the alternatives have been approved by the Food and Drug Administration for the particular indication, and therefore the outcomes will be equivalent. Given that assumption, reducing the cost of one of the inputs, drug therapy, should reduce the total cost of care. But that assumption may sometimes be false. Cost analysis should, therefore, also include *cost efficiency* of care.

Efficiency

Efficiency is the relationship of input to output, for example, (a) the cost per treated case, or (b) the degree to which the care has the desired effect with respect to the resources expended. Note that the cost of providing care is therefore not an outcome, but is associated with the inputs, i.e., the means of producing an outcome.

While effectiveness addresses how well a technology performs (in normal use), efficiency addresses the question of whether the technology is economically feasible or desirable.

Of course, for many diseases, different treatments actually differ in effectiveness. The assumption of equivalent outcomes is often unsupportable, and it is necessary to account for relationships between choice of a therapeutic alternative and other aspects of care.

People who are not achieving therapeutic objectives, e.g., who remain symptomatic, may receive additional care. For example, consider a typical but hypothetical treatment protocol for acute, uncomplicated urinary tract infections, as shown in Table 5.2 and Figure 5.1. The treatment protocol clearly suggests that differences in therapeutic effectiveness may result in different total costs of therapy. For example, fewer patients taking an antibiotic that is rapidly effective may need to return to the clinic after the 3-day follow-up. On the other hand, patients taking a drug with lower cure

TABLE 5.2

Hypothetical Treatment Guidelines for Urinary Tract Infection (see Figure 5.1)

Following a tentative diagnosis of AUTI:

1. Collect urine specimen for culture and sensitivity (C&S).
2. Begin therapy empirically with 6-day supply of recommended agent.
3. Follow up with patient or caretaker in 3 days.
   3.1. If patient is asymptomatic, patient completes initial therapy. No follow-up unless initiated by patient.
   3.2. If patient still has frequency, urgency, or pain on urination, patient returns to clinic.
      1) If C&S shows sensitivity to initial agent and reason for nonresponse can be corrected, order an additional 6 days of initial agent.
      2) If C&S shows resistance or equivocal sensitivity to initial agent, if reason for nonresponse is unknown or cannot be corrected, or if many bacteria (colony-forming units (CFUs)) are still present, change therapy to Megaflox.
   3.3. Follow up in 3 days.
      1) If patient is asymptomatic, continue therapy.
      2) If patient is symptomatic, refer to urology clinic.

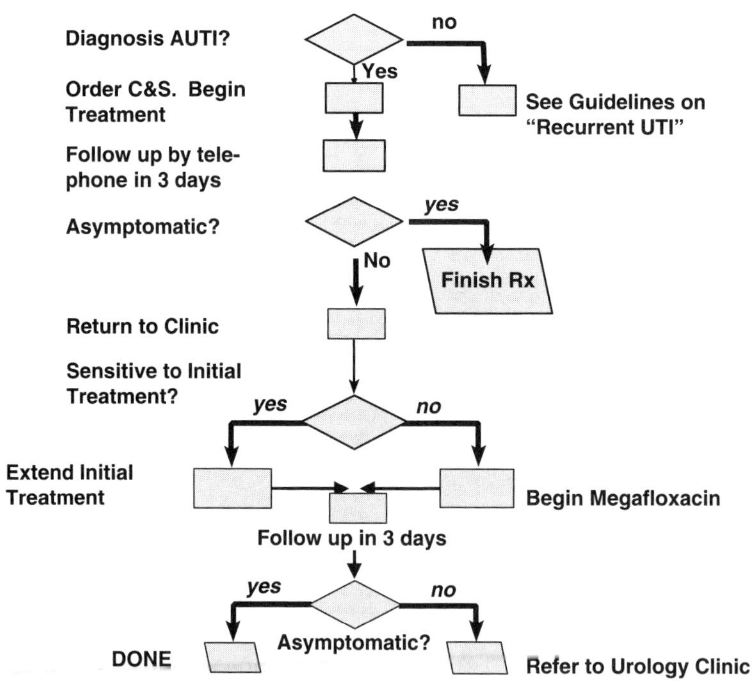

FIGURE 5.1
Flowchart of hypothetical AUTI treatment guidelines.

rates even after an extended course may be more likely to need a referral to the urology clinic.

The last three rows in Table 5.1 show three common efficiency measures in health care — cost-benefit, cost effectiveness, and cost utility. All are ways of expressing economic efficiency, cost per unit of outcome. In cost–benefit analysis (CBA), outcomes are converted to dollars. If there is a stream of outcomes far into the future, their respective values should be converted to present value. For example, suppose that the cost of an immunization program is $1000 per person, all to be spent this year (advertising, vaccine and administration, management of side effects, etc.). Suppose that the benefit of immunization is $100 per year (the annual cost of the chronic disease, weighted by the risk that a susceptible person would contract the disease). Assuming a 20-year horizon and a real discount (interest) rate of 2%, the benefit is not $2000 ($100 times 20 years), but rather $1600 (the present value of $100 per year for 20 years at 2%). The benefit/cost ratio is 1.6.

Cost-effectiveness analysis retains the natural units of the outcome, e.g., a treated case, and calculates the cost per outcome. An extended example is given below. In cost utility analysis, outcomes are evaluated in nonmonetary units, e.g., in terms of life span, quality of life, quality adjusted life years (QALYs), or another nonmonetary measure of the value of the outcome.

Calculating Efficiency

It is often possible to estimate, for each alternative therapy, the probabilities of the major steps in care. For example, see the flowchart in Figure 5.1. These data might be available as cure or remission rates from clinical studies. The clinical data that are extracted from clinical research literature are probably scientifically valid, but may only approximate true costs for a particular patient population. The costs of each step, e.g., the cost of a therapy, lab test, and clinic visit, can be estimated for the organization. These data may have the opposite problem of clinical data — they probably would apply to a particular health care organization but not be accurate (valid) because of accounting practices, market changes, etc. Given these data, one could calculate the expected total cost of therapy with each alternative agent.

Table 5.3 shows an example of the result of a cost-effectiveness analysis. (Appendix 2 illustrates the calculations that lead to Table 5.3.) Suppose that these drugs would all be alternatives for acute, uncomplicated urinary tract infection (AUTI). For example, the typical *drug product cost* for Megaflox is $80. (This could be the average price for a prescription for Megaflox or, more precisely, the average price of the number of doses required by a treatment protocol.)

Further, suppose that clinical research studies have shown that patients who received Megaflox for AUTI, in the dose we are considering, remained

TABLE 5.3

Comparison of Four Therapeutic Alternatives

Therapy	Drug Cost (D) $	Expected Effectiveness (E)[a]	Increment in E (ΔE)	Expected Total Cost of Therapy (C) $[a]	Increment in C (ΔC) $	Incremental CER (ΔC/ΔE)
Megaflox	$80.00	3.0	1.0	$82.00	$25.00	$25.00
SulfaX	$19.00	4.7	—	$70.00	$13.00	—
B-cillin	$35.00	4.0	0.5	$57.00	$7.00	$14.00
Cecycline	$25.00	4.5	n/a	$50.00	n/a	n/a

[a] From decision analysis. Cost does not include cost of initial visit or initial lab work (which is equal for all treatments).

Note: n/a = not applicable.

symptomatic for 3 days on average; so this effectiveness measure reflects the average number of days required until patients feel well enough to return to their normal activities. Note that a lower number indicates higher effectiveness in this example. (For other drugs, the effectiveness rating could reflect survival rate, average weight change in fitness program, quality-of-life measurements, patient or physician satisfaction measurements, etc.).

The *total cost of therapy* for each alternative includes nursing, pharmacy and medical care costs, initial visits, revisits, clinic referrals, additional therapies, etc. (This need not include costs that do not depend on choice of therapy — see footnote in Table 5.3.) For Megaflox, this cost is $82.

The alternative treatment regimens are listed in order of total cost of therapy (C). The lowest cost alternative therapy is Cecycline, for which a course of therapy costs, on average, $50 beyond the cost of the initial visit and lab work. Increments of effectiveness (ΔE) and of cost (ΔC) in a row are simply the differences from the corresponding value in the next row down. (Since *fewer* sick days show *more* effectiveness, we reverse the sign from negative to positive.) For example, ΔE for B-cillin equals 0.5, because symptoms resolve half a day sooner on average with B-cillin than with the next cheaper therapy, Cecycline.

SulfaX does not have a value listed for ΔE because its effectiveness measure is lower, while its cost of therapy is higher. Within the scope of this analysis, there is no basis for selecting SulfaX, even though it has the lowest drug cost. The technical term is that SulfaX is *dominated* by B-cillin. Therefore, we calculate the value of ΔE for Megaflox based on the next cheaper real alternative, which is B-cillin. Patients with AUTI who take Megaflox become symptom-free on average 1 day sooner than patients taking B-cillin.

The incremental cost-effectiveness ratio (ICER) is calculated by dividing ΔC by ΔE. In this example, the additional half day of effectiveness that we can expect from B-cillin compared to Cecycline will cost, on average, an additional $7. The incremental cost-effectiveness ratio for B-cillin is therefore $14 per day. Likewise, the ICER for Megaflox is $25. This is the cost per day of the more rapid resolution of symptoms.

Which Choice Is Optimal?

An input, such as the four therapeutic alternatives in Table 5.3, is optimal when it minimizes or maximizes the relevant output, within specified boundary conditions. The incremental cost analysis does not tell us which alternative is optimal, because it presents a variety of output variables. Choosing an optimal alternative depends on five basic issues, collectively called the *basis* of the decision: (1) the overall goal, (2) simplifying assumptions, (3) perspective and values, (4) decision rule, and (5) the basic environment in which the decision will be carried out. Normally, a decision maker will be unable to answer any of these precisely. This can sometimes be very complex. (That is why good decision makers are so valuable.)

1. Overall goal. This decision is surely part of a bigger picture. For example, this decision may form part of the drug therapy policy for a clinic or HMO. The decision maker needs to know the goal of that drug use policy — for example, should it promote optimally cost-effective care intended to maximize patients' health-related quality of life? Should it contribute to a marketing strategy based on low premiums, or a "provider bonding" program to attract physicians?
2. Perspective and values. Because of health insurance and other variations in the way that health care is paid for, two important questions are, "Who pays (and for what)?" and "Who benefits?" — in other words, "optimal for whom?" Purchasers (e.g., employers), payers (e.g., HMOs), and consumers have some common interests, but it would be naive to assume that their interests are identical.

   A "pharmacy benefit manager" charged with minimizing drug product expenditures might have been instructed to favor the lowest drug cost alternative. The top management of an HMO might favor the alternative leading to the lowest total cost. A patient or an employer that depends on its many highly skilled workers being productive every day might value speed of symptom resolution above all other considerations.

   This topic will be discussed more fully in Chapters 12 and 13. It is necessary to appreciate the difference between payer and consumer and the difference between fee-for-service (FFS) and capitation. A provider may have some patients for whom it is paid on a *fee-for-service* basis for each unit of care and each piece of goods, e.g., each clinic visit, each prescription. The same provider may also have patients for whom it is paid on a flat rate by *capitation* (e.g., fixed payment per member per month) or *episode* (e.g., fixed payment per hospital admission). The financial incentives are quite different for these two basic payment arrangements. In flat-rate payment, there is an incentive to control total costs.

3. Assumptions and calculations. The basis for deciding between alternatives is a calculated value of each alternative. In this example, the expected values of main interest are the expected total cost of therapy (C) and effectiveness (E) (see Appendix 2). The analyst usually has to make a number of assumptions when calculating expected value. In this case, the calculation assumed that therapy would follow the treatment protocol for AUTI.

   Average costs were used for each step in care. Published cure rates, etc., would have been used to weight the costs of each step in care to arrive at the expected value of an alternative. (See Appendix 2 for an example.) The analyst should recognize that these data are actually assumptions about the future. It may be necessary to check those assumptions when the decision is actually implemented.

   In addition, it is necessary to consider only feasible alternatives, eliminating those alternatives that cannot actually be selected, e.g., for contractual or political reasons. This is one example of "boundary conditions." In this example, all therapies are presumably real alternatives.

4. Decision rule. A decision rule or set of criteria should reflect the specified priorities, for example, how cost and effectiveness will be traded off if necessary. Sometimes a decision rule can be specified unambiguously. For example, "choose the alternative with the lowest total cost of care." Sometimes, however, a decision rule has to reflect factors that are not known for sure, for example, how robust one believes the assumptions are. Sometimes a decision rule will attempt to include factors that were not included in the analysis, such as stability of supply.

5. Environment. The basic question here concerns stakeholder response. Would the decision be accepted or resisted by stakeholders purely on its merits, or would they consider collateral issues that were not included in the decision analysis? Some decisions will receive support or resistance based on the stakeholder's goal, perspective, and assumptions. Others may involve quite different issues, such as political competition, horse trading, back scratching, favoritism, and patronage. For example, a drug policy decision made by an HMO may require cooperation from others, which may depend on issues that have nothing to do with the basis of the decision. Some stakeholders might support (or resist) any effort that seems to restrict prescriber choice.

   As shown in Table 5.3, SulfaX minimizes drug acquisition cost among these alternatives; Cecycline minimizes total cost of therapy when other aspects of care are considered; and Megaflox maximizes effectiveness. Which one is *optimal* depends on the relative importance of cost and effectiveness. The choice of SulfaX is said to be *suboptimal* because, even though it would minimize (contribute the least to) drug expenditures, it would increase total cost. Some other part of the institution or program would pay extra for that choice.

Hospitals and managed care organizations sometimes create conditions for suboptimization by giving narrow assignments to departments or other stakeholders. For example, a hospital with a large proportion of its care paid for by flat rate (capitation, or episode of care) may need to control its total costs of care, which it cannot pass on to payers. SulfaX would not be an optimal choice for that institution because the total cost per treated case is higher for SulfaX than for either B-cillin or Cecycline. If the hospital assigns its pharmacy department the job of minimizing *drug expenditures*, the pharmacy might favor SulfaX anyway. (If the hospital were paid on a cost-plus or fee-for-service basis, SulfaX is still not the best choice, because charges would be higher for Megaflox.)

To say that Cecycline is optimal because it minimizes the total cost of care to the institution makes more sense, if cost has been selected as more important than other criteria, e.g., revenues or effectiveness.

The incremental cost-effectiveness analysis shows that one additional unit (sick day) of effectiveness will cost $14 if we choose B-cillin over Cecycline, and an additional $25 if we choose Megaflox over B-cillin. We can, in effect, decide to purchase additional effectiveness for our patients at those prices, or offer those choices to them. This seems straightforward from a clinical or humanitarian point of view. Even from an economically oriented marketing viewpoint, a provider might prefer a more expensive therapy, if customers value effectiveness more than the higher cost. For example, a school system has to pay both a sick teacher and a substitute teacher. High-tech companies may need to get critical workers well and back on the job. Those advantages may outweigh a desire to save the insurance premium represented by the additional $25 for treating UTI.

Sensitivity Analysis

The input values used in a decision analysis calculation are assumptions that may or may not be correct. For example, the drug cost (D) of a course of therapy may change for one or all of the alternatives. Likewise, clinic costs, sensitivity rates, etc., are estimates that may not turn out to be exactly as expected. *Sensitivity* refers to how much a calculated value would depend on these assumptions.

In a one-way sensitivity analysis, one assumption is varied throughout a range that is considered relevant. For example, the cost of an initial course of therapy with Megafloxacin was assumed to be $80. How much would the cost of Megafloxacin have to decrease before a decision in favor of an alternative, say B-cillin, would change? It might be useful to know the break-even cost (threshold value) at which Megafloxacin and B-cillin would produce equal expected values for C (total cost of therapy), assuming every other variable stayed the same.

Since the relationship between C and D is linear in this model, it is necessary to compute only two values representing the extreme possibilities for D. This is illustrated in Figure 5.4 (see Appendix 2).

Finding a Common Ground for Deciding

After we have recognized the different perspectives, values, and criteria that may be involved in the use of medications, an important and fundamental question emerges. How should we account for the potential disagreements that may result from these apparently competing viewpoints?

Balancing Values

One classical way to account for competing values is to accept them as essentially irreconcilable and then to seek compromise. We could frame the problem as an ethical one. Then we could use ethical concepts (such as duty and responsibility) and ethical principles (such as beneficence and respect for persons) to find a balance between the short and long term, clinical outcomes and HQOL, cost and quality, etc.

Ethically sensitive policy that would balance the competing values might be quite useful, but the modern health care "enterprise" has not been able to accomplish this very often without legal or quasi-legal standards. On the contrary, policy makers seem to be hoping that market forces — which are largely amoral — somehow will substitute for ethical policy.

Often, as in the case of Donald Ashwell, and many patients in the New Hampshire Medicaid program, there is no timely opportunity to balance the perspectives of the patient, doctor, pharmacist, and third-party payer. Each participant simply represents his or her own perspective on what is best, and somebody loses. When the patient is old, poor, or mentally ill, he is likely to lose out. So, although the ethical approach of balancing competing values is philosophically stronger, it seems to fail in practice.

Suboptimization and Values

Examples like Mr. Ashwell and New Hampshire Medicaid may not show a callous disregard for the needs of people in order to reduce costs. In the New Hampshire example, the overall program paid much more than the cost of the denied prescriptions. More likely, the cause of problems like Mr. Ashwell's death is a misguided effort to control one part of the health care mix at the expense of others. (Such decisions are called *suboptimization.*) By now the point may be clear enough, but it seems elusive to so many managed care executives that it may bear a bit more discussion.

Trying to save money on one component of health care (say drug products and managing drug therapy) may be likened to a building contractor using cheap cement. It is likely that some walls, etc., will fall down or that more jobs will have to be done over sooner than they would if the job had been done correctly the first time (analogous to preventable adverse outcomes and treatment failures). The "bargain" work can hurt people, and the total cost can far exceed the savings on that one budget item. The concrete buyer may get bonuses, but the contractor — and his customers — would get inferior outcomes for a higher price.

The cost of drug therapy does not merely add to the other costs of care. The cost of treatment failures (as happened to Donald Ashwell) or correcting treatment failures (as happened to the displaced elderly in New Hampshire) is often much higher than the difference between needed therapy and least-cost therapy.

Perhaps the very first thing that the building contractor should do, to save his company, is change the assignment and especially the reward system for the concrete buyer. Perhaps the very first thing that managed care CEOs should do is integrate the assignment and especially the reward system for their pharmacy benefit managers.

Finding a Common Ground

In addition to making trade-offs, another classical approach would explicitly identify and emphasize *common values among competing perspectives.* For example, if a managed care organization knew that it would be obliged to pay for the consequences of ineffective treatment, there would be a large area of overlap among the interests of patients, caregivers, professionals, and payers. It should be possible to judge decisions according to this common interest. This approach might simplify the ethical analysis and lessen the pain of necessary trade-offs. An explicit agreed-upon objective is analogous to ethical policy, but might be more compatible with present market realities, and somewhat easier to develop. For example, a goal for a medications use system that partially unifies differing perspectives would be

> optimally cost-effective drug therapy intended to achieve explicit therapeutic objectives that are intended to improve a patient's clinical status and HQOL.

A small step toward this is the notion of efficiency, as illustrated in Table 5.3.

The second issue is the way that care is organized and carried out, and the way that providers are judged and rewarded. Even if the common goal is clear to all, it is possible to organize the delivery system in a way that makes the common goal much harder to attain. A common cause of institutionalized suboptimal decision making is to separate management of components without attending to the management of whole patients. Insurance uses a device called "carve outs," which separates, for example, the cost of drugs and dispensing from the rest of care. This allows the purchaser to control component costs, but sometimes this results in large reductions in efficiency.

Competing values will often remain to be balanced within this objective, e.g., clinical outcome and HQOL, long-term and short-term outcomes, collateral benefits and costs. However, intelligent application of such a decision rule would prevent many of the preventable injuries caused today by suboptimal decisions.

Quality of Care

According to the Institute of Medicine, quality of care is "the degree to which health services for individuals and populations increase the likelihood of desired health outcomes and are consistent with current professional knowledge."[7] The U.S. Office of Technology Assessment has defined *quality health care* as "the degree to which the process of care increases the probability of outcomes desired by patients and reduces the probability of undesired outcomes given the current state of knowledge."[8]

Quality is complex, but can perhaps be described according to three dimensions: domains, components, and methods (see Figure 5.2).

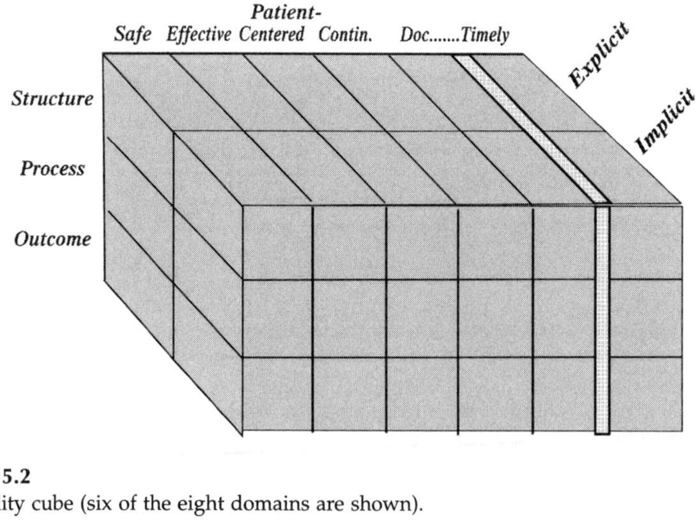

FIGURE 5.2
The quality cube (six of the eight domains are shown).

Quality Domains

Based on Joint Commission on Accreditation of Healthcare Organizations (JCAHO) publications and the IOM's recent *Crossing the Quality Chasm*, quality can be broken down into eight quality domains, as follows (the quoted passages are from the IOM):[9]

1. **Safe:** "avoiding injuries to patients from the care that is intended to help them"; the degree that the care is free from physical, social, and other hazards, including violation of confidentiality
2. **Effective:** "providing services based on scientific knowledge to all who could benefit and refraining from providing services to those not likely to benefit (avoiding underuse and overuse, respectively)"; the degree to which the care
   a. Meets the need for which it is intended
   b. Improves the patient's health
   c. Prevents disease
   d. Is selected and provided correctly, given the current state of scientific knowledge and skill
3. **Patient centered:** "providing care that is respectful of and responsive to individual patient preferences, needs, and values, and ensuring that patient values guide all clinical decisions"; the degree to which the patient is informed about, participates in, and is satisfied with the care
4. **Continuous:** the degree to which the care needed by a patient is coordinated among practitioners, and across organizations and time
5. **Documented:** the degree to which information about care is recorded for purposes of communication, continuity, and review (evaluation)
6. **Efficient:** "avoiding waste, including waste of equipment, supplies, ideas, and energy"
7. **Equitable:** "providing care that does not vary in quality because of personal characteristics such as gender, ethnicity, geographic location, and socio-economic status"
8. **Timely:** "reducing waits and sometimes harmful delays for both those who receive and those who give care"

Quality Components

Each of the eight domains of quality can be applied to each of three components of quality (structure, process, and outcome). Each can be assessed by explicit, implicit, or structured implicit methods. (See next section.)

Avedis Donabedian, perhaps the most famous American writer on health care quality, has proposed three evaluable and interrelated components of quality: structure, process, and outcome.[10,11] *Structure* concerns the type, number, and characteristics of resources. It includes such things as physical facilities, written policies and procedures, and qualifications of staff. *Process* concerns how those resources are actually used to provide or support patient care, i.e., the activities of governance, management, and clinical and support personnel. Process refers to what actually happened. *Outcome* concerns the results of process, occurring within structure. Donabedian defines outcome as a change in health status attributable to health care (i.e., process carried out within a structure).

Structural components of quality are, in many ways, much easier to assess than are process and outcome components. For example, descriptions of physical facilities, and written policies and procedures, are relatively easy for evaluators to obtain and evaluate. Processes are somewhat more difficult to observe than are structures. However, if structural requirements include appropriate documentation of care, evaluators can sometimes use documentation to represent the processes of care. It is said that "if you did not document it, you didn't do it." (Obviously, this was coined by a frustrated quality assessor.) Examples of structural quality indicators for medications use are qualifications (credentials) of professionals, policies regarding drug product selection, therapeutic guidelines, drug use evaluation, and other quality review policies.

Process evaluation is by far the most common approach for evaluating prescribing. To be valid measures of quality of care, there should be evidence that desired outcomes are more likely when certain processes are done than when they are not. Without such evidence, process measures may reflect mere adherence to a meaningless custom or accepted practice. Sometimes, "drug of choice" criteria used in such assessments are supported by evidence connecting prescribing to patient outcomes, sometimes not. Examples of process and outcome evaluations are given below.

Outcomes are obviously the most important component of quality. Both the IOM and OTA definitions of quality refer to desired outcomes. However, a patient's outcome is often difficult to define precisely, especially in chronic diseases, and is more difficult to evaluate than process. Outcomes may occur some time after the processes of care. Moreover, it can be problematic to attribute outcome to any particular cause — some patients will receive good outcomes despite poor quality of care, and vice versa. Outcomes — especially outcomes data — may be influenced by a variety of seen and unseen factors in addition to the provision of care. A vivid example was the short-lived idea of publishing hospital death rates as a rough measure of hospital quality. This seems intuitively reasonable. And there are rather dramatic differences in hospital death rates. Unfortunately, a large part of these differences could be explained by the fact that some hospitals operate hospice programs. Of course, hospice patients could be removed from the statistics, but there is a virtually endless list of other patient variables, such as socioeconomic status, diagnosis, and age distributions, that may influence outcomes but are probably not related to quality of care.[12]

Quality Standards

Quality standards are enforced through professional associations; accrediting bodies like the Joint Commission on Accreditation of Healthcare Organizations; health care financing programs and other health care networks, e.g., Medicare and Medicaid; and state licensing boards, e.g., boards of pharmacy and hospital licensing boards. Hospital accreditation is a good example of how quality standards were instigated and how they have evolved.

Joint Commission on Accreditation of Healthcare Organizations

In 1910, Ernest Codman proposed an "end result system of hospital standardization." Under this system, a hospital would track every patient it treated to determine whether the treatment was effective. If the treatment was not effective, the hospital would then attempt to determine why, so that similar cases could be treated more successfully in the future. Although he is credited as the father of the hospital accreditation movement, Codman's outcome-oriented "end result method" was rejected during his lifetime. This is easy to understand, given the state of hospital quality in 1917.

In 1917, the newly founded American College of Surgeons (ACS) developed a "minimum standard for hospitals," based on structure and process standards. It began on-site inspections of hospitals the next year. Only 89 of 692 hospitals surveyed met the minimum standard. By 1950, more than 3200 hospitals had met an enlarged version of the standard.

In 1952, the ACS transferred its Hospital Standardization Program to the 1-year-old Joint Commission on Accreditation of Hospitals, which began offering accreditation to hospitals in January 1953.* Today, the Joint Commission on Accreditation of Healthcare Organizations evaluates and accredits more than 18,000 health care organizations and programs in the United States. Joint Commission evaluation and accreditation services are provided for general, psychiatric, children's, and rehabilitation hospitals; health care networks, including health plans; home care organizations; home infusion and other pharmacy services; durable medical equipment services; hospice services; nursing homes and other long-term-care facilities; dementia programs and long-term-care pharmacies; behavioral health, drug dependency, and mental health care organizations; ambulatory care providers, including outpatient surgery facilities, rehabilitation centers, and infusion centers; and clinical laboratories.*

In the Joint Commission's early days, quality criteria largely concerned structure (literally such things as cleanliness and fire safety) and basic processes, such as infection control. The development of hospital accreditation has progressed to include structure and process, and finally structure, process, and outcome.[37] Today, the emphasis is on more sophisticated quality improvement processes and consideration of outcomes management.

---

* http://www.jcaho.org/about+us/index.html

Example of Quality Improvement

For example, a chapter on improving organization performance from a 1998 JCAHO accreditation manual for long-term-care pharmacies states that the objectives of improving pharmacy organization performance are to design processes well and to systematically monitor, analyze, and improve performance. The goal is to improve patient outcomes. It defines performance improvement as including:

- Designing of processes
- Monitoring of performance through data collection
- Analyzing of current performance
- Improving and sustaining of improved performance

The manual goes on to say that continually monitoring, analyzing, and improving clinical performance and other processes are at the heart of the standards. Examples of recommended improvement efforts include designing a new service, flowcharting a clinical process, collecting performance measures or data about patient outcomes, comparing the pharmacy's performance to that of other pharmacies, setting priorities, and experimenting with new procedures.

This example illustrates that quality improvement (QI) represents an integration of quality assessment and quality management. Managing to improve quality according to an accepted set of criteria represents a fundamental shift in the basic conception of quality, from a more or less permanent property of a system to a more fluid attribute. It emphasizes the formative, that is, diagnostic and corrective, use of quality assessment.

The significance of the QI approach is evident in the way that QI uses measurement. A *quality indicator* is a quantitative measure that can be used to monitor and evaluate the quality of clinical and support functions that significantly affect patient outcomes. Quality indicators have been used for many years as explicit criteria for "final" (summative) quality assessments. For example, quality indicators can be used during a JCAHO survey (site visit) to make a decision whether to accredit a hospital.

The fundamental conceptual change is the *formative* use of indicators. Formative evaluations are done by local management, not by outside assessors. They are done to identify and correct problems in shorter time cycles (days, weeks, months), rather than every 5 years or so when the institution is up for reaccreditation. Quality improvement is discussed more fully in Chapters 7, 8, and 11.

Tracking process and outcome indicators over time can make it possible to relate changes in structure to changes in process or outcome. For example, the effect of a new procedure or staff training program can be followed up to see if it had the expected effect on process and, in turn, whether the changed process was associated with intended outcome improvements.

Also, performance can be tracked over time, and degradations in quality can be detected and corrected early. Quality improvement is the basic theme of many of the remaining chapters.

Coming Full Circle

Evaluation of outcomes was, in essence, Ernest Codman's original 1913 proposal. His end result system, with some major measurement refinements, is reflected in the Joint Commission's Agenda for Change. The 60 years, roughly from 1917 to 1977, that were required for health care quality assessment to return to its original outcome orientation should provoke curiosity. Why did it take so long? Have we simply arrived now at where Codman started? The process probably was not quite as glacially slow as it might appear. It first laid a necessary foundation for a systematic means to improve the quality of care.

In the near future, corresponding process and outcome indicators may complement clinical research as the basis of valid process and outcome standards for medications use. Perhaps the information needed to develop quality standards for medications use systems will come in part from randomized clinical trials and in part from the users themselves.

Quality Assessment

Quality assessment procedures may be grouped under two main headings: implicit and explicit.[13] The two approaches differ according to the definiteness or clarity of the standards or criteria that they use. In an implicit assessment, the assessor (reviewer) compares the structure, process, or outcome being assessed to his or her personal knowledge, opinion, and beliefs, and may emphasize various aspects according to his or her own values. This may understate the situation in some implicit reviews. Some reviewers may not even consider aspects that other reviewers consider to be very important. Implicit reviews may be idiosyncratic and may differ from assessor to assessor.

To counteract this unreliability,* implicit reviews usually require *peer review*. That is, each assessor should be a qualified expert in the activities being assessed, and often more than one expert carries out a review. Reviews with implicit criteria may be somewhat more reliable if a reviewer's expert judgement is based on a common body of knowledge, training, and experience, e.g., specialty board certification in a relevant field. Peer review can also be flexible, because a well-informed, attentive, and fair expert can take more complex circumstances into account. Implicit reviews may also be necessary when there are no clear quality standards, or when their exact

* Reliability (also called inter-rater reliability) refers to the amount of agreement among different assessors or assessments of essentially the same thing. Low agreement) among reviewers means that assessments are unreliable. See below.

applicability is not settled, which is often the case in judging the medications use process. Except for the PDRM indicator studies, all of the studies reviewed in Chapters 2 and 3 used peer review with implicit criteria. In contrast, most drug use evaluation (DUE) uses explicit criteria, but considers only one aspect of the medications use process.

Explicit criteria provide operational definitions of high-quality structure, process, or outcome. They may specify what to look for, how to judge it, and how much importance should be given to each aspect. The advantage of explicit assessment is high reliability; ideally, explicit assessments are nearly independent of who did the assessment.[13] Explicit criteria require expert reviewers less than implicit criteria, as the need for judgment is less. They are open to review themselves. Complicated subjects or data sources, e.g., medical records, can be abstracted by nonexperts according to explicit guidelines. The PDRM indicators described in Chapters 2 and 3 are examples of this approach.

However, explicit reviews tend to be inflexible. Explicit criteria may not address seldom-occurring, yet important aspects of quality, e.g., instances where the usual conditions for high quality did not apply or were not sufficient. There may be aspects of diagnosis or treatment that require professional judgment, which cannot be described objectively in advance. In short, the reliability of explicit review may be higher than that with implicit review; however, if the explicit criteria include only some aspects or dimensions of quality, the accuracy (validity) of the explicit assessments may be lower.

Guided or *structured* implicit review occupies a middle ground. It attempts to combine the advantages of implicit and explicit criteria without also combining their disadvantages. In this approach, the assessor would receive explicit criteria concerning what to look for, relative importance, etc. However, he would be asked to apply the criteria according to professional judgment. He might be directed to consider information for which quality can be judged but not stated in advance.[13]

Six Methods of Quality Assessment

Suppose an investigator (e.g., researcher or quality improvement manager) has identified a group of patients who were recently treated for urinary tract infections. He has access to data about their care, e.g., medical records or summaries of their care. According to Table 5.4, he could assess the quality of their drug therapy by six basic methods. Table 5.4 is based on a list by Brook et al. of five specific approaches for assessing health care quality (methods 1 through 5).[14] Table 5.4 classifies these approaches according to their use of process or outcome data, and implicit or explicit criteria or review procedures. The table is completed by a sixth approach (explicit process and outcome criteria). The table also includes some examples to illustrate how each approach can be applied to assessments of the quality of medications use.

TABLE 5.4

Approaches to Quality Assessment

	Implicit Criteria	Drug Therapy Example	Explicit Criteria	Drug Therapy Example
Process	**1.** Was the process of care adequate?	Was the drug therapy received by this patient appropriate for his needs at the time?	**4.** How well did the process of care meet defined quality criteria?	Did the drug therapy received by this patient meet (defined) treatment guidelines?
Outcome	**2.** Could better care have improved the outcome?	Does this treatment failure or recurrence occur when care was adequate?	**5.** Were the outcomes in a defined population consistent with outcomes obtained from scientifically validated processes of care?	Is the adjusted failure rate higher in this population than in a population of patients who received high-quality care?
Both	**3.** Were both the process and the outcome consistent with quality?	Would better prescribing and drug therapy management have avoided the problem in this patient?	**6.** Were both the process and the outcome consistent with defined criteria?	See examples from MacKinnon and Faris in Chapters 2 and 3.

Source: Brook, McGlynn, and Cleary, *N. Engl. J. Med.*, 335, 966, 1996.

The investigator could assess *process* quality with either method 1 or method 4. The question with implicit criteria (method 1) is general: Was the drug therapy received by this patient, as documented in the record, appropriate for his needs at the time? The question asked under method 4 is more focused and refers to guidelines.

Drug use evaluation is a process of assessing the quality of prescribing according to explicit criteria for appropriate and inappropriate prescribing. (Drug use evaluation is discussed in Chapter 6.) From the perspective of quality-of-care assessments, most DUE activities would fit into method 4. Often, drug use evaluation employs drug choice criteria exclusively, although DUE criteria can, in principle, encompass dosage, appropriateness for a patient, etc. Still, prescribing is only a part of the medications use process.

From a quality assessment perspective, DUE is usually somewhat limited in scope. For example, process evaluations as described by Brook et al.[14] require patient information. A common form of DUE is done, however, without diagnosis or any other patient information. For example, DUE may compare actual prescribing to a list of approved drugs, while the indication for the drug is assumed. This procedure would misclassify, as acceptable prescribing, all instances where a drug of choice had been prescribed, even if the drug had been unnecessary or in an *inappropriate* (nonindicated) therapeutic class. This method would also miss completely all instances where an indicated drug had not been prescribed.

Despite its name, DUE does not assess the quality of drug use, just prescribing. Furthermore, most ambulatory care DUE is done from prescriptions dispensed and submitted for payment. Occasions when the prescription was not needed, when a prescription should have been written but was not, or when the order was never carried out (e.g., where the patient should have filled the prescription but did not) would often be ignored. DUE ordinarily does not consider drug administration, consumption, or effects, and sometimes does not consider dose. DUE is a useful, but very limited assessment tool, even for prescribing. It should be supplemented by one or more methods useful for evaluating medications use, e.g., as listed in Table 5.4. DUE data may be useful for identifying potential problem areas in prescribing, but decisions based only on DUE data should be appropriately limited.

Methods 2 and 5 use outcome evaluations. With method 2, the review would ascertain whether the outcome was consistent with the reviewer's opinions, beliefs, and judgments about quality of care. In method 5, explicit outcome criteria would be used to review either individual records or population data. Outcomes are difficult to assess independently of process. Method 5 might be best for (a) identifying cases that should be followed up with another method, e.g., method 3; or (b) outcomes that are exceptionally good or bad. A *sentinel event* is defined as an outcome or other important occurrence that does not happen in the presence of adequate care. The question under method 2 asks, in effect, if an outcome was a sentinel event. In method 5, this approach is more explicit. It asks whether the prevalence of an outcome in the population being reviewed is consistent with the corresponding prevalence in a reference population.

With methods 3 and 6, the assessor attempts to assess process and outcome together. Method 3 requires a case-by-case review. The reviewer might, for example, identify patients with undesired outcomes, such as treatment failures or symptom recurrences, and then ask if the process of care caused the outcome, or if the outcome could have been better if the process of care had been more appropriate, according to the reviewer's opinions. This approach was the method used by most of the studies summarized in Chapters 2 and 3.

Method 6 uses explicit criteria to evaluate both process and outcome. This approach was not included by Brook et al., but it is a logical consequence of the arrangement in Table 5.4. This is the approach of the PDRM indicators described in Chapter 3, which includes many examples. (This will be discussed in more detail in Chapters 7, 8, and 11.) Review of both process and outcome, using explicit criteria, allows assessments of populations and could be used to identify patients for follow-up by another method. It could also be used to produce explicit *process* criteria with a wider scope than DUE criteria.

Two Remaining Issues in Quality Assessment

Two major issues in quality assessment remain: the use of evidence vs. professional consensus, and the recent trend to rely on consumerism and market forces to solve problems in quality, cost, and access.

Evidence vs. Professional Consensus

From 1917 until the early 1990s, accreditation standards emphasized structure and process, perhaps for practical reasons in the evolution of accreditation. In contrast, patients have tended to evaluate quality according to the outcomes of care, as represented by the OTA definition given above. (This contrast is illustrated in the ironic proverb, "The operation was a success but the patient died.")

Medical societies and the American Hospital Association traditionally dominated the Joint Commission. During this time, professional consensus was the predominant source of quality standards. Many requirements were based in common sense, such as fire retardant floor coverings and fire escapes. Some were based on professional opinion, for example, documentation of patient care. Few, however, had research to confirm their relationship to outcomes.

Managing quality based on formally validated measures and standards is an ideal that has still not been achieved, and may not be achievable. The complexity of health care, compounded by a rapid rate of change in available technique and equipment, introduces a large element of judgment, and therefore disagreement. Given such circumstances, evidence-based professional consensus standards seem to be the next best alternative to formally validated standards. This is, so to speak, a generalized version of the idea that peer review is the gold standard for quality assessments.

There are two real problems involved in the issue of evidence-based vs. professional consensus standards. First, large, inexplicable "practice pattern variations," especially in surgical rates, call into question the validity of professional consensus standards. Second, some of the research evidence linking procedure to outcome does not itself meet scientific standards. If professional consensus is an unreliable basis for quality standards and well-done scientific studies are unavailable, it is not clear how quality can be defined and measured.

Practice Pattern Variation

A review by David Eddy and colleagues gives a number of examples of the first problem.[15–17] In one study, four cardiologists were asked to assess patient status based on some good-quality angiograms. The cardiologists differed by 40% in deciding whether there was 50% or more blockage (which could be a criterion for angioplasty or bypass). In another study, cardiologists changed their opinions about blockage in up to 37% of cases just from seeing the angiogram a second time.

In his series of studies, Wennberg[20–22] found up to 3-fold differences in procedure rates from practice to practice for heart bypass, thyroid, and prostate surgery; 7-fold differences in knee replacement rates; and 20-fold differences in carotid endarterectomy rates. These differences do not support the assumption that medical quality standards (and decision making) have a common scientific basis.[18–22]

In the field of medications use, it is commonly required that health care organizations maintain lists of approved drugs and conduct drug use evaluations to screen prescribing for compliance with the approved agents. (Chapter 6 will discuss this topic in more detail.) Formulary restrictions, however, have little scientific support, and some studies suggest that the requirement can have unintended (negative) consequences not only on outcome, but also on total costs of care.[23]

Validity of Clinical Research

The second problem is the empirical basis for consensus in clinical research. It has two aspects. First, even when professional consensus is based on clinical research, the research may have severe limitations. One common problem is lack of scientific controls. Sometimes this is a difficult problem to overcome, since one cannot blind a surgeon to the identity of the procedure he is providing. The ethical problems involved in randomizing patients to a placebo group can be insurmountable. Placebos are commonly used in new drug research; in fact, such studies are required for marketing approval. However, studies comparing a new drug to standard therapies are not legally required and often unavailable for years after a new drug is marketed. Further, drug efficacy is only one dimension of safe and effective medications use. The evidence base for quality standards in other aspects of care, e.g., medications use management, is limited.

The second aspect of the evidence problem is that clinical research may not address outcomes that matter from a patient's perspective, e.g., changes in patient's quality of life. Adar et al. reviewed 39 studies of a surgical procedure intended to open popliteal or femoral arteries, to relieve leg pain, and to restore patients' ability to walk. These studies usually evaluated the success of surgery according to whether the artery remained open. Not one study measured pain relief or whether patients could walk after recovery from surgery.[16] Studies of corneal transplantation measure visual acuity (with an eye chart), but not patients' ability to see in everyday situations.

Market Forces

The second problem may result from the first. Suppose that quality standards have often not been validated (i.e., that scientific studies on a certain practice are incomplete or inconclusive). Further suppose that professional opinion may rest on tradition, untested assumptions, or even occupational self-interest.

Then on what basis should patients and third-party payers judge the quality of the care they purchase?

A trend is clearly discernable toward reliance on consumers and managers in a marketplace to decide on appropriate care — a marketplace of managed care, where insured second parties receive care purchased for them by third parties — managed care organizations, and health insurance companies. Perhaps some professionally approved procedures without scientifically demonstrated value are a waste of money, or even dangerous. If so, the reasoning seems to go, third parties have a right, if not a duty, to restrict professionals' choices — or at least the choices that health insurance will pay for.

This begs two important questions: (1) What is the scientific basis for managed care policy? and (2) Who will watch the watchers? If medical science (or medical practitioners) really do not know, for example, whether a depressed patient needs drug therapy, psychotherapy, or changes in diet and exercise, should managed care employees decide? On what basis? If health care professionals do not always have an empirically valid basis for their decisions, and if their standards may sometimes be self-serving, might not managed care suffer from the same shortcomings? These are rhetorical questions, but the rhetoric is not directed against managed care as such, but rather in favor of evidence-based practice and quality standards. However, when scientific (population) standards are insufficient to guide policy and decision making, local standards based on performance indicators should be mandatory. New standards are needed, and they should require all health care payers and providers to maintain QI programs that are able to identify, resolve, and document important quality problems.

Summary on Quality

This section has defined quality with respect to a "quality cube" comprising three components (structure, process, and outcome), eight domains (effectiveness, safety, patient orientation, continuity, documentation, efficiency, equitability, and timeliness), and two methods (implicit and explicit criteria). The metaphor of a cube is intended to imply the idea of a unity that can present different aspects.

Quality can be measured by means of criteria, indicators, and standards. The use of these tools has changed from periodic quality assurance exercises, as symbolized by ACS and JCAHO surveys, to continuous quality management, as symbolized by the JCAHO Agenda for Change and the HEDIS (Health Plan Employer Data and Information Set) program of the National Committee for Quality Assurance (NCQA).

Despite questions about the validity of some quality standards, there is reasonable evidence that enforcement of quality standards has dramatically improved the quality of health care in America, especially the quality of physical facilities and standard procedures. Such questions do not depreciate the value of structure, process, and outcome criteria. They should, however, provide a constant reminder that quality is an extremely complex subject that cannot easily be captured in one or two approaches. The relevance of professional quality standards to outcomes that have real value to people should be continually questioned. Quality is a journey, not a destination.

Patient Satisfaction with Care

Patient satisfaction with care is related to quality of care. Some would say that it is part of quality. However, it is not settled just how, exactly, satisfaction and quality are related. To some, patient satisfaction is a sine qua non of quality. According to one author, " … care cannot be of high quality unless the patient is satisfied."[24] From another perspective, however, satisfaction is only a part of the patient orientation and acceptability quality dimension.

Satisfaction is defined in normal usage as fulfillment of a need or want, or as a person's subjective evaluation of that fulfillment. Satisfaction with care is neither a clinical outcome nor an HQOL outcome. It is, instead, a person's *response* to certain aspects of clinical outcomes, processes of care, and physical facilities — namely, the aspects that the person could experience. Furthermore, since these are perceptions, they can be influenced by the patient's expectations and emotional state. Satisfaction with care can be managed; however, the methods for managing satisfaction might overlap only somewhat with quality management.

Table 5.5 provides the dimensions of satisfaction proposed by Parasuraman et al.[25,26] This structure adds precision to the casual definition and use of the term.

Why the Interest in Satisfaction?

A number of issues have converged in recent years to make patient satisfaction with care an important criterion measurement and tool for quality improvement. These are, in summary:

TABLE 5.5

Dimensions of Satisfaction (Service Quality)

Tangibles	Appearance of the physical facilities, equipment, and personnel
Reliability	Dependable and accurate service performance
Responsiveness	Staff willingness and ability to help customers and provide prompt service
Assurance	Customer confidence and trust in the competence of staff
Empathy	Staff's apparent understanding of the customers' feelings

1. The health care consumer movement. This movement is, in part, a reaction to medical paternalism, and a perception that professional definitions of quality were, at best, incomplete. It includes a demand for professional accountability.
2. The use of market forces and managed care as allocation and distribution methods, which would increase consumer influence through choice of provider. In an open market, the consumer is assumed to be sovereign, and his satisfaction is assumed to have paramount importance.
3. The increasing emphasis on outcome-based definitions of quality. Since satisfaction is not itself an outcome, the connection seems to involve an assumption that the consumer would know when his needs were satisfied and therefore be able to judge the quality of an outcome.
4. Increasing emphasis on chronic and other diseases that require cooperation by patients in their own care. Satisfaction with care may improve patient cooperation. Furthermore, it is possible that some outcomes of some diseases depend on patient attitudes in addition to clinical science.
5. Finally, patient satisfaction with care is an intuitively appealing objective.

Satisfaction with Drug Therapy

Satisfaction with drug therapy may seem a somewhat narrow aspect of satisfaction with health care. However, given the importance of drug therapy in managing many diseases, satisfaction with drug therapy could significantly influence medication taking by patients and therefore outcomes, not to mention overall satisfaction with care. In particular, patients may attribute certain changes in their HQOL to drug therapy, as illustrated in the story of Mr. Diehl in Chapter 4. They may then increase or decrease their cooperation in care based on that satisfaction or dissatisfaction. This may directly link satisfaction with drug therapy to outcomes, especially in patients with chronic diseases.

So, patient satisfaction is important, in part because of its contribution to outcomes and in part because satisfaction surveys are becoming an obligatory part of the evaluation of care. However, there are serious philosophical and scientific issues to be addressed in conducting and evaluating the results of satisfaction surveys.

Critique of Satisfaction Measures

Consumer Focus

Dissatisfied people may not keep appointments or cooperate in care. They may find another provider. However, there are some logical limits to the interpretation of satisfaction data. First, a consumer relationship with a health care professional is only one of at least three possible relationships, as described in Chapter 4. Although patients may have wants, they may also have needs that they do not fully recognize. They may also be unable to understand the real choices involved in satisfying their needs.

It is easy to imagine cases where initial satisfaction, based on fulfillment of wants, gives way to subsequent dissatisfaction based on nonfulfillment of needs. Dissatisfaction must be avoided, but satisfaction cannot be the only, or even the main, objective of professional service.

The value of wellness and the fact that costs are usually offset by insurance payments make health care purchase decisions different from usual consumer behavior. Consumers may not have access to information needed for deciding what medical services to buy and from whom to buy them. Satisfaction may not have a realistic basis independent of the care received from a specific provider. As a result, consumers may learn what to expect as they receive care, and satisfaction measures may fluctuate as consumer expectations change.

In a Danish study of pharmaceutical care in a community pharmacy, patient satisfaction rose in the first 6 months and then fell to the original level. Patients' expectations of pharmacy service had changed. Also, some resentment developed that the higher level of pharmaceutical service was the subject of a study and not standard care.

Measurement Issues

For satisfaction to have any practical use as a criterion for managing the quality of drug therapy, it is necessary to know what people mean when they say they are satisfied and to deduce why they are satisfied. Brian Williams has concluded that we do not know these things. Rather, we make simplifying assumptions with little real basis.[27] Interest in satisfaction seems ultimately to depend on the assumption that satisfaction measures reflect patient values or that they reflect how well service has met a patient's expectations. However, on average, patient values explain only about 8% of measured variation in patient satisfaction. Expectations explain about 10%.[27] So, people evidently indicate on surveys that they were satisfied with a service when the service had neither produced an outcome that they had said they valued nor had met their expectations.

It is possible that both expectations and values may change during the process of care, as patients learn about the possibilities and clarify their priorities. This suggests a dynamic (as opposed to a static) model of satisfaction in which snapshots of average satisfaction measures are much less meaningful than changes in an individual's satisfaction over time.

Patients may not be able to evaluate quality on a basis *they* would consider valid. They may defer to the expertise of the professional (despite the assumptions of health care consumerism). Finally, satisfaction with care may come from outside of the immediate process of care, e.g., from past encounters and the experience of others.

Measuring patient satisfaction with pharmaceutical care may be useful and appears to be a practical necessity. It is also necessary, however, to question the apparently safe assumptions that support current interest in patient satisfaction surveys. Inferences from them should be made cautiously.

Drug Law: Quality of Drug Products as Legal Requirements for Safety and Efficacy

Drug law provides the principal quality controls on drug products in the United States and most other developed nations. As problems with medications have become evident, the federal Food and Drug Administration has come under pressure to improve drug use. This approach is attractive to some people, because of the power of the federal government and because the legal apparatus already exists. This section will address the limitations of legal controls on the marketing of drug products when the objective is to improve the outcomes of medications use. A key to this understanding will hinge on the distinction between the concepts of *drug efficacy* and *drug effectiveness*, and the corresponding distinction between product safety and safe use of a product.

As articles of commerce, marketing of drug products is subject to state and federal laws and regulations. Furthermore, as they apply to drug products, the terms *safety* and *effectiveness* (or *efficacy*) are legally defined in the United States and other nations. On the one hand, drug products are only a part of drug therapy. On the other hand, drug licensing includes regulation of labeling (legal indications for use) that may influence drug use. The demarcation between drug product regulation and the management of drug use is not clear.

Regulatory Perspective on Drug Product Quality*

Drug product quality is a matter of law in most countries. Commerce in drug products in the United States is controlled by the U.S. Food and Drug Administration, the Drug Enforcement Administration (DEA), the Federal Trade Commission (FTC), and state law.[28] Federal laws tend to be product oriented, while state laws tend to regulate professional practice. However, there is overlap both in law and in practice.

The FDA administers the U.S. Food, Drug, and Cosmetic Act (FDCA) of 1938, as amended. Among the provisions of the 1938 act was a requirement that drugs must have proof of safety before being introduced into interstate commerce. Under the Durham–Humphrey Amendment of 1951, the FDA

* Legal information in this section is based generally on Brushwood, op. cit.; however, he is not responsible for the examples and opinions, or for any errors committed by the author.

could designate some drug products as prescription-only and others as over the counter (OTC). The Kefauver–Harris Amendments of 1962 added a requirement for proof of efficacy.

The FDA decides whether a drug product can be marketed in the United States at all, and if it may be marketed, whether it can be sold without a prescription (over the counter). The constitutional authority of the FDCA is the regulation of interstate commerce. It excludes regulation of professional practice, which falls under the police powers reserved to the several states by the U.S. Constitution.

According to the FDCA, a *drug* is (1) an article listed in official drug compendia; (2) an article intended for the diagnosis, cure, mitigation, treatment, or prevention of disease in man or other animals; (3) an article intended to alter the structure or function of the body (except for food); or (4) a component of an article described in (1), (2), or (3).[28]

A *new drug* is any drug not generally recognized as safe and effective among experts qualified by scientific training and experience. A previously approved drug may become a "new" drug if its composition, directions, or dosage forms are modified.

Before a new drug can be legally marketed in the United States, a New Drug Application (NDA) must be submitted by a sponsor (usually the originator, manufacturer, or licensee). For minor changes in a previously approved drug, or for a new manufacturer of a previously approved drug, an abbreviated NDA (ANDA) may be submitted. The NDA or ANDA must be approved by the FDA prior to marketing.

The basis for FDA approval is not as simple as it may appear. The phrase "generally recognized as safe and effective among experts qualified by scientific training and experience" has been construed to include the quality of the evidence that the experts must use. Unlike standards based on professional consensus in other subject areas, NDAs must include results of formal clinical trials. The FDA does consult experts, but only after rigorous research in three phases: Phase I tests are based on animal studies and are carried out among small groups of healthy volunteers to determine approximate dose–response relationships and toxicity. In phase II, the drug is given to small groups of people who have the condition in which the drug is proposed for use (the drug's indication). In phase III, the drug is given to much larger groups of people with the indication. The purpose is to learn more about the efficacy and safety of the drug. Whenever possible, phase III tests are randomized, double-blinded, clinical comparisons of the drug against a placebo (usually called randomized clinical trials (RCTs) for short).

RCTs are carried out under research and treatment protocols that describe in exacting detail who is eligible for inclusion in the study, who is not, how the drug is to be used (dosage, duration, monitoring), and how its use will be evaluated.

Clinical trials are carried out after the FDA grants an Investigational New Drug (IND) exemption, which permits an unapproved drug to be shipped for use in research. An IND requires evidence of safety, to permit research that might show a drug's effectiveness. In addition, the FDA can grant compassionate INDs on request from health care professionals or providers for the therapeutic use of investigational drugs. Normally, a new drug has a commercial sponsor to pay for the very expensive clinical trials and record keeping required for an approvable NDA. However, some drugs have too little commercial appeal to attract a commercial sponsor, for example, because their potential market is too small, because they are not patentable, or because they represent public relations problems that a major manufacturer would prefer to avoid. These are the so-called orphan drugs discussed earlier, under "Physical Access."

A pharmacist who compounds an approved product pursuant to a legal prescription for a patient does not come under the new drug requirements.

Major Provisions

The major concepts in the FDCA are *adulteration* and *misbranding*. The introduction of an adulterated or misbranded drug into interstate commerce and the adulterating or misbranding of a drug after it is in interstate commerce are prohibited. This limits the FDCA, and the FDA's authority over the practice of health professions; however, these limits are somewhat open to debate.

According to the law, *adulteration* has occurred when a drug product does not conform to standards of purity and potency or standards governing the facilities and manner in which it was produced, packaged, and stored. A drug is deemed to be *misbranded* if its labeling is false or misleading in any particular. Labeling includes the label affixed to the package, brochures enclosed within the drug package (package inserts), advertising, and virtually any information provided by a drug manufacturer about a product. A major use of the prohibition of misbranding is to control the therapeutic claims and recommendations for use of a drug product. This is the connection between the FDCA and medications use.

Worthless Drugs

One objective of the food and drug act is to prevent the marketing of worthless and unsafe drugs. Examples of drugs without proven therapeutic value are purported cancer cures like krebiozen and laetrile. However, drugs being promoted for nonscientific uses include more than these well-recognized examples. Prior to the 1962 Kefauver–Harris amendments to the FDCA, reputable pharmaceutical manufacturers promoted many drugs based on evidence of effectiveness that could not withstand scientific review. After the 1962 amendment, the FDA contracted with the National Academy of Sciences/National Research Council (NAS/NRC) to review the scientific evidence supporting the efficacy of drugs marketed between 1938 and 1962. Approximately 360 prescription drugs (about 7% of the drugs reviewed) were rated as lacking substantial evidence of effectiveness by the NAS/NRC review and were removed from the market. Of 16,000 therapeutic claims made for these products, 66% lacked a substantial scientific basis. Products of many major U.S. pharmaceutical manufacturers were included. Often the removals involved considerable controversy, including appeals to the U.S. Supreme Court.[29]

Unsafe Drugs

Thalidomide is perhaps the most notorious example of an unsafe drug. It illustrates a number of interesting aspects of drug product regulation, and the story is worth summarizing. The following brief account is taken primarily from Silverman and Lee.[4]

Thalidomide was introduced in 1958 by Chemie Grünenthal as a sedative. It appeared to be one of the safest sedatives available, and was approved in many nations around the world, even for sale without a prescription. In contrast to the barbiturates and other sedatives commonly used at the time, thalidomide caused no sedative hangover, appeared nonaddicting, and was useless for attempted suicide. The Merrill Company obtained a license from Chemie Grünenthal to market thalidomide in the United States and Canada, and applied for governmental approval in both countries.

In 1960, approval of a New Drug Application in the United States was automatic at the end of 60 days, and could be denied only if a drug was not generally accepted as safe. In September 1960, the application was assigned to Dr. Frances O. Kelsey, a new medical officer at the FDA. Dr. Kelsey repeatedly delayed the approval process. She neither approved nor rejected the thalidomide NDA, despite pressure from Merrill, who argued that she was interfering with its legal rights to market the drug in the United States.

Then, a rare birth defect, phocomelia, in which children are born with flipper-like limbs, began to appear with increasing frequency. The increase was noted first in Germany, then in Australia, Japan, and other countries. A German physician warned Grünenthal of the possible connection between phocomelia and thalidomide in November 1961. Within 2 weeks, Grünenthal had withdrawn the drug from the market and warned its licensees. The West German government issued a warning. Merrill continued to market the drug in Canada until March 1962. Perhaps 10,000 babies were afflicted by thalidomide-caused phocomelia in 20 countries. Although the drug had never been marketed in the United States, free samples had been widely distributed to physicians by Merrill, and American women had obtained the drug while living abroad or from friends.

The thalidomide disaster seems to have rescued the 1962 Kefauver–Harris amendments from legislative limbo. This is ironic in a number of contradictory ways. On the one hand, thalidomide was not approved in the United States because of the 1938 requirements for drug safety, but on the other hand, safety testing requirements prior to 1962 were not adequate to detect the drug's teratogenicity. The problem with thalidomide appeared after marketing and would not have been discovered in clinical trials. On the one hand, efficacy was not an issue for thalidomide, but on the other, the scandal seemed to open the door to the FDA's argument that safety cannot be assessed without considering efficacy. Thalidomide led to passage of efficacy requirements in the 1962 amendments in the U.S., and it led to radical revisions of German drug law.

Unapproved and Off-Label Uses

A second objective of the food and drug act is to prevent a manufacturer from promoting inappropriate uses of a drug after it has been approved for marketing (based on other uses). The issue of unapproved use is discussed further below. The criterion for FDA approval of an NDA or an ANDA is whether the benefits of a drug for its specific uses outweigh the risks for the same uses. Thus, thalidomide, originally proposed for use as a sedative and antinauseant, was deemed an unsafe drug and was banned from the U.S. market until recently. The benefits of approving another sedative did not outweigh the risks that it may cause birth defects if used accidentally by pregnant women.

Thalidomide (as a sedative) can be contrasted to isotretinoin (Accutane). Isotretinoin also can cause severe, sometimes fatal, fetal malformations and is absolutely contraindicated in pregnancy or in women who may become pregnant within a month of using it. However, its value in treating severe cystic acne and other severe skin diseases gives it a favorable balance of risks and benefits, and it is marketed in the United States.

The new drug approval process requires judgment in the gray areas left by scientific data. The process is also political, although not necessarily in a partisan sense. Beyond scientific questions of risk and benefit, for example, there are questions of who benefits and who takes risk, and the context within which such judgments are made. Thalidomide again provides an example. Despite the experience with thalidomide in the 1960s, about 30 years later the FDA did quietly grant orphan status to thalidomide and approve a number of INDs. Then it was approved for limited U.S. marketing in July 1998 because it has shown potential therapeutic benefits in a number of conditions related to HIV and leprosy. Its approval was subject to unprecedented restrictions, such as restriction of prescribing to certain physicians.

Organizations of AIDS patients pushed hard for approval of thalidomide. However, others fought against approval. Randolph Warren, representing thalidomide victims, wrote that they "will never accept a world with thalidomide in it." Nonetheless, he recognized that AIDS patients were illegally importing the drug for use in the United States and that legal regulation would be safer than a black market. "Medical experts and social scientists predict that no amount of regulation and precaution can prevent the birth [of] at least a few 'thalidomide babies' now that the drug is legal."*

---

* FDA Approves Thalidomide, Daily Briefing, Tuesday, July 21, 1998, www.policy.com.

Drug Enforcement Administration

The Drug Enforcement Administration administers the Controlled Substances Act (CSA). The objective of the CSA is to regulate the distribution of substances with a potential for addiction, including many with legitimate medical purposes recognized by the FDA. The federal law cannot regulate which drugs may be prescribed, the quantity prescribed, or the frequency of prescriptions. Nonetheless, the DEA's War on Drugs does sometimes inhibit medically necessary use of controlled substances, in particular control of severe chronic pain. A physician who treats many patients with narcotic analgesics in high doses and the pharmacist who fills those prescriptions may attract the attention of the DEA and may need to defend against criminal or professional charges.

Nonprescription Drugs and Nutritional Supplements

The FDA decides whether a drug product may be sold without a prescription or over the counter. The legal basis is the misbranding provision of the FDCA. A prescription-only drug must bear the *prescription legend*, limiting sale to prescription only. The substantive basis for this decision is, briefly, whether the product can be labeled adequately for a layman to recognize indications for the drug, to understand its directions for use, and to use it safely.

Appropriate indications for use of a nonprescription medicine are self-limiting problems, such as coughs and colds. The FDA decides whether a layperson should be able to discriminate these from serious diseases that may have similar symptoms in their early stages. So, for example, labeling of nonprescription cough preparations includes warnings to consult a doctor if the cough is accompanied by certain other symptoms or if it persists.

The FDA has authority to regulate advertising of prescription medications to professionals and laymen, but only limited authority over the advertising of nonprescription drug products. Advertising of OTC drugs is actually under the authority of the Federal Trade Commission. Claims made for nonprescription drugs should have a scientific basis, and corrective advertising can be required by the FTC. For example, Warner-Lambert once claimed that Listerine mouthwash prevents colds and sore throats. The FTC found this claim to be unsubstantiated and required Warner-Lambert to include a corrective message in subsequent advertising.

Nonprescription medicines are important aspects of medications use for a number of reasons. First, OTC status is not limited to the safest drugs available. An international comparison of which medicines are available without a prescription in various nations of the industrialized world shows that legal, ethical, and political considerations may be as important as safety data. For example, asthma is a dangerous, non-self-limiting disease that requires medical attention. Epinephrine, a potent drug, was approved by the FDA in 1939. Most epinephrine products are prescription-only. However, epinephrine administered by a metered-dose inhaler is available without a prescription for treatment of asthma. (The FDA has expressed concern regarding OTC status for this dosage form.)

Penicillin is very safe (apart from occasional, possibly severe, allergies). It is almost without pharmacological effects in humans. But it is a prescription-only medicine almost worldwide. The conditions that are to be treated with penicillin almost always need medical attention. There would be no reliable means to limit the OTC sale of penicillin in the United States to those few indications that patients can manage for themselves.

A relatively safe drug like famotidine or ranitidine may be classified as prescription-only in one country because experts in that country consider its indications (gastric ulcers or esophageal reflux) to be dangerous for people to treat without medical attention. In another country this issue may not be considered as important, and the drug may be classified as nonprescription.

Second, nonprescription drugs can cause toxicity, side effects, and drug interactions. Aspirin is sold OTC in practically every country, and other more potent drugs in its class are available OTC in most countries. These drugs can cause severe, even fatal, gastrointestinal bleeding. Aspirin affects blood coagulation and interacts with the anticoagulant effect of the prescription drug warfarin. Cimetidine is a safe enough drug to be sold OTC in the United States, but it can interact with a number of other OTC and prescription-only drugs. Perhaps they are OTC because their labeled indications are self-limiting.

In general, in the United States an OTC medicine can be sold in any retail outlet. There are, however, a few exceptions in the United States — schedule V controlled substances and insulin. Controlled substances in schedule V are those with the least potential for abuse. Most are cough suppressants containing codeine or antidiarrheal preparations. They must be sold by pharmacies because of DEA record-keeping requirements.

Federal law provides that insulin can be sold without a prescription. However, many state laws require that it be sold only in pharmacies. A possible third group of pharmacy-only medications in the United States are products that a manufacturer wishes to restrict to sale through a pharmacy or that a pharmacy keeps "behind the counter." Some eyedrops are sold only in this manner. Some other countries maintain a category of pharmacy-only nonprescription drugs that can be sold only in pharmacies or only by pharmacists or trained pharmacy assistants. Some countries do not enforce legal requirements, and prescription-only medications are freely available in pharmacies or even other shops.

Nutriceuticals

Dietary supplements can be legally marketed in the United States without an NDA, if the manufacturer and distributor do not make therapeutic claims for the product that would cause it to fall under the definition of a drug. So-called *nutriceuticals* are marketed under the Dietary Supplement and Health Education Act of 1994 (DSHEA). Because nutraceuticals are not regulated as drugs and do not require the research needed to support an NDA, scientific data supporting claimed benefit(s) are not always as available for nutraceuticals as for traditional pharmaceuticals. Also, rigid quality control standards are not required for nutraceuticals, and substantial variability can occur in both potency and purity.

There is considerable vagueness about the difference between an article *intended* for use as a drug and one that is *promoted* for use as a drug. The phrasing of the law in passive voice leaves wide open who would be doing the intending or promoting.

For example, St. John's wort is used by many people in the United States and Europe as an antidepressant. There is clinical literature available to support its use as an antidepressant, with specific dosage recommendations, precautions, etc. Companies that manufacture and distribute it in the United States make claims that it can improve mood. Certainly some people who buy it in the United States intend to use it as a drug under the legal definition. Until the FDA decides that these claims have become therapeutic claims, it can remain a dietary supplement.

State Law

The main impact of state law on medications use is in regulating entry to and practice of professions. For example, states could establish laws and regulations enforcing professional quality standards. States also may enact their own laws regulating drug distribution, and there is some latitude for reclassifying drug products from prescription-only to OTC status. For example, Florida allows a pharmacist to "prescribe" certain drug products that were designated as prescription-only by the FDA. This is theoretically an area where state and federal law may collide to create constitutional questions of state vs. federal jurisdiction. Some states allow physician's assistants, clinical nurse practitioners, and pharmacists to prescribe prescription-only medicines under certain restrictions.

Drug Products vs. Drug Use

To summarize, the terms *safety* and *effectiveness* have narrow legal meanings when they are used to describe drug products. A drug can be deemed effective in comparison to a placebo for specific uses enumerated in the NDA and evaluated in the clinical trials that supported the NDA. Likewise, a drug can be deemed safe for those specific uses. However, it is necessary to clarify the distinction between the evaluation of drug products in controlled clinical trials and the everyday use of drug products after marketing.

Two issues may help to clarify this distinction: so-called off-label use and evaluative comparisons, not to placebos but to real therapeutic alternatives.

In its narrow sense, off-label use refers to unapproved uses of drug products, that is, for indications other than the ones for which the drug was approved.

Sometimes, as with the over 250 drug products that were forced off the market after 1962, it would be necessary to prevent some manufacturers from making unwarranted claims for their products. For example, a manufacturer of PETN, a drug once commonly used for angina pectoris, claimed that it was useful to prevent coronary heart attacks until the FDA alleged that those claims misbranded the drug and seized shipments in a number of states.

On the other hand, some off-label uses are generally supported by research, but remain off-label until further research is done, an ANDA is submitted, and the FDA has completed the review. There can be orphan uses as well as orphan drugs, when no sponsor will push a new use for a drug.

Interesting examples of unapproved uses that later became approved uses are propanalol, a beta-blocker, for use in migraine headache; methotrexate, an anticancer drug, to treat psoriasis or arthritis; and lidocaine, a local anesthetic, to treat cardiac arrhythmia. Each of these products was commonly used for these unapproved uses before approval. The use of lidocaine for arrhythmias is particularly interesting, because it became a de facto standard of care while its use was still unapproved by the FDA.

The FDA cannot control medical research or the publication of evidence that an approved product is effective for an unapproved use. Neither can it regulate the practice of medicine. So physicians can read about a new (unapproved) use of an approved agent and prescribe it for that use. FDA has argued unsuccessfully that unapproved uses by physicians constitute misbranding of a drug product after it has entered interstate commerce.

This disagreement is instructive as a conflict of perspectives — what would be misbranding from a regulatory perspective can be a standard of practice from a clinical perspective. This is not, however, an irreconcilable difference. FDA eventually approved these unapproved uses.

By analogy, there are many other kinds of off-label uses, for example, use of a drug in the presence of comorbidities that were not represented in the clinical trials; in children or elders, or other classes of patients who were not included in clinical trials; in doses above or below the labeled recommendations; with other therapies; and so on.

Furthermore, after a drug is marketed, patients rarely receive the level of supervision and monitoring received by patients in drug trials. Considering indication, dose, concurrent diseases, supervision, and patient age, most postmarketing drug therapy may be off-label in one way or another. In simple language, the idea of approved use suggests a legal view in which actions not specifically approved are prohibited. This is clearly at variance with the realities of professional practice and is clearly unmanageable. Attempts to control drug use through the FDA's market regulation approach would be difficult at best, and often unsuccessful.

Effectiveness and Efficacy

The performance of a drug product after marketing may be so different from its performance in clinical trials that one needs a vocabulary that can reflect the distinction. Despite the language used in the food and drug act, the performance of a technology under ideal conditions (e.g., a controlled clinical trial) is usually called *efficacy*. *Effectiveness* usually refers to beneficial effects of a drug product or other therapy in actual use under everyday conditions.

Drug safety also can differ from clinical trial to postmarket use. For example, Schiff et al. studied the toxicity of theophylline, a drug once a mainstay of asthma therapy. They found many errors in its use and concluded that "theophylline's overall risk benefit ratio for inpatients may be less than that measured in well-controlled studies of the drug's efficacy because of these ... errors."[30]

Evaluating Effectiveness and Safety in Use

The assessment of safety and effectiveness after marketing is commonly termed *postmarketing surveillance* or, more commonly in Europe, *pharmacovigilance*. Adverse effects from drugs that have demonstrated safety and efficacy in controlled clinical trials are relatively rare in statistical (epidemiological) frames of reference. Therefore, controlled clinical trials are useful mainly to compare newly marketed products to placebos or to older products (effectiveness and safety relative to alternative agents) and for efficiency (cost-effectiveness) studies.

The research approaches generally used to assess safety are observational epidemiologic studies (cohort, case-control, cross-sectional), drug utilization surveys, spontaneous reports, and automated databases linking medications and disease.[31,32]

In adverse drug reaction surveillance, a cohort of patients may be followed in order to detect adverse drug reactions (see Chapter 3). Then hypotheses can be generated about the drug products implicated in causing these reactions. In a case-control design, patients receiving a drug product may be matched to patients with similar diagnoses and other attributes (e.g., age, sex, comorbidities), and their outcomes, adverse reaction rates, etc., may be compared, or patients with a particular adverse outcome may be matched to patients who did not have that outcome.

Manufacturers are required to actively seek instances of adverse drug reactions for years after drug approval and to report periodically to the FDA. From time to time, a drug product will be implicated in too many adverse outcomes, and the product's approval will be reconsidered. In some cases, the product labeling may be limited, the manufacturer may voluntarily withdraw the product from the market, or the FDA may rescind its approval and force a product withdrawal.

Drug Product Withdrawals

Drug product withdrawals occur when a manufacturer or sponsor and the FDA decide that the benefits of an approved drug product no longer outweigh its safety risks. They follow, in effect, the reversal of a formal regulatory decision, based on expert opinion and rigorous scientific proof of safety and efficacy.

Drug product withdrawals cause problems for patients and their doctors, the FDA, and pharmaceutical manufacturers. Some withdrawn products are useful for many patients and have no easy replacement therapy.[33] Sometimes the drugs prescribed to replace a withdrawn product are also risky. Ross Degnan et al. found that zomepirac prescribing substituted for use of other nonsteroidal anti-inflammatory drugs (NSAIDs) and propoxyphene. After the product's withdrawal from the market, a cohort of frequent zomepirac prescribers increased prescribing of other NSAIDs by about 7%, propoxyphene by 2%, and analgesics containing barbiturates by about 3%. The authors concluded that the sudden withdrawal of zomepirac from the market resulted in substitutions not only of other NSAIDs, but also of alternative analgesics with risks of habituation and adverse effects. They advised that "apparent gains in patient safety resulting from market withdrawal of medications must be evaluated in comparison with risks of medications likely to be substituted."[34]

Drug product withdrawals represent a public relations and regulatory problem for the FDA. The new drug approval process is exacting and stringent, but drug product withdrawals show that "the pre-approval process cannot expose all potential risks associated with a drug."[35] Some critics argue that product withdrawals also show that the fast-track approval system, funded by user fees from drug manufacturers, applies pressure to approve drugs more rapidly. Others allege that withdrawals may be associated with inappropriate behavior by the FDA and manufacturers.

We have seen that a manufacturer often has hundreds of millions of dollars invested either in drug development, testing, or product license fees. Product withdrawals are financial catastrophes that may damage a company's profitability and reputation. It matters little whether the withdrawal was voluntary or not. A major, profitable drug product is seldom, if ever, withdrawn without compelling evidence that contradicts and outweighs the earlier compelling evidence. Some drug product withdrawals from the market are also highly significant events from a systems perspective.

Noah and Brushwood have discussed the FDA regulatory process and the problem of drug product withdrawals broadly and in considerable detail.[35] Their paper would serve as a useful resource for further information on the regulatory aspects of this topic. They described various types of information relevant to drug withdrawals, distinguishing between withdrawals caused by adverse drug reactions (ADRs) and those caused by adverse drug events (ADEs). They proposed a systems approach to ADR detection. This would be a postmarketing feedback system based on information about the effects of newly marketed drugs. The information would be gathered by pharmacists from patients. If the pharmacist suspected that a patient was having an adverse drug reaction from a newly marketed drug, he could recommend that the patient see his physician. The pharmacist would upload the data into the FDA MedWatch program. The FDA could then pool and analyze the reports and use the information to focus regulatory attention, postmarketing studies, etc., on problem areas. This proposal was framed as a quality improvement system, as introduced earlier in this chapter. (Subsequent chapters will explore further applications of quality improvement in detail.)

Furthering Noah and Brushwood's distinction between drug withdrawals caused by ADRs and those caused by ADEs, I would propose three basic scenarios that lead to withdrawal of a profitable drug product. Most actual withdrawals seem to involve more than one scenario. Often, however, one scenario will predominate. In the first scenario, information about an adverse drug reaction takes longer to accumulate than the time required by a clinical trial or even the phase III process itself. This can happen for a number of reasons, some of which are controversial. Some ADRs take longer to develop than the typical duration of a premarketing clinical trial. Some ADRs tend to occur in people who are underrepresented in (or excluded from) clinical trials, like the very young, very old, or people with multiple diseases. Some ADRs are rare and, during clinical trails, simply do not appear to be associated with the drug or to be severe or frequent enough to warrant withholding approval.

Some critics, for example, newspaper columnist Joe Graedon ("The People's Pharmacy") and Dr. George Susens, then president of the San Francisco Medical Society, argue that the "fast track" is too fast, that it misses some ADRs and that some promised postmarket studies are never done. Some critics quoted by Dr. Susens go further, charging that the FDA has caved in to pressure from Congress, changing its role from regulator of the pharmaceutical industry to partner.* This echoes some FDA officials quoted in Alicia Mundy's book about diet drug withdrawals. Some critics go even further yet, charging that sponsors may suppress information about adverse effects.[5]

Nomifensine (Merital®) is an example of the first withdrawal scenario. Nomifensine is an antidepressant. It was known to cause serious hypersensitivity reactions, including hemolytic anemia in some patients, based on clinical data from Europe. These ADRs were believed to be reversible; however, as experience with the drug increased and postmarketing surveillance studies were reported, the estimate of severity was revised and the drug was voluntarily withdrawn from the U.S. market by its sponsor in 1985, 3 years after approval. According to the FDA, "nomifensine illustrates that the safety profile of a drug evolves over its lifetime on the market. Even after [years of experience] new information … can be detected." This withdrawal scenario may illustrate weaknesses in the drug approval process, as critics have charged. It clearly illustrates the real and the potential value of postmarketing surveillance as a supplement to the drug approval process. It is, however, drug related rather than drug use related, and does not necessarily reflect specific weaknesses in the medications use system.

A second drug product withdrawal scenario does reflect weaknesses in the medication use system. In this scenario, a drug has recognized preventable contraindications, side effects, or toxicities. These are essentially pre-

* Graedon, J., FDA's Risk-Management Efforts Sometimes Fall Short (www.s-t.com/daily/09-01/09-04-01/b03li069.htm); Susens, G., The FDA Has Failed Us (www.sfms.org/sfm/sfm301k.htm).

ventable drug-related morbidities, as defined in Chapter 3. The PDRM associated with a drug may have been suggested by animal studies or in early phases of testing in humans, may have been recognized during clinical trials, or may have come to light after the drug was marketed.

If it had been recognized prior to the completion of clinical trials, the clinical research protocols would properly have been written to avoid the problem. In fact, the IND could not be approved if the protocols did not make provision to protect subjects from known risks. For example, the protocols might have provided careful dosing or drug regimen guidelines and may have limited the kinds of patients who were included in the studies, the diseases for which the drug was tested, the comorbidities of the research patients, the duration of the trial, or the way the drug was monitored. Used according to protocol, the drug was safe, effective, and approvable.

When the drug was marketed, or whenever serious PDRMs became known after marketing, precautions and contraindications would appear in labeling, advertising, promotions, etc. Sometimes they could even appear prominently in what are called "box warnings" in advertising and in the package insert. Sometimes, as more cases of the particular PDRM appeared, the FDA or the manufacturer would issue a "Dear Doctor" letter reminding health professionals of the problem and how to avoid it. But, since this is a drug withdrawal scenario, inexorably more and more cases of the problem would appear until the drug lost its presumption of safety and effectiveness and was withdrawn from the market.

Many drug withdrawals include elements of this scenario. For example, Dennis Ross Degnan et al. examined changes in the prescribing of analgesics after the market entry and subsequent withdrawal of zomepirac sodium, a nonsteroidal anti-inflammatory drug. Zomepirac was withdrawn after reports of zomepirac-related deaths. They compared prescribing in two cohorts of primary care physicians from July 1980 through September 1983. The physician cohorts comprised 260 primary care physicians who provided 10 or more prescriptions for zomepirac (cohort A) and 308 who provided 10 or more prescriptions for NSAIDs other than zomepirac (cohort B) during the study period. They found that zomepirac accounted for a stable 11.0% of analgesic prescribing among the A cohort. Label changes and manufacturer product risk warnings 11 months before the product's market withdrawal had no impact on use.[34]

Among recent withdrawals, cerivastatin (Baychol®), troglitazone (Rezulin®), terfenadine (Seldane®), bromfenac (Duract®), mibefradil (Posicor®), alosetron (Lotronex®), and cisapride (Propulsid®) each shared this scenario to some extent. Most relevant to the topic of medication use systems, in each withdrawal the FDA and sponsor went through the scenario of recognizing necessary precautions or contraindications, clarifying and amplifying them, and ultimately failing to control use.

Cerivastatin is an effective statin, a class of drugs that helps to reduce cholesterol levels and prevent coronary artery disease and stroke. It was withdrawn in 2001, 3 years after U.S. licensing, following 31 deaths in the

United States, caused in part by (a) excessive dosage, (b) concurrent use with a contraindicated drug, gemfibrozil, another lipid lowering drug, and (c) nonresponse to early symptoms of muscle damage, which led in some patients to probably avoidable kidney failure and death. It was withdrawn in every country but Japan, where gemfibrozil was not marketed and where cerivastatin was licensed only in lower strengths.

Troglitazone had an essential place in the management of non-insulin-dependent diabetes, but caused liver damage in some patients. The FDA changed its indications, dosage, and monitoring guidelines, and its sponsor, Parke-Davis, issued warning after warning. It was eventually withdrawn, in part because some doctors either did not order the recommended liver function tests or did not take appropriate action in response to them.

Mibefradil is an antihypertensive and anti-anginal drug. It was contraindicated in patients taking certain other drugs, e.g., statins and beta-blockers. In a press release announcing its withdrawal, its sponsor, Roche, said, "In principle, drug interactions can be addressed by appropriate labeling; however, with respect to Posicor, Roche believes that the complexity of such prescribing information would make it difficult to implement." This is an interesting statement. It could mean (among other things) that Roche decided that, for mibefradil, the medications use nonsystem was beyond its capacity to correct.

Terfenadine was associated with severe risks when patients took it along with certain antifungal drugs, antibiotics, mibefradil, some antidepressants, cisapride, and grapefruit juice. It was withdrawn in part because the efforts of the FDA and its sponsor, Hoechst Marion Roussel, to promote its safe use were unsuccessful.

A similar scenario seemed to operate in the FDA's reluctance to approve clozapine, an antipsychotic drug for schizophrenics in whom other therapies had failed. Clozapine requires frequent monitoring of the white blood cell count (WBC) to avoid serious, sometimes irreversible and fatal, drops in WBC. Despite its therapeutic necessity, the FDA approved clozapine only after the sponsor developed, on its own, a way to ensure that regular WBC monitoring would be done for patients taking the drug.[36]

The third group of reasons for withdrawal may augment the other two. In this scenario, a drug in a therapeutic class appears to be more dangerous (or perhaps less effective) than available alternatives. The FDA proposed the withdrawal of terfenadine in part on this basis. The reason for withdrawing cerivastatin and mibefradil may have included the recognition that safer alternatives were available. Conversely, the world's most notorious unsafe drug, thalidomide, is back on the market (with precautions and contraindications) for Hansen's disease because of therapeutic necessity (see Appendix 1). Another teratogenic drug, Accutane® (isotretinoin), remains on the market (also with prescribing restrictions) for the same reason.

Two major points should be evident from this discussion. First, many drug product withdrawals include major elements of the second scenario. Such events add to the evidence presented in earlier chapters that medications use is often defective. This type of drug product withdrawal involves PDRM. On a broad market-wide scale, such withdrawals often represent pure, preventable waste, as do PDRMs on a clinical scale. Just as one feels that something should be done to prevent PDRMs on a clinical level, one wonders why the pharmaceutical industry has been so ineffective in promoting the safe use of its products, or at least in promoting an infrastructure that would support the safe and effective use of its products. Finally, drug product withdrawals and PDRMs have a common denominator. Although drug product withdrawals may embarrass the FDA and may reduce a manufacturer's revenue, ultimately it is the patient who suffers the injury and then pays for it again through higher drug prices, insurance premiums, and taxes.

Second, scenarios 1 and 2 illustrate the important distinction between the safety and efficacy of *drug products* and the safety and effectiveness of *medications use.* The premarket testing of drug products may sometimes be effective when the problem is inherent in the drug product, but often ineffective when the problem is with the unsafe use of a safe drug. The authority of the FDA is based in the control of interstate commerce (drug products as articles of commerce). This authority can only stretch so far into control of how those products are used by physicians and patients. The FDA is prohibited by statute (and arguably, the U.S. Constitution) from controlling the practice of medicine, and by extension, pharmacy. Expecting the FDA to improve medication use through control over drug products seems unrealistic. Such an approach might cause more problems than it corrects (for example, from centralized decision making and imposition of standardized guidelines).

Postmarketing surveillance is an underutilized tool for improving the quality both of drug products and drug use. It should, however, include more than just recently marketed drug products. As we have seen in Chapter 2, many old familiar drugs like digoxin and warfarin are major causes of PDRM. Postmarketing surveillance should include valid epidemiological studies, but it should also use indicator and other methodologies to identify areas for epidemiological research.

For example, the patient data collected in the QI systems approach of Noah and Brushwood[35] are indicators. They would compensate for any lack of scientific rigor by greatly broadening the scope of postmarket clinical feedback. Further, some surveillance should be directed at patient outcomes rather than drug products. Patient-oriented information from many sources is needed to improve the quality of medications use, and the quality improvement systems that use the information should exist on many levels. The systems described later in this book are like that. They are decentralized and based on information about structure, process, and outcome, especially the last two.

The purpose of this section on drug law was to make these two points, not to provide a comprehensive dissertation. However, I have now opened the question of how federal drug law and regulation might promote pluralistic, multilevel medication use quality improvement systems. I offer three premises and a proposal. The first premise is that the American health care delivery system is heterogeneous regarding the quality of care. Some medication use systems are safer and more effective than others, and one FDA decision does not fit all. Just as some patients can safely benefit from drugs that are withdrawn, some health care provider networks could safely manage the use of those drugs.

The second premise is that therapy with some drug products is more difficult to manage than with others. Make this more concrete by saying that a "difficult" drug is (a) a new drug that the FDA is very reluctant to approve, or (b) a drug already on the market that the FDA wants the manufacturer to withdraw.

The third premise is, as Alvin Toffler said, that change requires the intersection of ideology and economic interest. Regarding ideology, the evidence is overwhelming that health care in general and drug therapy in particular often fail to deliver their potential to patients. Quality improvement is well accepted as the best way to change that.

Regarding the economic part, perhaps the FDA could find a legal basis for restricting the distribution of difficult drug products to systems in which they can be used appropriately. This seems to have begun already with FDA requirements setting certain preconditions for the use of drugs like clozapine, isotretinoin, and reapprovals of alosetron and thalidomide. This would affect manufacturers' sales and providers' access to some of the tools of their trade.

The FDA has described requirements for good manufacturing practices (GDPs). Perhaps it can also describe a safe and effective medications use system (SEMUS). Health care providers would not be legally required to develop a SEMUS. A SEMUS would, however, be a precondition for the purchase and distribution of certain drugs on the "difficult" list.

The requirements for a SEMUS could be simple: in addition to normal requirements for a trained and organized professional staff, etc., a SEMUS would need (a) an information system to describe how a difficult drug product should be used, (b) process indicators to monitor use and ascertain whether use is according to guidelines, and (c) outcome indicators to detect adverse events and correct the system. Such a description would allow a provider network to show that it had the necessary information system to manage and monitor the use of potentially valuable but difficult-to-manage drug products.

Manufacturers and wholesalers would be prohibited from selling certain drug products except to a SEMUS. A provider would have to certify to the manufacturer that it met the SEMUS definition or minimum standard. If so inclined, the manufacturer could help the network reach compliance as a part of its promotion of the product. Accrediting bodies also could certify SEMUS compliance as part of their more general accreditation process. Perhaps my enthusiasm is running rampant, but I could imagine that eventually states might implement such provisions under their constitutional authority to regulate the practice of professions.

Chapter Summary

This chapter has introduced three concepts essential for thinking critically about health care services in general and drug therapy in particular: access, cost, and quality. A patient's access to drug therapy is the end of a chain, beginning with research and drug marketing and ending with an ability to afford the medicine and use it correctly.

One can think about drug cost in various ways. Product cost is obviously the one that preoccupies managed care executives, politicians, and the press. From a systems perspective, however, drug products are inputs or instrumentalities. While buying the right drug regimen as cheaply as possible would usually make sense, drug cost should be evaluated in terms of its marginal contribution to the total cost of care. The New Hampshire studies show the unintended consequences that can happen when this point is ignored and providers try to control drug costs in isolation from their purpose in care. Donald Ashwell is the symbol of this fallacy. This should be so well known by now that the bad consequences of driving down component costs can scarcely be called unintended.

Quality is perhaps the most complicated of the three. The quality cube suggests that quality has 24 components, each of which can be measured by implicit or explicit criteria. The trend toward quality improvement seeks to integrate quality into routine management. Indicators are essential for quality improvement. Medications use lends itself very well to the use of indicators and to quality management.

From a legal perspective, drug products are articles of commerce as well as professional instruments of care. The regulatory perspective may result in an overemphasis of drug *products* as the most important aspect of medications use. However, an important distinction must be drawn between drug product efficacy (as required by drug laws) and drug use effectiveness.

Some drug product withdrawals illuminate the distinction between the quality of drug products and the quality of drug use. They illuminate the interface between control of drugs as commercial articles and control of drugs as therapeutic instruments. They demonstrate the need to reconceptualize medications use from a systems perspective. Federal authority is powerful in regulating drug products as articles of commerce. How that authority may be used to regulate drug use remains an open question.

References

1. Soumerai, S.B. et al., Effects of limiting Medicaid drug-reimbursement benefits on the use of psychotropic agents and acute mental health services by patients with schizophrenia, *N. Engl. J. Med.*, 331, 650, 1994.
2. Soumerai, S.B. et al., Effects of Medicaid drug-payment limits on admission to hospitals and nursing homes, *N. Engl. J. Med.*, 325, 1072, 1991.

3. Eberhardt, M.S. et al., *Urban and Rural Health Chartbook, Health United States 2001,* National Center for Health Statistics, Hyattsville, MD, 2001.
4. Silverman, M. and Lee, P.R., *Pills Profits and Politics,* University of California Press, Berkeley, CA, 1976, p. 1.
5. Mundy, A., *Dispensing with the Truth: The Victims, the Drug Companies, and the Dramatic Story behind the Battle over Fen-Phen,* St. Martin's Press, New York, 2001.
6. Eisenberg, J.M. et al., What is the cost of nephrotoxicity associated with aminoglycosides? *Ann. Intern. Med.*, 107, 900, 1987.
7. Kohn, L.T., Corrigan, J.T., and Donaldson, M.S., *To Err Is Human: Building a Safer Health System,* National Academy Press, Washington, D.C., 2000.
8. Angaran, D.M., Quality assurance to quality improvement: measuring and monitoring pharmaceutical care, *Am. J. Hosp. Pharm.*, 48, 1901, 1991.
9. Institute of Medicine, *Crossing the Quality Chasm: A New Health System for the 21st Century,* National Academy Press, Washington, D.C., 2001.
10. Donabedian, A., The role of outcomes in quality assessment and assurance, *Qual. Rev. Bull.*, 356, 1992.
11. Donabedian, A., The quality of medical care, *Science*, 200, 856, 1978.
12. Lohr, K.N., Donaldson, M.S., and Harris-Wehling, J., Medicare: a strategy for quality assurance: V. Quality of care in a changing health care environment, *Qual. Rev. Bull.*, 18, 120, 1992.
13. Ashton, C.M. et al., A method of developing and weighting explicit processes of care: criteria for quality assessment, *Med. Care*, 32, 755, 1994.
14. Brook, R.H., McGlynn, E.A., and Cleary, P.D., Part 2: measuring quality of care, *N. Engl. J. Med.*, 335, 966, 1996.
15. Eddy, D.M. and Billings, J., The quality of medical evidence: implications for quality and care, *Health Aff.*, 19, 1988.
16. Adar, R., Critchfield, G.C., and Eddy, D.M., A confidence profile analysis of the results of femoropopliteal percutaneous transluminal angioplasty in the treatment of lower-extremity ischemia, *J. Vasc. Surg.*, 10, 57, 1989.
17. Eddy, D.M., Clinical decision making: from theory to practice, *JAMA*, 263, 287, 1990.
18. Welch, W.P. et al., Geographic variation in expenditures for physicians' services in the United States, *N. Engl. J. Med.*, 328, 621, 1993.
19. Roos, N.P. et al., Therapies for benign prostatic hyperplasia, *JAMA*, 268, 1269, 1992.
20. Wennberg, J.E., Unwanted variations in the rules of practice, *JAMA*, 265, 1306, 1991.
21. Wennberg, J.E., Population illness rates do not explain population hospitalization rates: a comment on Mark Blumberg's thesis that morbidity adjusters are needed to interpret small area variations, *Med. Care*, 25, 354, 1987.
22. Wennberg, J.E., The paradox of appropriate care, *JAMA*, 258, 2568, 1987.
23. Horn, S.D., Unintended consequences of drug formularies, *Am. J. Health Syst. Pharm.*, 53, 2204, 1996.
24. Vuori, H., Patient satisfaction: an attribute or indicator of the quality of care? *Qual. Rev. Bull.*, 13, 106, 1987.
25. Parasuraman, A., Zeithaml, V.A., and Berry, L.L., A conceptual model of service quality and its implications for future research, *J. Mark.*, 41, 1985.
26. Parasuraman, A., Berry, L.L., and Zeithaml, V.A., Empirical examination of relationships in an extended service quality model, Report 90-122, Marketing Science Institute Research Program Series, 1990.

27. Williams, B., Patient satisfaction: a valid concept? *Soc. Sci. Med.*, 38, 509, 1994.
28. Brushwood, D.B., *Medical Malpractice: Pharmacy Law,* Shepard's/McGraw-Hill, Colorado Springs, CO, 1986.
29. Bowles, G.C., Jr., N.A.S.-N.R.C. reports efficacy of drugs released before 1962, *Mod. Hosp.*, 115, 108, 1970.
30. Schiff, G.D. et al., Inpatient theophylline toxicity: preventable factors, *Ann. Intern. Med.*, 114, 748, 1991 (see comments).
31. Edlavitch, S.A., Postmarketing surveillance methodologies, *Ann. Pharmacother.*, 22, 68, 1988.
32. Waller, P.C. et al., Review of company postmarketing surveillance studies, *Br. Med. J.*, 304, 1470, 1992.
33. Lechat, P., Problems raised by the withdrawal from the market of drugs in therapeutic use, *Therapie*, 42, 403, 1987.
34. Ross Degnan, D. et al., Examining product risk in context: market withdrawal of zomepirac as a case study, *JAMA*, 270, 1937, 1993 (see comments).
35. Noah, B. and Brushwood, D.B., Adverse drug reactions in elderly patients: alternative approaches to postmarket surveillances, *J. Health Law,* 33, 383, 2000.
36. Hepler, C.D., Clozapine and the outmoded drug use process, *Am. Pharmacy,* NS30, 39, 1990.
37. Nadzam, D.M., Development of medication-use indicators by the Joint Commission on Accreditation of Healthcare Organizations, *Am. J. Hosp. Pharm.*, 48, 1925, 1991.

Appendix 1: Orphan Drug Law

For years, patients suffering from orphan diseases such as Gaucher's disease, rare cancers, hemophilia, multiple sclerosis, and Parkinson's disease simply were out of luck. Without financial incentives, pharmaceutical companies said they could not risk the time and money to develop orphan products. Other possible drug developers, such as universities or research hospitals, lacked the capital or business acumen to develop treatments for small patient groups.

Congress passed the Orphan Drug Act in 1983. This law gives tax breaks, special monopoly protections, and other incentives to companies who support research and sponsor New Drug Applications for orphan drugs, i.e., existing chemicals that are at least believed to be effective for orphan diseases, but lack a sponsor.

By the year 2000, the FDA had approved 182 orphan products — including drugs and biologicals. Sponsors had submitted 1252 applications for orphan designation, of which the FDA had granted designation to 917. Examples include:

- Crohn's disease — Remicade (infliximab), approved in August 1998, was the first approved specific (i.e., more than symptomatic) treatment for this chronic, incurable inflammatory bowel disease.
- Hansen's disease (leprosy) — The FDA cleared thalidomide to treat a serious inflammatory symptom seen in Hansen's patients. Because of its well-known potential for causing birth defects, the drug was approved with tight restrictions on its use. Thalidomide also has received orphan designation, though not approval yet, for treating primary brain tumors and Karposi's sarcoma, an AIDS-related cancer.
- Sickle cell anemia — Under the orphan program, a decades-old cancer drug, hydroxyurea (Droxia), was approved to treat adults who suffer from this inherited blood disorder that causes chronic anemia and periodic episodes of pain.
- Cutaneous T-cell lymphoma — Ontak (denileukin diftitox) treats this slow-growing form of non-Hodgkin's lymphoma when other therapies have not worked.
- Pneumocystis carinii pneumonia (PCP) — Mepron (atovaquone) treats this infection that strikes high-risk, HIV-infected patients.

"How encouraging it is that a medical tragedy [thalidomide birth defects in the 1960s] led to a medical breakthrough that will likely help people with many diseases. Nobody would have done research on this aspect of thalidomide without the Orphan Drug Act."*

* Henkel, J., Orphan Drug Law Matures into Medical Mainstay, FDA Consumer Magazine, May–June 1999.

However, there is controversy about the incentives provided by the Orphan Drug Act. According to James Love, "What is needed are more targeted incentives to conduct essential medical research, with greater public accountability."* In his view, the Orphan Drug Act has been written to qualify a very wide range of drugs as orphans, including, for example, all AIDS medicines in the United States, plus drugs for countless other severe illnesses. He feels that the Orphan Drug Act is a very blunt instrument that is often wasteful, costly to consumers and taxpayers, and sometimes counterproductive (by discouraging investments by rivals once markets become legally exclusive).

* Love, J., Brief note on the abuse of Orphan Drug programs in creating monopolies, http://www.cptech.org/ip/health/orphan/.

Appendix 2: Steps in Cost-Effectiveness Analysis

Calculation of Table 5.3 is complicated and is best described as a series of steps:

1. Outline the steps in therapy that are associated with costs relevant to the analysis. This may be descriptive of existing treatment guidelines or prescriptive of proposed treatment guidelines. Table 5.2 and Figure 5.1 are examples of the result of this step.
2. Identify the costs and probable outcomes for each therapeutic alternative. Cost information would usually be specific to a particular institution, while probable outcomes, e.g., cure rates and side effect rates, would come from clinical literature. Sometimes a review article (or even a report of a decision analysis) will provide most of the clinical information required in a useful format.
3. Prepare a decision tree based on step 1. The decision tree is different from a treatment flowchart because it shows the logical possibilities rather than the time course. See Figure 5.3. A decision tree has two kinds of nodes: choices (decision) and chances (results of choices). In Figure 5.3, there is one choice node, shown as a square. Chance nodes are shown as circles, and the associated probability is given. (Note that the probabilities at a node add up to 1.)
   a. Assign probabilities to chance nodes and costs to choices.
   b. Probabilities of all outcomes from one branch must total 1.0. Example: Choice of Megaflox ($80 per course), chance that patient is symptomatic in 3 days is .010, or asymptomatic (.990).
4. To calculate the expected value of treatment costs (C in Table 5.3) for each treatment alternative:
   a. Sum the costs associated with each possible path through the treatment guideline (flowchart) or decision tree. This gives the total cost for that path. For example, the total cost for a patient who is symptomatic at the second follow-up after B-cillin, with a sensitive organism, is $420 ($35 drug cost + $75 return to clinic + $35 for alternative therapy + $275 for additional care — urology clinic referral).
   b. Multiply the probabilities along each path. This gives the probability of each outcome. For example, the probability that a patient will be symptomatic at the second follow-up after B-cillin, with a sensitive organism, is .01.
   c. Multiply the cost of each outcome by the corresponding probability. This gives the expected total cost for each outcome. To finish the example, the contribution to the expected value of B-cillin of an outcome with a probability of .01 and a cost of $420 is .01 times $420.

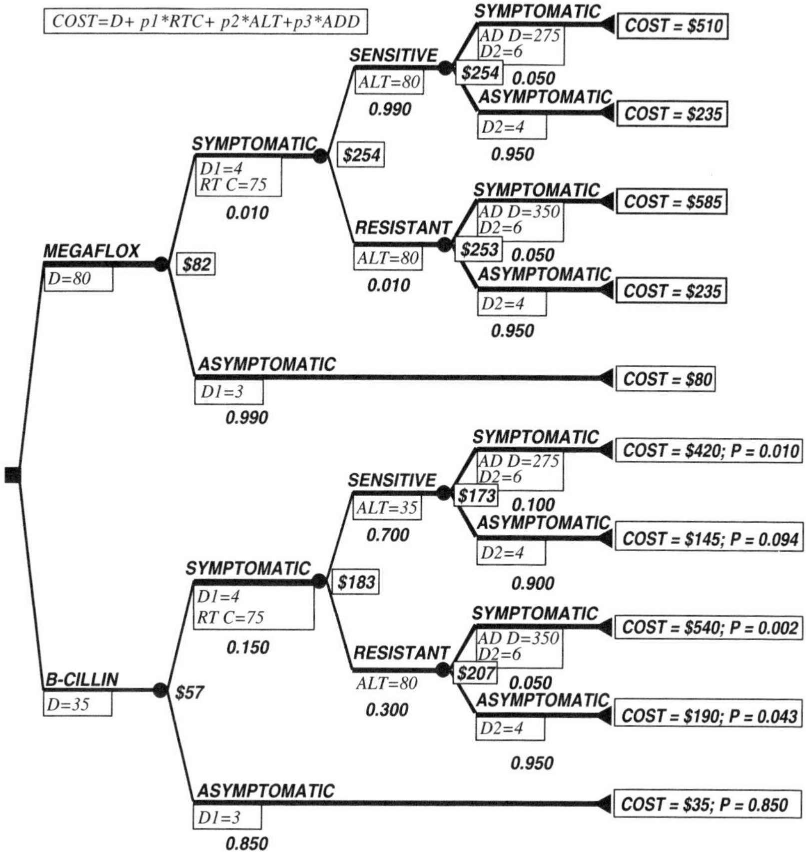

FIGURE 5.3
Decision tree for two alternatives from Table 5.3.

d. Add the expected total costs for all of the outcomes for a given treatment. The sum is the expected value of this alternative. It reflects drug costs and other costs of care that depend on choice of drug therapy.

e. Repeat for each therapeutic alternative. (Alternatively, calculate the probability of reaching each chance node and multiply by the cost of that node. This formula is shown at the top of the figure.)

5. Repeat step 4 for effectiveness measures, e.g., sick days.

Sensitivity Analysis

It might be useful to know how much our assumption about the cost of Megafloxacin would affect our final decision. One way to do this is to calculate the break-even cost (threshold value) at which Megafloxacin and

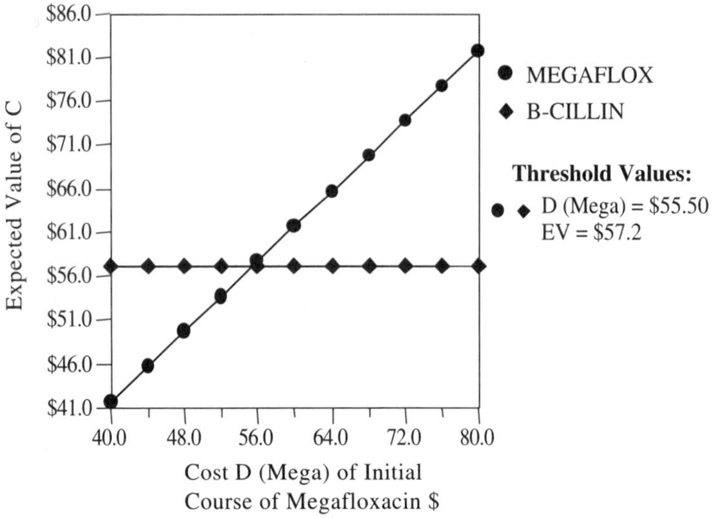

FIGURE 5.4
One-way sensitivity graph. Total cost C vs. cost of initial course of Megafloxacin. Total cost is equal when D(Mega) is $55.50.

an alternative, say B-cillin, would produce equal expected values for C (total cost of therapy), assuming every other variable stayed the same.

Since the relationship between total cost C and drug cost D is linear in this model, it is necessary to compute only two values representing the extreme possibilities for D. This is illustrated in Figure 5.4. The expected value of C for Megafloxacin would equal that for B-cillin if the cost of an initial course of Megafloxacin was $57.20 or less and all other values stayed the same. This result suggests that a decision to recommend use of B-cillin would not be considered very sensitive to likely drug cost changes. Also, the C vs. D relationship might be useful in recalculating incremental costs and in negotiating with the vendor of Megafloxacin.

6

Prescribing and Prescribing Influence

Prescribing has been a topic of substantial research and practical interest for many years.

Inappropriate prescribing has been implicated as a possible cause in most studies of preventable drug-related mortality (PDRM). Furthermore, the published literature includes literally hundreds of studies that raise serious questions about prescribing appropriateness. This interest goes beyond medicines use per se. Some authors have seen the use of drugs, especially drugs like antibiotics and psychoactive medications, as a barometer of the quality of health care or even as a proxy for medical decision making and the (mis)use of technology. Interest in prescribing also extends into the cost of prescribed medicines.

The philosophical gulf separating those who buy drugs from those who use them was introduced in Chapter 5, in the discussion of optimizing drug product cost with respect to the total cost of care. This gulf is also very important for understanding prescribing influence activities, as they are usually carried out by governmental and private managed care programs.

To a clinician, drug products are instruments: primarily, they are instruments of therapy, sometimes a means to communicate power or caring. From a clinical perspective, the purpose of prescribing influence is to improve clinical outcomes or to make care more cost-effective (see Chapters 4 and 5).

To those who sell or buy drug products, however, drugs are articles of commerce. Drug costs are seen, rightly or wrongly, as major contributors to the cost of health care. From this perspective, prescribing assessment and influence can become separated from clinical objectives. The story of Donald Ashwell (Chapter 5) may not be an aberration. What happened to Mr. Ashwell is but one example of a widespread problem that contributes significantly to the prevalence of adverse effects and treatment failures.

Philosophically, as prescribing is seen less as a part of a medications use system, it can become increasingly self-referent, seen as an end unto itself. "Drug of choice" product-oriented drug use evaluation (DUE), described in Chapter 5, is a manifestation of prescribing as an end. If neither specific patients' needs nor outcomes are considered in a prescribing assessment, prescribing is obviously being viewed as an end rather than a means. Such product-oriented prescribing assessments set the stage for prescribing influences that are intended to lower drug expenditures, again, as an end in itself.

A program may promote the use of certain (cheaper) drug products even if, as a consequence, many patients may not achieve their therapeutic objectives and even if total costs of care increase. Examples were given in earlier chapters to explain possible origins of PDRM. Here is another example. In their review of prescribing for asthmatic patients in East London, Naish et al. concluded:

> Pressure to reduce the cost of asthma prescribing may lead to a lowering of the ratio of prophylactic to bronchodilator treatments. However, reducing prophylactic prescribing would run contrary to the British Thoracic Society guidelines and might worsen the quality of asthma care.[1]

Incidentally, asthma is not expensive to treat correctly. Furthermore, the total cost of treating asthmatic patients is usually less when they are treated correctly, because undertreatment usually results in expensive emergency department visits and hospitalizations.

This chapter will address three main topics: the place of prescribing in drug therapy, including prescribing quality or appropriateness and the proposition that changing prescribing quality can change patient outcomes; a theoretical foundation for prescribing influence activities; and a critical appraisal of common methods for prescribing influence, and a systematic approach to improving the quality of drug prescribing.

Furthermore, we will use the "story" of prescribing restrictions as a case study or analogy to the larger problem of improving the overall medications use process. Other inputs to medications use may also be self-referent, manipulated without due regard to the consequences. Other simple solutions may be implemented without checking to see whether they improve outcomes.

Prescribing in Medications Use

Prescribing influence activities are diagramed in Figure 6.1. Figure 6.1 shows two subsystems. The prescribing influence system is the focus of interest in this chapter.

A prescribing influence system actually can comprise both prospective and retrospective prescribing assessments. Prospective prescribing evaluation and influence are patient and time specific. They occur before or during drug therapy. Therefore, prospective prescribing influence is properly part of the medications use process or pharmaceutical care system, which will be described in Chapters 8 and 10 and elsewhere throughout the remainder of this book.

Most prescribing influence activities are retrospective and encompass many patients over a long period of time. Note that the arrow from "prescribing influence" in Figure 6.1 does not pierce the box surrounding the medication

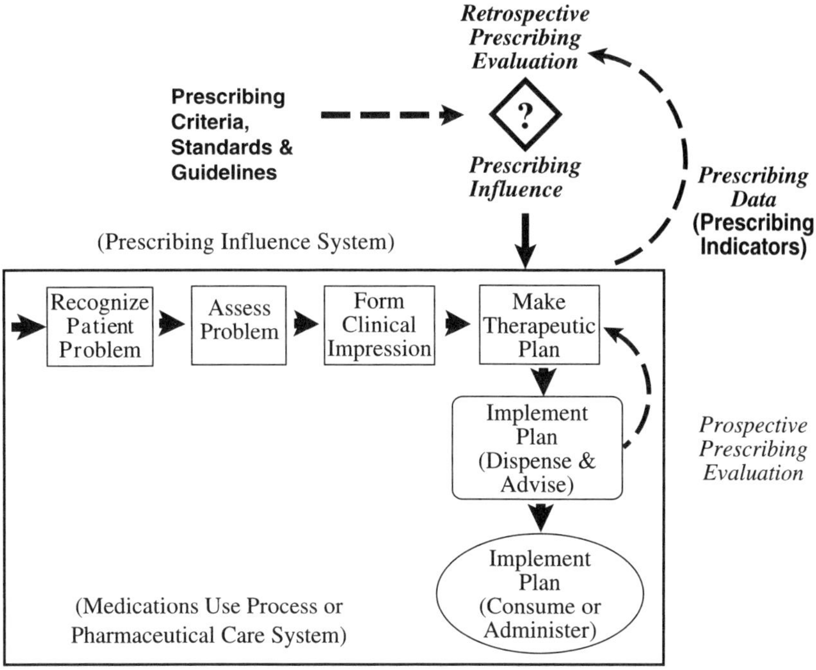

FIGURE 6.1
Prescribing improvement and medications use processes.

use process diagram. That is intended to illustrate the general nature of retrospective prescribing influence, which should not address the therapy of individuals. This process is often called *retrospective drug use evaluation* (RDUE) or *retrospective drug use review* (RDUR). (The term is overly broad in most applications, which review only certain aspects or types of prescribing.)

The process of retrospective prescribing review or evaluation can be understood as three steps, as follows:*

1. **Prescribing review:** collecting *data* that describe prescribing in ways that are relevant to the criteria.
2. **Prescribing evaluation** or assessment: comparing data to the criteria and identifying *discrepancies*.
   2.1. **Problem definition:** defining the prescribing problem and finding root causes.
   2.2. **Understanding** (modeling) the prescribing process and the causes of quality variation. Considering alternative improvement interventions, and the likely effect of each, using the prescribing model.
3. **Implementation:** selecting and implementing the interventions.

* This process is similar to the FOCUS-PDCA quality improvement process described in Chapter 11.

The effect of each intervention should be followed up with continued prescribing review.

Criteria for Prescribing Appropriateness

Beforee prescribing review can go forward, it is necessary to establish (or adopt) *criteria* based on the purpose of prescribing, i.e., to decide what constitutes appropriate prescribing. These criteria establish the basis for prescribing assessment.

Criteria for prescribing appropriateness should logically depend on the function of prescribing in health care. In the system models described in Chapters 8 to 10, drug prescribing is the initiation of therapy, a consequence of a therapeutic plan, intended to address a patient problem or a clinical assessment. Furthermore, the components of a drug prescription are many: the drug product (chemical entity, formulation, and dosage form), the dosage, route of administration (oral, parenteral, or topical), dosage frequency, and duration, collectively called a drug *regimen*. So, choice of a therapeutic agent or drug product, which seems to receive so much attention, is only one of many necessary steps in a long and complex medications use process.

Philosophical Basis of Prescribing Quality

Medical philosophers have stressed the ideas of medicine as the application of science to solve practical problems that affect people's lives. Gatens-Robinson, a medical philosopher, emphasizes the humanistic nature of scientific application in medical practice. She wrote, "Medicine … is a practical human science … its rational orientation is one that applies general knowledge to particular situations."[2]

Thomasma considered therapeutic appropriateness under three senses of "rationality": consensual, scientific, and ethical. He concluded that a theory of medical therapeutics based only on objective scientific standards is "wrongheaded." Even therapeutic plans based on medical indications alone should be understood as "inherently consensual and … governed by a logic of proportionality."

> A rational treatment plan combines scientific standards, collegial consensus, preferential indications by the patient or guardian, and the burdens/benefits calculus, including a judgement of the proportion between the proposed intervention and the current condition of the patient (the patient's quality of life) through which a consensus is reached.[3]

The purpose of drug therapy, generally, should be to improve the patient's health-related quality of life by curing, controlling, preventing, or diagnosing disease or by controlling symptoms. This is logically consistent with the mandate claimed by all health professions. The purpose of a prescription should be to initiate drug therapy, whenever possible for a definite therapeutic objective, e.g., "remission of symptoms in three days, or return to clinic."

There may be reasonable scope for disagreement about some aspects of this purpose, e.g., the relative values attached to clinical outcome (e.g., cure) and humane outcomes (i.e., improved quality of life), and about the exact definitions of those terms — and how to measure them. However, there does not seem to be much scope for reasoned disagreement about the overall purpose.

This may seem to belabor the obvious. However, the jargon of prescribing and medications use is confusing. First, some authors have used the term *medication use* or *drug use*, as in "drug use review," when the real subject was only prescribing, often only one aspect of prescribing, i.e., choice of therapeutic agent. This seems to make prescribing an end in itself, to disconnect it from its purpose and place in a medications use system. The usage may merely reflect professional parochialism, but whatever its causes, it creates confusion and impedes discussion.

There is another respect in which prescribing seems to be considered as if it were an end in itself: the concept of prescription "carve-outs," and the use of certain prescribing restrictions without concern for the effect on patient outcomes or total costs of care. This may be related in part to professional parochialism and in part to the commercial value of drug products.

Proposed Criteria for Appropriate Prescribing

Prescribing is a part of medications use, which in turn is a part of patient care. Therefore, prescribing criteria and medications use criteria should reflect all applicable domains of health care quality, for example, the eight quality domains listed in Chapter 5. These can perhaps be consolidated into four medications use criteria. The following criteria (whose letters spell TESS if rearranged) reflect the clinical, economic, and humane purposes of drug therapy. They constitute a working definition of *prescribing appropriateness.*

Scientific appropriateness — Consistency with current scientific evidence and professional consensus regarding safety, effectiveness, and efficiency; optimality with respect to the risks and benefits of alternative therapies. This is the general, scientific foundation of appropriate therapy.

Specificity *(patient appropriateness)* — How well a prescription addresses a patient's clinical, social, economic, and other needs, including (a) appropriateness for the therapeutic objective; (b) patient, prescriber, and co-therapist abilities to use (or manage the use of) the medicine correctly; (c) financial and physical accessibility and acceptability to the patient; and, especially, (d) the effect of the therapy on the patient over the course of therapy.

Equitability — Consistency with principles of fair allocation of limited resources available for drug therapy (distributive justice). This should include (a) attention to outcome optimality, as described in Chapter 5, so that expenditures for drugs reach clinical objectives as efficiently as possible and the just distribution of medications among members of a population; (b) proportionality to the likely benefit of therapy and the dangers of the disease.

Timeliness — Whether the medicine was prescribed (provided) when needed, available without significant interruptions, and adjusted to meet changing patient requirements (requires appropriate monitoring).

The *scientific* criterion acknowledges the need for a basis in evidence. The *specificity* criterion acknowledges patient needs and circumstances in clinical and other realms. The *equitability* criterion is meant to recognize the economic realities of modern health care, the ideal of just distribution of goods, and the need for a reasonable balance of costs, risks, and benefits. The *timeliness* criterion means that prescribing should be subject to requirements for *continuity of care*. Prescribing can sometimes be appropriate without monitoring of its effects on the patient, but that would be a matter of luck. Prescribing that produces unrecognized drug therapy problems cannot be fully appropriate in this view.

As shown in Figure 6.1, medications use consists of many steps, e.g., patient assessment, prescribing, dispensing, and medication (self-)administration. Problems at many of these steps were identified as possible causes of PDRM in Chapter 3. Logically, the purpose of prescribing is to initiate drug therapy as an instrument of patient care. Therefore, prescribing should be evaluated according to how well it supports drug therapy or medications use, as a part of patient care.

Prescribing assessment and drug use evaluation, however, are the only routine medication-related assessment activities mandated by accreditation bodies and federal Conditions of Participation. Perhaps for this reason, prescribing is the only step in the medications use process that is routinely evaluated by hospitals, managed care organizations, and third-party payers. (Many hospitals may operate adverse reaction programs, but few operate them as management functions, for "internal" use.) Criteria for prescribing seem therefore to be a practical necessity. However, they should reflect, as much as possible, the objectives of medications use.

The validity of prescribing assessments depends on the validity of the criteria and the quality (accuracy, completeness, and patient specificity) of the data. The validity of prescribing assessment criteria should depend in part on their demonstrated connection to medications use and to patient outcomes. Prescribing data, e.g., from administrative databases used for payment purposes, are often quite accurate and patient specific, but lack patient data.

These criteria should guide the design of prescribing evaluations and the interpretation of results. They should also demonstrate the limitations of many accepted approaches to prescribing evaluation. Some of these criteria are inconvenient to measure, especially in large samples. However, if one or more criteria were not reflected in a prescribing evaluation, that evaluation would be incomplete as a summative evaluation, convenience notwithstanding.

For example, nearly every prescribing assessment emphasizes the *scientific* criterion. *Specificity* is rarely evaluated, because it is inconvenient to obtain specific patient information to judge it. In some instances, surely, specific patient needs or limitations caused a prescriber to choose a drug that was not the drug of choice according to the scientific criterion. In others, perhaps the scientific choice was invalidated by patient factors that the prescriber should have taken into account but did not.

An assessment that judged only the scientific basis of prescribing should not be accepted as a complete evaluation. It is possible that assessment of other dimensions, e.g., specificity, would change a summary judgment. Medications use is so important in people's lives that its full purpose should take precedence over the convenience of evaluating it. New methods of prescribing assessment should be developed to make assessments of specificity and practicality more feasible for routine use. Many authors have proposed both implicit and explicit process criteria for evaluating prescribing. (Some basic frameworks for quality assessments were discussed in Chapter 5.) Certain criteria are easier to apply in certain data sets than in others, and so the literature includes a variety of differing criteria and methods.

Implicit criteria, including the hybrid called structured implicit criteria, can address many of the criteria listed above. Such criteria usually require the application of professional judgment. The usual method for implicit review of prescribing is medical record review — either of entire records or of abstracts. This method is more expensive to use and less reliable, because a human has to be able to find the necessary information in a record and apply judgment to it. This is less consistent than applying explicit definitions, especially with a computer. However, judgments made with implicit criteria may be more valid; i.e., they may be more consistent with the real purpose of drug therapy. Indeed, medical record audit done by experts, using structured implicit criteria, is widely accepted as the gold standard for judging many kinds of medical appropriateness. (See Chapter 5.)

Explicit prescribing criteria, such as "long-acting benzodiazepines should be avoided in the elderly," can be scientifically sound, i.e., theoretically plausible and well supported by epidemiological evidence. Their merits can be discussed, and expert consensus can be reached. For example, Beers used an expert consensus panel to develop a list of drugs that should be avoided in the elderly.[4] Explicit criteria are easy (inexpensive) to apply to large data sets.

Samsa, Hanlon, Fitzgerald and their co-workers have developed this concept further.[5–7]

Explicit criteria usually have high measurement reliability, especially if used in computerized screening programs. This means that their application is predictable. They would tend to yield similar or identical results from similar or identical populations, regardless of who applied them.

The validity of implicit review can be combined with the efficiency of explicit assessments. Buetow et al. address the issue as follows:

> … evaluations of "appropriateness" have sought to supplement incomplete evidence with professional opinion.… We suggest that appropriateness is the outcome of a process of decision-making that maximises net individual health gains within society's available resources. This definition distinguishes between (in)appropriate prescribing, as an outcome, and (ir)rational prescribing as a process. To assess appropriateness, we advocate combining explicit criteria with independent review in cases of uncertainty and disagreement. Refinements based on reviews using implicit criteria should draw on shared professional knowledge.… The Medication Appropriateness Index is … a solid foundation for identifying dimensions of prescribing appropriateness.[47]

Given criteria, data collection and prescribing assessments (e.g., application of prescribing criteria) are carried out in various combinations of methods. Many studies use Beers' or Hanlon's criteria. Data are typically drawn from administrative databases (e.g., those used by providers and third-party payers), from questionnaire or interview surveys, or from medical record review. Some studies are cross-sectional (all subjects in one episode of care of a short time frame), and some are longitudinal (subjects observed over many episodes of care). Some examples are included in the chapter appendix.

Prescribing assessments done as part of a prescribing influence system should be *formative* assessments, meaning that they should be useful for identifying problems and choosing corrections. Formative assessments require information that may help to explain why inappropriate prescribing takes place, or at least suggests what could be done to improve it.

After the assessment steps, the remaining task is choosing and implementing improvement actions. These fall generally into two broad groups: direct (administrative or coercive) and indirect (educational or persuasive) interventions. These will be discussed further below.

Understanding the Prescribing Process

A rational approach to prescribing influence would be modeling of causes and solutions, that is, an understanding of the prescribing process. Three basic models have been proposed to explain the prescribing process and to account for variation in prescribing. These are prescriber characteristics or personal attributes, psychology of prescribing (including education and decision making), and sociology of prescribing.

Characteristics of Inappropriate Prescribers

An early (and unsuccessful) attempt to explain inappropriate prescribing was to identify characteristics of inappropriate prescribers. One example from this early literature was the study by Stolley et al., which looked for demographic correlates of incorrect beliefs about drugs.[8] The study suggested that inappropriate prescribers tended to be older, with less busy practices. Although this approach may have some intuitive appeal, useful demographic markers are difficult to replicate and do not withstand critical analysis. For example, prescriber age or recency of education may be statistically correlated with incorrect drug knowledge. However, if the appropriateness criteria happen to reflect agreement with academic opinion about drugs of choice, the bias in favor of more recently trained physicians would be obvious. "Modern medicine" would favor the recently trained, and the reasoning would appear to be rather circular.

Personal attributes such as age could be empirical risk factors, i.e., correlates of inappropriate prescribing. Then, if they were demonstrated to be valid and reliable, they could be useful for targeting "high-risk" prescribers. However, risk factors offer no theoretical insight into why prescribers with a particular attribute tend to prescribe inappropriately. This approach seems to be a dead end. It is perhaps equally likely that older prescribers rely more on experience than younger prescribers, who may rely more on consensus or training. Considering only the scientific criterion would bias studies against professional acumen or wisdom that some older prescribers may possess.

The Social Psychology of Prescribing

The social psychology of prescribing seeks to describe the mental processes used by prescribers to choose drug products in response to the stimulus presented by a patient presentation. This approach does not emphasize prescriber personal characteristics such as prescriber age, practice type, etc., but rather prescriber beliefs and values and problem-solving or decision-making processes. Problem solving and decision making are closely related, but the distinction can be important. Strictly speaking, problem solving includes generative processes to discover and develop "new" alternatives. Decision making refers to cognitive processes used in evaluating and choosing from among alternatives that are known to the decision maker. Problem solving includes decision making, but not vice versa.

Schwartz et al. identified physicians from state Medicaid prescribing records who were moderate to high prescribers of therapies that the investigators considered to be inappropriate, e.g., cerebral or peripheral vasodilators or propoxyphene.[9] These physicians were visited by clinical pharmacist educators as part of an academic detailing prescribing improvement program. Physicians' motivations for their prescribing patterns were discussed in an informal, interactive manner; all responses were recorded in detail by the pharmacists immediately following each visit.

The most common reason offered by physicians for use of these medications was patient demand (51 (46%) of 110 statements). Physicians also frequently attributed their prescribing of these drugs to an intentional use of placebo effect (24%). Equally often, prescribers asserted that their own clinical experience indicated that these drugs were acceptable, even desirable for the conditions presented (26%), despite contrary research evidence. Such indications included the use of vasodilators for senile dementia or peripheral vascular disease, cephalexin for viral upper respiratory infections, and propoxyphene instead of acetaminophen or aspirin for mild pain. Inappropriate prescribers in this study tended toward the following belief and value profile:

- Incorrect beliefs about clinical pharmacology
- Skepticism about theoretical evidence
- Acceptance of commercial sources of information
- Risk aversion (with some drugs)
- Orientation toward certain outcomes, e.g., patient satisfaction

Other researchers have taken a more theoretically based and systematic approach to the psychology of prescribing. Figure 6.2 shows a comprehensive drug choice model (DCM). The DCM shown in Figure 6.2 is based on a model developed by Denig and Haaijer-Ruskamp after a long series of investigations.[10,11]

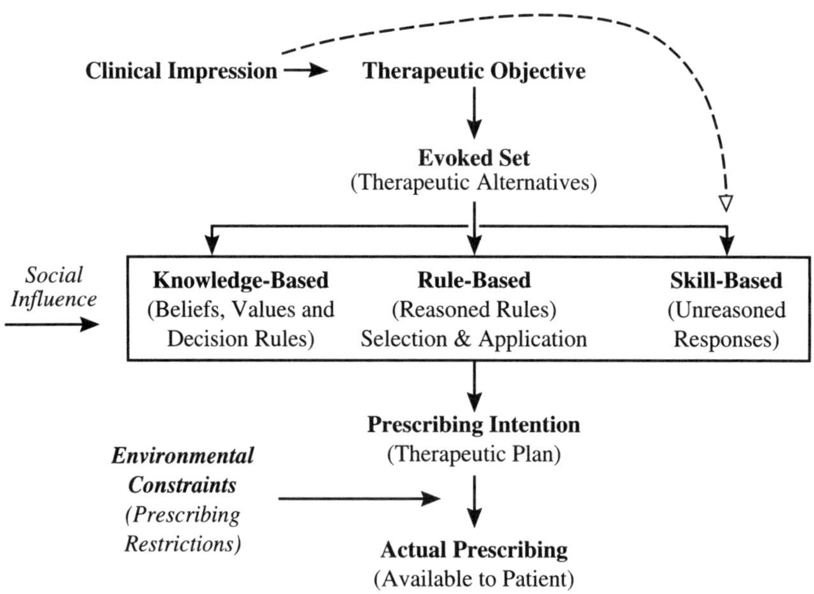

FIGURE 6.2
Drug choice model (after Denig et al.[12]). Dotted line shows alternative pathway for unreflective prescribing from habit.

According to the DCM, a prescriber would process information obtained during a clinical visit to form a *clinical impression*. (For a discussion of a process leading to clinical impression, see "Professional Dialog" in Chapter 10.) In this model, a clinical impression is seen as a psychological stimulus (or set of stimuli). The prescriber might respond by (a) considering therapeutic alternatives in direct response to the clinical impression, or (b) setting one or more explicit therapeutic objectives before identifying therapeutic alternatives. Theoretically, whether the clinical impression or the therapeutic objective leads to the evoked set might lead to different decisions. For example, a clinical impression of essential hypertension (previously untreated with drugs) might lead to a different evoked set than would a therapeutic objective (for the same patient) to reduce diastolic blood pressure by 10 mm within a month.

An evoked set of therapeutic alternatives — for short, *evoked set* (ES) — is the collection of alternative therapies that come into the prescriber's mind in response to the therapeutic objective or clinical impression. A drug's presence in a prescriber's ES is necessary but not sufficient for its actually being prescribed. The ES is roughly the same as the list of therapies that a physician might produce in response to a question following a case presentation, e.g., "What drugs would you usually consider to begin drug therapy of this patient's medical problem?" The ES may occur to the prescriber according to priorities, such as frequency of use, and may change over time as new information enters from outside the model, in particular awareness of new potentially useful therapies. Also, seldom-used drugs may drop out.

For example, Denig et al. asked hospital physicians which alternatives they might consider for patients with eight indications.[12] The number of alternatives in the evoked set ranged from 1 to 8. The indication with the lowest mean number was platelet inhibition after surgery (1 to 4 alternatives, average 1.7). The indication with the largest number of alternatives was infections of unknown origin (3 to 7 alternatives, average 5). Note that if there were no acceptable alternatives in the evoked set, then problem solving (search) would occur. If there were only one acceptable alternative in the evoked set, decision making would be automatic, because there would be no alternatives to compare.

Given an ES, the process described by the DCM may follow one of three pathways: *active problem solving*, application of *reasoned rules*, and application of *unreasoned rules* or habits.

Active Problem Solving

Active problem solving processes knowledge. This is shown in Figure 6.2 as the knowledge-based path to the left. Active problem solving corresponds to the knowledge-based (KB) activities described in Chapter 3. Active problem solving may be a course of last resort, taken only when a prescriber recognizes an unfamiliar or unique problem, or when he recognizes that the outcome may involve unusually important values. This part of the DCM has good theoretical and empirical support.

Outcomes

The DCM proposes that a prescriber can foresee outcomes or results of therapy. In a number of studies, when prescribers were asked to list possible outcomes and results of drug therapy, they mentioned biomedical, social, and personal consequences.[12]

- Biomedical
    - Therapeutic effect
    - Rate of onset
    - Serious side effects
    - Resistance
- Social
    - Cost of therapy
    - Affordability to the patient
    - Acceptability of therapy to patient or caregivers
    - Prescribing or treatment norms — opinion of colleague, patient, etc.
- Personal
    - Acceptability to self (experience, confidence, familiarity)

Values and Beliefs

Prescribers may value various outcomes differently. Prescribers studied in research projects could express their subjective values both in general terms and for specific diseases, therapeutic classes, or patients. Values may differ among outcomes for the same prescriber and among prescribers for the same outcome.

Furthermore, prescribers have beliefs about the connections between therapeutic alternatives and each outcome. For example, a prescriber may say that treatment A has a nearly 100% chance of being effective, while treatment B has an 80% chance. That does not automatically mean that the prescriber will prefer treatment A, because he may also have beliefs connecting each treatment to other outcomes, such as side effects. Beliefs may or may not be based on data or accurate information.* They are subject to change based on social processes such as education and the diffusion of new information (see below). A person's values also can change, but the process of values change may involve more complicated social and psychological processes than beliefs.

Decision Rule

Before we can predict which alternative the prescriber will select, we need to know (or assume) his decision rule. In decision theory, a *decision rule* is the

* The decision rule is called *knowledge* based, but said to depend in part on *beliefs*. The distinction is subtle, but occasionally important. Usually, knowledge implies a basis in reality. Beliefs may sometimes have no basis in reality.

mental process by which a decision maker reduces more complex data to information that can be the basis of a decision. In the example, it would be the way that the decision maker processes (simplifies) the information about the two alternatives into a form that is more useful as a basis for choosing. Decision rules can be broadly classified as noncompensatory and compensatory, depending on whether disadvantages are weighed against advantages.

Noncompensatory Decision Rules — Noncompensatory decision rules picture the prescriber as trying to find an alternative that is consistent with his values and beliefs, but without weighing all the pros and cons of each alternative. The two best known are *satisficing* and *elimination by aspects.*

Satisficing — According to a satisficing decision rule, a decision maker sets up a minimum set of criteria and then selects the first alternative that satisfies those criteria. Suppose a prescriber just wants a treatment that is effective more than 75% of the time and has minimal side effects, say 20% or less. According to the satisficing decision rule, the prescriber will choose the first drug in his or her evoked set that meets this simple rule. The prescriber would not go on to consider whether another alternative actually has a balance of outcomes that suits him better.

Elimination by aspects — A decision maker may sequentially evaluate the attributes (aspects) of an alternative and eliminate that alternative if some attribute does not meet minimum standards. If attributes differ in importance, the final choice may depend on which attribute is evaluated first. Decision makers may therefore consider their most valued outcomes first. For example, in the list above effectiveness is most important, followed by side effects. Any agent not exceeding a minimum effectiveness would be eliminated before the prescriber considered side effects, and so forth.

Compensatory Decision Rules — According to compensatory decision-making rules, the decision maker weighs all advantages and disadvantages of the known alternatives and chooses the one that maximizes the overall impact of desired and undesired outcomes. In other words, he balances total advantages against total disadvantages and chooses the alternative with the best balance. Three points should be made to clarify the significance of compensatory decision rules to prescribing.

First, the model is painstakingly rational. It is a *normative* model because it states how prescribers should choose therapies if they want the best possible outcomes, according to their own beliefs and values. The model predicts that a prescriber will select a therapy that he believes will be most likely to obtain the outcomes that he values the most.

Second, the model is *predictive* for some prescribers, some of the time. It is not literally descriptive. There is no reason to believe that prescribers actually do calculations as described above. However, these models are frequently used in studies of prescribing. In research studies, prescribers often are observed to make the choice predicted by these models, based on the prescriber's own values and beliefs. It is clear from this research that prescribers can, and sometimes do, reason in ways that reach the ideal rationality of the compensatory model. (This does not mean that they literally do these calculations, just that they arrive at the result.)

Third, this model satisfies the specificity criterion for appropriate prescribing, because the prescriber is using beliefs and values about the patient and the alternatives to reach an objective. However, it would fail the scientific criterion if the prescriber's beliefs about drug effectiveness, safety, cost, etc., were not correct. This is important, because the cause of inappropriate prescribing may not be the decision rule, but rather incorrect beliefs that can be (easily) corrected.

Reasoned Policy and Rules

The second way of choosing a therapy from the alternative in the ES is the middle pathway in Figure 6.2. This is equivalent to the rule-based (RB) activities described in Chapter 3. (This type of rule is a principle or generalization, different than a decision rule, which is actually a thought process.) Obviously, prescribers might not take the time required to work their way through even a noncompensatory decision rule every time they see a patient with a given diagnosis (clinical impression) and therapeutic objective. After making a decision a certain number of times, a prescriber may form a generalized prescribing rule or guideline that says, in effect,

> For patients with characteristics [X] and with therapeutic objective [Y], prescribe therapy [Z].

These are called reasoned rules because the prescriber chooses and applies them through a process that may be somewhat similar to decision making. Prescribing guidelines are an important example of reasoned rules. A prescriber may receive information or formal prescribing guidelines from outside (as shown by social influence in Figure 6.2) and may incorporate them into his practice with (or without) modification.

Unreasoned Rules and Habit

Some prescribing seems to result without application of rules that have a detectable relationship to definite clinical outcomes intended to improve a patient's quality of life. This is the right-hand pathway in Figure 6.2. It corresponds to psychomotor skill-based (SB) production discussed in Chapter 3. The prescriber may set a therapeutic objective and consider an evoked set, or the clinical impression may be a sufficient stimulus to choose a therapy, as shown by the curved, dotted line in Figure 6.2.

The theoretical distinction between reasoned and unreasoned rules is clear, but observing those differences in practice can be quite difficult. The mechanics of this pathway have not been well elucidated. The study by Schwartz et al., cited above, provides examples of reasons that seem to have very little connection to patient need or logical drug selection.

Sometimes, prescribing seems to result simply from a desire to take some therapeutic action when confronted with an obviously sick patient. Hepler, Clyne, and Donta[53] studied so-called empiric antibiotic prescribing by house staff in a teaching hospital. Empiric antibiotic prescribing occurs in response to symptoms but without bacterial culture and sensitivity studies. It was nearly universally discouraged in that hospital at that time.

Clyne interviewed residents to elicit their reasons for empirical prescribing. Explanations given by residents included such themes as "how I was trained," clinical experience, and conformity with expectations set by a senior resident, or even (falsely) by the chief of service. None of those explanations, however, demonstrated reasoning toward starting therapy, choice of agent, or choice of dose. Review of that prescribing by the chief of Infectious Disease Service found no instances of appropriate prescribing.

Some prescribing may result from an attempt to emulate the (perceived) prescribing of others. Explanations for prescribing such as "how I was trained" or "what the senior resident said to do" suggest that emulation of others' behavior may sometimes substitute for a decision rule.

Psychological Models and Prescribing Improvement

It happens that these three prescribing pathways correspond closely to James Reason's discussion of error types (see Chapter 3): knowledge based (reasoned), rule based (reasoned rules), and skill based (habit or unreasoned patterns). So, a parallel may exist between types of inappropriate prescribing (prescribing errors) and the prescribing processes that have been elucidated in research. James Reason points out that people who prefer the SB level will resort to RB when they see that they have no SB solution, and will actually think through a problem only when they can find no acceptable RB alternative.

The phrase "prescribing habit" was once common and is still occasionally used.[13] Much routine prescribing may be SB, and some may be RB. This type of prescribing might be amenable to change through prescribing restriction programs, e.g., restrictive formularies. There is little research to show that SB and RB prescribing are preferred by prescribers or frequently used. Most of the research evidence, on the contrary, documents that physicians use the KB (reasoned) pathway. This may be an artifact of the research methods themselves. If a prescribing research study assumes KB pathways and asks prescribers about their beliefs and values, the prescriber may "switch" to a KB pathway to answer the questions, even if that is not how he or she usually makes those decisions when not in a study. Of course, it may also show that physicians often do reason their way to a prescribing decision. Restrictions would not theoretically be an effective way to change KB prescribing.

On the one hand, most studies confirm that prescribers can and do reason. If they prescribe unacceptably, it might be that their beliefs are incorrect, that they have not recognized salient outcomes, that their decision rule was inappropriate, or that the values they attach to outcomes are different than those of the people who wrote the prescribing criteria. Some apparently inappropriate prescribing, especially that found by routine drug use evaluation, may reflect reasonable differences in opinion or values. For example, some drugs that are considered inappropriate for use in elderly people can still be used safely if they are monitored carefully.

This suggests some general, theoretical contributions of prescribing psychology to designing prescribing improvement efforts. First, appropriate prescribing requires correct knowledge of therapeutics and recognition of important consequences of therapy, including not only drug effects and safety, but also cost and acceptability. These can be taught by a variety of educational methods.

Second, a prescriber needs a repertoire of decision rules and the ability to choose the appropriate decision rule for the decision being made. This is a skill that can be acquired through education and training.

Third, value disagreements about the relative importance of consequences can be somewhat resolved through discussion, but in some instances, the prescriber's values should perhaps be accepted as representing a reasonable balance of perspectives.

Prescribers have a patient perspective that differs from the population perspective of clinical effectiveness studies. Also, the realities of practice may differ from the ideals of a pharmacy and therapeutics committee. To mention just one example, in a market, prescribers may need to satisfy patient expectations more than the opinions of those who review prescribing. This is not to justify inappropriate prescribing, but rather to illustrate the need to recognize differing values and perspectives as a means to improve prescribing.

Finally, no published studies have directly addressed the psychological consequences of administrative and coercive interventions, e.g., prescribing restrictions (see below). However, psychological theory, supported by studies done in other fields, suggests that coercion and punishment may produce evasive and defensive behavior and negative emotions. It is unlikely that coercion would change prescribers' beliefs and values about clinical outcomes or improve decision rules. The literature reviewed below suggests that although prescribing restrictions are often effective in changing prescribing, they are counterproductive with respect to patient outcomes and the total cost of care.

Sociology of Prescribing

The sociology of prescribing addresses the effect of interpersonal relationships and mass communications on prescribing. Some research on this topic has considered only sources of information used by prescribers, e.g., which sources they use and how they assess them. However, the main line of research concerns the flow of information related to prescribing and drug therapy through formal or informal social groups or networks. The sociological view is a necessary complement to the psychological model described in the preceding section. Where the psychology of prescribing addresses the manner in which knowledge is processed by a prescriber, the sociology of prescribing addresses how knowledge and values are acquired by many prescribers.

The framework for leading studies in the sociology of prescribing is diffusion of innovation (DoI).* The basic idea of innovation diffusion is the "absorption" of an innovation in a population that is composed of social networks, i.e., people with some sort of social relationship. In this view, information about an innovation is understood to flow *to* a social network or peer group and then *through* the social network to its individual members.

Diffusion is the process of communicating an innovation (actually, any new information or idea) via various media, over time, among the people in a social group. It is often measured either by asking people questions about their stage of adoption (e.g., whether they have heard of the product or idea) or by observing adoption behavior (e.g., prescribing rates or sales).

DoI studies usually concern the aggregate of all individual decision processes and observe (measure) the pattern and rate at which a new product or idea catches on and is adopted by the population. They see the rate of flow, as observed by adoption behavior, as depending on the structure of communications between and within networks.

Networks and Relationships

Perhaps the simplest social group in occupational sociology is a *clique,* defined simply as a small, exclusive group of friends or associates. *Social distance* is the perceived unlikelihood of interpersonal communication between two people or two categories of people. Naturally, social distances among members of a clique are small (see Figure 6.3).

Many socially close relationships, e.g., within cliques, are also *homophilous,* meaning that the people in the relationship share important values and beliefs and see themselves as similar. The opposite is a *heterophilous* relationship, in which the people have important differences in their values and beliefs. Specifically, a heterophilous information source is one that the adopter sees as being different from himself in some significant way, especially as having different beliefs and values.

Differences in type of occupation would be one source of social distance or heterophilous interactions. A drug salesman and a physician would be an example of a heterophilous relationship that carries news of an innovation. Communication between heterophilous individuals requires more effort, is less rewarding, and is more likely to produce dissonance (e.g., skepticism and disagreement).

---

* This section includes information generally from Rogers, E.M., Diffusion of Technological Innovations C&J 473/595, Department of Communication and Journalism, University of New Mexico. See also Rogers, E.M., *Diffusion of Innovation,* 4th ed., Free Press, New York, 1995.

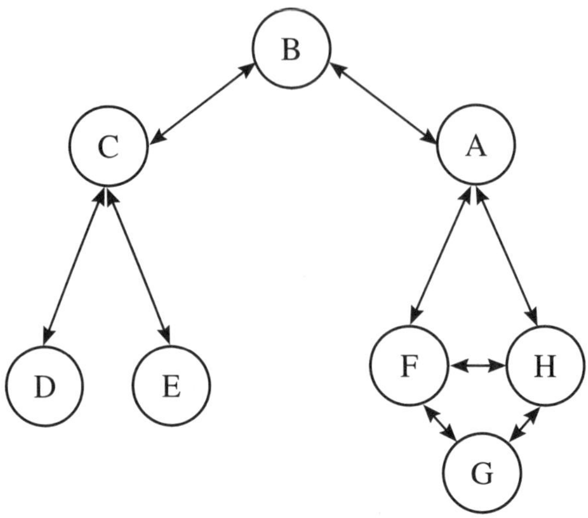

FIGURE 6.3
Simple sociogram. A, F, G, and H are a clique. B is a change agent representing C, D, and E. C is an opinion leader for D and E. The social distance between D and E is greater than the distance between F and G.

By definition, information that is new to a group enters from the outside, e.g., through a change agent. It follows that diffusion is necessary initially *between* networks or cliques. Heterophilous communication is therefore necessary to spread innovations, even though it may often be more difficult and less enjoyable than homophilous communications. Research has tended to bear this out — early phases of adoption, i.e., awareness, are more likely than later stages to have been influenced by heterophilous or socially distant sources, including mass media.

A *change agent* is an individual who influences clients' attitudes or behaviors about innovation in a direction deemed desirable by a *change agency.* The change agent is the link between the client and the change agency. (This terminology may be a carryover from agricultural studies involving agricultural extension offices and county agricultural agents.) A pharmacy and therapeutics committee or other group seeking to influence prescribing would be an example of a change agency. The change agent could be, for example, a pharmacist. Other examples include pharmaceutical representatives and teachers.

Later stages of adoption (and from a population view, higher penetrations) require social interaction and therefore social closeness and homophilous relationships. Information is spread within a social group by more homophilous relationships, e.g., between members of a clique and an opinion leader.

A member of a social group is an opinion leader to the extent (amount or frequency) that he is able informally to influence other individuals' attitudes or adoption behavior in an intended direction. In studies of professional systems, the term *opinion leader* is reserved for members of the social group (profession or clique). For example, a physician who often influences other physicians in his clique to adopt new therapies would be an opinion leader.

An important point of this discussion of change agents and opinion leaders is the strategy by which change agents identify opinion leaders as the recipient (target) of their communications. Developing friendly (i.e., less heterophilous) relationships and credibility with opinion leaders may facilitate the communication of innovative ideas by reducing dissonance and is much simpler than developing relationships with the whole group. Addressing many opinion leaders at once within a network will accelerate awareness and therefore, perhaps, adoption of innovation.

Pharmaceutical products achieve market penetration through DoI. Anecdotally, effective pharmaceutical representatives are accomplished change agents. They know who the opinion leaders are in their target group, for the main therapeutic uses of their products, and maintain relationships with those opinion leaders.

Credibility is the capability or power to elicit belief. There may be two dimensions to credibility — competence and safety. *Competence credibility* is the degree to which a communication source or channel is perceived to possess accurate knowledge and expert information. *Safety credibility* is simply trustworthiness, which depends on shared values and consistency. If a source is not high on both dimensions, then it might not be sufficient to initiate the adoption process. For example, a manufacturer's representative (detail man) might be seen as competent, but biased toward his employer's products. A colleague might be trusted, but his competence credibility may be limited by his personal experience.

Different innovations require different relationships. For example, an innovation that is consistent with the values and assumptions of a group might require a less homophilous information source and less credibility than an innovation that is more revolutionary. This is related to the concept of *adaptive potential* discussed below under "Issues Influencing Adoption."

Stages of Adoption

The theory of DoI proposes that a prospective adopter, for example, a prescriber, goes through a sequence of identifiable stages when presented with a new product or idea. Different prospective users would be at different stages of the decision process at any given time and would differ in the time it takes to complete that process.

1. **Knowledge of the innovation:** Knowledge of the innovation is seen as consisting of three substages:

   Awareness of the innovation

   Learning how to use it (practices)

   Learning how it works (principles, e.g., mechanism of action)

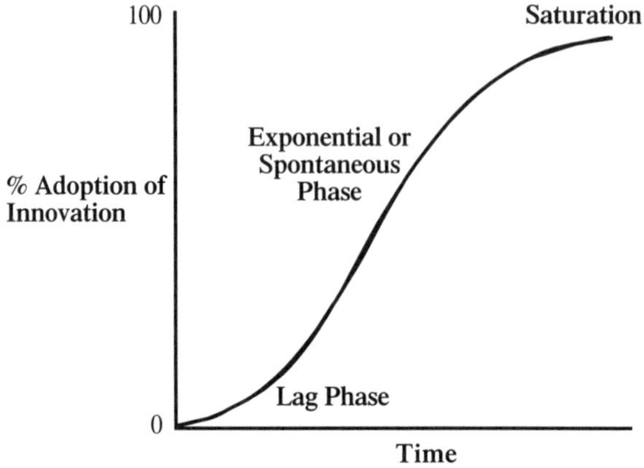

FIGURE 6.4
Cumulative adoption curve for an integrated network.

2. **Persuasion:** Persuasion occurs in two substages: awakening of interest (motivation to try) and actual trial (evaluation). Evaluation is a decision-making process, so it connects sociological DoI models and psychological decision-making models. A potential adopter would acquire information about an innovation through a network, and then form instrumentality beliefs about that innovation. Presumably, these would be referred to the adopter's existing values, but it is possible that those values could be altered somewhat by the social contacts that brought the innovation.

   For example, the same sources that brought information about a new and safer class of nonsteroidal anti-inflammatory drugs for use in osteoarthritis might also change a potential adopter's awareness of, and concern about, gastrointestinal bleeding from these drugs. It seems possible that an adopter might consider advantages and disadvantages according to a variety of decision rules, from compensatory through imitation (e.g., "how I was trained"). Furthermore, an adopter's evaluation of an innovation may depend, in part, on his position in the network. For example, a leader, if he is aware of his leadership, may factor that into his decision.[14]

   There is an odd dilemma in this analysis, which may represent the collision of academic disciplines. Psychological researchers rarely draw much of a distinction between personal experience and vicarious learning from teachers, books, journals, etc. However, Coleman, Katz, and Menzel[54,55] accepted physicians' claims that they could not trust scientific results because scientific evidence might not apply to their patients. Roy Mapes[56] argues that adoption is inevitably an "irrational" adventure because the adopter by definition has no personal experience with the innovation. This is interesting in light of Schwartz et al.'s[9] finding that *inappropriate* prescribers tend to place their clinical experience before research evidence. This is an area for further research. Perhaps experiential vs. scientific knowledge plays into the rationale of drug sampling (giving doctors free drug samples to try out on patients).

3. **Decision:** After favorable evaluation, perhaps gradually, a potential adopter may decide to adopt the innovation (and relinquish the "defender"). There is another connection to the psychology of prescribing here. Adoption appears to be equivalent to the entry of a new therapeutic alternative into a prescriber's evoked set.
4. **Implementation:** If a potential adopter has decided to adopt, the next step is to implement the decision, possibly with modification, adaptation, and reinvention before or immediately after adoption.
5. **Reevaluation:** With the passage of time, an adopter may confirm or disconfirm his adoption, and continue to use the innovation, modify its manner of use, or relinquish it.

Issues Influencing Adoption

Published research about the factors that influence adoption of a therapeutic innovation is somewhat limited, although one supposes that pharmaceutical manufacturers may have volumes of private information. Most of the published research in this area has been in consumer behavior and in agricultural practices. The following are factors that are commonly suggested to encourage or discourage adoption. Their application to prescribing seems plausible.

Individual Issues

Needs or problems that are easy to recognize tend to encourage adoption of an innovation that may meet the need or help solve the problem. Conversely, innovations that seem to involve risks of change tend to discourage it.

Product Issues

Five product attributes that tend to encourage adoption are: (1) relative advantage of the innovation, i.e., the degree to which an innovation is perceived as better than the idea it supersedes; (2) the compatibility of an innovation with an adopter's current values and practices; (3) simplicity, the perception of how easy the innovation is to understand and use; (4) divisibility, i.e., perception of how easy an innovation would be to try without irreversible changes or major commitment; and (5) observability and communicability, i.e., how easily the potential adopter can observe and discuss an adoption and its consequences, how easily others can observe the adoption.

Some innovations involve practices perceived as private or personal in nature. Common consumer examples are sexual practices and recreational drug use. Professional examples could be trade secrets.

Environmental Issues

An adoption is encouraged if an innovation is consistent with a potential adopter's social, cultural, and religious values and beliefs. Becker (quoted in Burt[14]) has proposed the concept of *adaptive potential*, i.e., consistency with the values or norms of the group. Innovations that do not conflict with group norms are said to have high adaptive potential (HAP). Low-adaptive-potential (LAP) innovations do conflict with group norms. Becker suggested that early adopters of LAP innovations may often not be closely integrated in their social network. He speculated that such early adopters innovate to obtain prestige in their communities rather than within their network.

In contrast, early adopters of HAP innovations tend to be well integrated and socially central in their networks. They adopt early to obtain admiration of peers. Opinion leaders, who are at the center of a social structure, tend to be normatively innovative.

In other words, connected people, who are integrated in a social structure, tend to learn of innovations via relations with others in the group, which reduces the time to adoption, but only for innovations that are consistent with group norms. People at the periphery of the social structure tend to discover innovations on their own, but they are less influenced by norms and so may be the entry point of more radical innovation.

Willingness to Adopt

Individual members of a network are sometimes classified according to the point in the cumulative adoption (market penetration) curve where they adopt an innovation. Figure 6.4 shows such a curve. This idea is sometimes expressed as if relative speed of adoption were a stable, personal attribute. Readiness to adopt may be related to stable manifestations of personality, e.g., confidence and need for social acceptance. However, there is little justification to assume that, for example, an early adopter of a new surgical technique would also be an early adopter of drug therapies or other new technologies. The characterizations listed below are common in textbooks of DoI. Although it may be accurate to define the earliest and latest people to adopt a certain innovation as innovators or laggards, the terms are properly applied to groups of people with respect to a certain innovation. These are not known to be personal attributes of those people. Threshold, however, may be an individual characteristic. Threshold is the number of other individuals who must be engaged in an activity before a given individual will join that activity.

Innovators (first 2.5% of population to adopt): Innovators introduce a new idea to their network by importing innovation from outside. Innovators are said to be venturesome risk takers who can cope with high uncertainty. They tend to be motivated by ideas and to have relationships with people outside their network or peer group. They may or may not be highly respected by peers.

Early adopters (next 13.5%): Potential adopters look to early adopters for advice and information about the innovation. Early adopters are more respectable, more socially integrated into the network than are innovators. Like innovators, they are motivated by ideas, but seem to make more careful innovation decisions. Opinion leaders are most often early adopters.

Early majority (next 34%): Members of the early majority are thought to provide an important link to late majority. They are deliberate and follow others. They tend to be motivated by what others are doing.

Late majority (next 34%): The late majority adopts slightly later than average. They tend to adopt for reasons of peer pressure, competition, or economics rather than the possible utility of the innovation. They often point out costs and disadvantages of innovation, and say that they are reluctant to risk scarce resources. They are skeptical and want most of the uncertainty about a new idea to be removed before they will adopt it.

Laggards (last 16%): Laggards are the last group to adopt. They are thought to be risk averse, and to see themselves as protectors of the status quo. They may hold conservative (traditional) views, and expect foolproof and proven ideas. They can be very influential, but they adopt so late that they have almost no opportunity to provide opinion leadership.

Sociological Models and Prescribing Improvement

As an innovation penetrates a population, some people posit a *critical mass*, the number or proportion of adopters in a group sufficient for the innovation's further rate of adoption to become self-sustaining. (See Figure 6.4.) For some innovations, e.g., e-mail, a minimum number of people have to adopt before the innovation can even become useful. Critical mass is an attribute of an innovation in a network rather than the network itself or its members.

In the DoI perspective, we try to understand the process by which a new idea or practice spreads throughout a population or network, e.g., health care. DoI suggests strategies for targeting certain types of innovations at well-chosen members of a network. Perhaps different types of clinical problems have different opinion leaders.

Members of some hospital pharmacy and therapeutics committee would include opinion leaders, especially if representatives are elected by their peers. Senior residents in teaching hospitals are probably opinion leaders among other house staff. In the United Kingdom, many primary care group practices have designated one of the partners as "prescribing lead." This may be a formal equivalent of the usually informal status of opinion leader.

Furthermore, different innovations may require different approaches. For example, to influence choice of agent within a well-accepted therapeutic paradigm, say one beta-blocker for hypertension rather than another, a change agent should perhaps target opinion leaders, or early adopters who are well integrated into their peer groups. To introduce more radical innovations, say those involving new therapeutic classes or unfamiliar approaches to managing drug therapy (see Chapter 11), it might be necessary to target less integrated members, even if they are not normally opinion leaders.

DoI theory emphasizes the importance of communications about the innovation and about who is using it. The actions and opinions of opinion leaders may influence others more powerfully than the quality of the evidence about an innovation. The Hepler, Clyne, and Donta study[53] suggested that at least for some house staff, imitation of opinion leaders may be a substitute for a decision rule for some prescribing.

DoI theory sees objective rational benefit as less important than does the psychological view. This contradicts some assumptions of scientific medicine, but may reflect reality for some adoptions.[14]

Methods of Influencing Prescribing

The prescribing influence methods and programs described in the literature appear to fall along a continuum of permissiveness–restrictiveness. Another distinction depends on whether they emphasize changing prescribing *indirectly* — by influencing knowledge, belief, or decision rule — or *directly*. Indirect methods would affect prescribing *intention* (which might indirectly change prescribing behavior), while direct methods would not affect intention.

Indirect programs use educational (psychological) or sociological approaches. Direct approaches tend to force or restrict access to drug products, sometimes without apparent attention to prescriber beliefs and values or to peer group dynamics.

Educational Approaches to Prescribing Influence

Many educational programs are implicitly or explicitly based in cognitive psychology and educational theory. They are usually directed at (a) changing prescribers' evoked sets, (b) changing prescribers' beliefs about outcomes (e.g., safety, effectiveness, patient acceptability), or (c) publicizing recommendations from a pharmacy and therapeutics committee, promulgating voluntary rules or guidelines.

Mass Communications

Perhaps the most familiar example of mass communication intended to influence prescribing would be drug product advertising in journals, by direct mail, and at meetings. On a local level, the most common example might be a nonrestrictive formulary.

Educational formularies are characterized by their attempt to influence rather than restrict prescribing. The simplest kind of educational, nonrestrictive formulary presents recommendations from a committee of local physicians and pharmacists. Some formularies or therapeutics newsletters publish locally written (or at least locally endorsed) monographs with recommendations regarding the use of these therapeutic agents. Such formularies change prescribers' evoked sets. If monographs and recommendations are included, they may change prescribers' beliefs about therapeutic alternatives. Educational formularies may be part of a formulary system that includes provision for obtaining (and tracking) new and nonformulary agents, e.g., nonformulary drug request forms.

Prescribing newsletters are another form of mass communications that can change the evoked set and beliefs about drug effectiveness and safety. Studies of their effectiveness show that effectiveness is unpredictable and may depend on the topic, the source of the information, and perhaps relationships with prescribers.[15–18]

Individual and Small Group Education

Face-to-face education appears theoretically to be the most powerful means of changing prescribing. It would have a number of strengths from both psychological and sociological perspectives. One form of face-to-face education, academic counterdetailing of prescribers by physicians, pharmacists, or nurses, has been shown to be effective in controlled trials. Academic counterdetailing uses essentially the same methods and tools to influence prescribing as pharmaceutical manufacturers. There is little doubt that it is effective and that its effects are persistent.[19–25]

Academic detailing is usually laborious, however, drug by drug and prescriber by prescriber. Also, studies of academic detailing were intended to measure effect on prescribing rather than medications use, and they provide little evidence that academic detailing actually changes patient outcomes or costs of care. Academic detailing has most often been used with identified problem prescribers. An interesting variation would be further emulation of pharmaceutical detailing: to use a variety of face-to-face educational approaches with *opinion leaders*, on the theory that an investment of time and effort to change their beliefs and behaviors will have far-reaching effects within their networks.

Other forms of face-to-face education are theoretically promising. They have been less well studied than academic detailing. These include:

- Drug information service
- Active consulting on working rounds or in conjunction with prospective prescribing evaluations (prospective DUE and drug regimen review)
- Cooperative practices

Consulting, including referral clinics and cooperative practices, has been shown to improve prescribing and, in some studies, to improve patient outcomes. These activities often include drug effect monitoring, and so they go beyond the scope of this chapter. Examples of cooperative practice studies are described in Chapter 9.

Prescribing Restrictions

Prescribing restrictions (PrRs) may be the most frequently used form of prescribing influence. In managed care networks, prescribing restrictions are administrative policies that restrict payment for unapproved drug products. In hospitals, physical access may be restricted directly if the hospital pharmacy does not provide "non-formulary" (i.e., locally unapproved) drug products or requires prior authorization. Common examples of PrRs are (a) formularies that list acceptable choices and exclude or limit access to other agents, (b) prior approval requirements for access, (c) specific limits on number of prescriptions or total prescription expenditure per person per month, and (d) specific limits on prescriber drug expenditures.

Prescribing restriction is qualitatively different than educational approaches to influencing prescribing, e.g., academic detailing. PrR rules usually exact some penalty from noncompliant prescribers, for example, the inconvenience of being interrupted by the pharmacist and perhaps either changing a prescription or making special application for an unapproved drug.

A range of inconvenience may exist in how long a patient or prescriber must wait for approval of a nonformulary drug application or prior authorization, or in the amount a patient must pay as copayment for unapproved drug products. Further, some enforcement can be coercive, for example, refusal to pay for an unapproved drug, threat of terminating a noncompliant prescriber's participation in a program, or a hospital pharmacy's refusal to provide a nonformulary drug.

This section will review published literature on prescribing restrictions, mainly in ambulatory care. Some issues in interpreting this literature include vague terminology, vague or conflicting objectives for prescribing restrictions, and invalid assumptions. The balance of evidence, however, seems clearly against the cost-effectiveness of PrRs in primary care, especially in managed care organizations.

Review of Literature on Prescribing Restrictions

More than 42 studies have been published on this topic. Two major reviews have summarized this literature: Jang[26] and Kozma et al.,[27] who reviewed literature on four prescribing influence methods.

Restrictive Formularies

As the term is commonly used, *formulary* can denote a wide range of prescribing influences. At one extreme is a simple list of drug products approved for use in a health care organization or for payment by a third party. (These are more accurately called *drug lists*.) At the other extreme is a primarily educational program of recommended drug products with one or more provisions for a prescriber to obtain nonformulary drugs. (These were described above.)

In his review article, Jang found that where restrictive formularies are used in ambulatory care, other drugs or services tend to be substituted. The substitutions often cost more than drug product savings. For example, using restrictive formularies, Louisiana Medicaid reduced its drug expenditures by $4 million, but spent $15 million more on nonprescription expenditures, e.g., hospitalizations. Furthermore, Jang questioned the therapeutic appropriateness of some substitute therapy. He concluded, " ... restricted drug lists appear to save money but the savings are illusory. They cost ... other services or represent a reduction in benefit to participants."[26]

Kozma et al. found that formulary restrictions often succeed in affecting drug choices and program expenditures for targeted drugs. However, restrictions may have unintended economic effects. They note that the literature shows a complex relationship among formulary restrictions, overall program costs, and therapeutic effects.[27]

Susan Horn et al. studied the relationship between formulary restrictiveness and utilization of other health care services in six managed care organizations (MCOs) located in six states.[28,29] The study included 13,000 patients over 1 year and used prospective data collection and multiple regression analysis. Formulary restrictiveness was associated with higher rates of emergency department visits and hospital admissions for all included diagnoses except otitis media, and was associated with higher drug cost, more prescriptions, and more office visits for some diagnoses. The range of effect was approximately twofold; i.e., the most restrictive formulary tended to be associated with twice the utilization of the least restrictive formulary.

Bloom and Jacobs studied the cost effects of prescribing restrictions on peptic ulcer disease (PUD) in the West Virginia Medicaid program during 1982, using a before–after comparative design.[30] They found that total Medicaid costs for PUD treatment were 15% lower during a period when a restrictive formulary was in effect than during a period when an "open" formulary was in effect. However, this overall 15% savings was explained by a sharp decline in the number of patients receiving care under the Medicaid program for PUD. The cost per member per month (PMPM) for PUD patients actually increased 9.4%. Furthermore, although pharmacy costs fell by 80%, physician costs increased by 3.1% and inpatient hospital costs increased by 24%.[30]

Cromwell et al. studied the effect of moderate prescribing restrictions on PUD in Florida. They found that restricting payment to only one PUD agent at a time, allowing only one refill per prescription, and imposing time limits for high-dose therapies were associated with a significant reduction in prescription expenditures without a significant increase in PUD-associated hospitalizations. Use of other ambulatory care services, e.g., office visits, was

TABLE 6.1

Effects of Hospital Formularies

Author, Year (reference no.)	Principal Result
Riffenburg et al., 1996 (32)	Degree of formulary restrictiveness (FR) was related to cost shifting
Sullivan and Hazlet, 1995 (33)	Restrictive formulary was related to 26% lower drug cost per patient day, with no increase in length of stay
Sloan et al., 1993 (34)	Degree of FR was related to cost shifting
Hazlet and Hu, 1992 (35)	Restrictive formulary was related to 10–13% lower drug cost per patient day

not included in the analysis. It is noteworthy, however, that the use of six alternative PUD therapies was reimbursed under this policy.[31]

Hospital Formulary Studies

Table 6.1 summarizes four studies of the financial effects of hospital formularies. One unpublished study (Sullivan and Hazlet[33]) suggests that restrictive hospital formularies are associated with reduced drug cost without increasing length of stay (a surrogate for total cost per admission). The others show that reductions in drug cost associated with hospital formulary restrictiveness result in part from cost shifting, i.e., reducing expenditures in one account (the drugs budget) at the expense of another, e.g., the nursing budget.

Prescription Limits

Some managed care programs may limit the number of prescriptions that they will pay for per month, or their monthly expenditure per capita. Soumerai et al. studied the effects of a limit of three prescriptions per patient per month, established for an 11-month period by the New Hampshire Medicaid program. As intended, the limit caused substantial reductions in both prescriptions and expenditures for drugs.[36,37] However, the limit seemed to lower prescribing of both ineffective and effective drug products. In addition, the study found significant adverse consequences for poor elderly patients and chronically mentally ill patients. For elderly patients who had been using more than three prescriptions per month, there was a 35% reduction in prescription expenditures, but this was offset by a twofold increase in the risk of nursing home admissions and a 20% increase in the risk of hospital admission. Furthermore, many elderly poor who had entered nursing homes or hospitals during the period of the prescription limit were permanently dislocated from their communities. For chronically mentally ill patients, the average increase in total cost of care was $1530, 17 times the drug cost savings.

Years after the publication of these works, prescription caps continued to be used by state Medicaid programs, among others. (See the discussion of Donald Ashwell in Chapter 5.)

Prior Authorization

Prior authorization (PA) is a type of prescribing restriction that is related to a formulary or drug list, and often is a supplemental provision. "In essence, PA is an administrative tool that requires a prescriber to get a pre-approval for ... a drug ... before reimbursement...."[38] In essence, the prescriber must apply for coverage of a nonformulary drug product. The payer, usually on advice of a pharmacy and therapeutics committee, may agree to provide (or to pay for) the drug product on a case-by-case basis, subject to advance review and approval. In the usual example of hospital restrictions on antibiotic use, a consultation with the Infectious Disease Service is required to use certain antibiotics.

Kozma et al. reviewed a number of studies showing that prior approval programs are highly effective in reducing antibiotic prescribing and overall drug costs for hospitalized patients. However, they recommend caution when applying results from institutions to health care systems. Some state Medicaid programs report substantial savings in drug costs, but according to Kozma et al., their study methods are questionable.[27]

MacKinnon and Kumar reviewed the literature on PA in 2001. They concluded,

> Overall, PA programs appear to be effective at reducing drug-related costs. There is some evidence that they reduce nondrug-related costs but little evidence that they have a positive impact on clinical or humanistic outcomes. None of the studies had a randomized, controlled design; most of the studies had severe methodological limitations.[38]

Drug Use Evaluation as Enforcement

DUE is described above as a prescribing evaluation procedure rather than a restriction. A critical issue involves the criteria used for DUE when the method is used for management (rather than research). There are no comparative studies to show the kinds of criteria used in management DUE. However, the DUE literature suggests that management DUE often is used only to measure compliance with a formulary or other list of approved drug products. Kozma et al. concluded that there is a strong need for more clinically meaningful criteria for selecting drug products and therapeutic classes for DUE. In particular, they point out that quality of care has not been incorporated routinely into DUE programs operated by third-party payers and that valid outcome measurement tools are needed to determine the true impact of DUE programs.[27]

DUE may be followed up with administrative enforcement of prescribing restrictions or with educational programs to change prescribing. Consistent with the prescribing focus of DUE, the prescribing physician is usually the target. One comparative study of *patient-oriented* DUE suggests that DUE directed at physicians did not increase the efficiency of prescribing for asthmatic patients (Table 6.2). However, DUE targeted at physicians and pharmacists significantly decreased prescription expenditures, with a smaller (although not statistically significant) total outlay for care per member per month.[39]

TABLE 6.2

Average Monthly Cost per Patient for Asthma Medications by Study Group

	Before Mean $ (SD)	After Mean $ (SD)	Difference (Before – After)
Letter and Fact Sheet to Physician	158 (94)	139 (124)	19
Only (45 Patients)	239 (354)	362 (815)	–123
Letter and Fact Sheet to Physician	153 (96)	132 (91)	21[a]
and Pharmacist (35 Patients)	201 (138)	171 (127)	30

[a] Indicates statistical significance.

Source: Sleath et al., *Am. J. Health Syst. Pharm.*, 54, 2197, 1997.

Conclusion from Literature Review

The evidence clearly shows that PrRs influence prescribing, which presumably is their primary objective. There is, however, little support for the belief that PrRs increase the cost-effectiveness of drug therapy, i.e., that they either reduce total cost per capita or improve patient outcomes. On the contrary, there is considerable evidence that PrPs may have unintended consequences. In particular, despite its limitations (and the controversy that surrounded its publication), the Horn[28,29] study cited above is not an aberration. It is consistent with the majority of evidence. There is no countervailing evidence in the literature.

The ostensible intention of prescribing influence programs is to replace inappropriate prescribing with evidence-based prescribing. However, the balance of evidence is that prescribing restriction programs may actually reduce the appropriateness and cost-effectiveness of care, when patient outcomes and total costs PMPM are considered. There is no obvious explanation for why this happens. Perhaps prescribing restrictions and DUE overemphasize the scientific appropriateness of prescribing at the expense of other issues, e.g., suitability to patient need. Perhaps prescribing restrictions interfere with appropriate decsion making in some way.

Remarkably, selection of prescribing restrictions appears to be perverse, as the least supported techniques, e.g., formularies, seem to be used the most often. This interesting anomaly should receive attention from health service researchers and students of organizational policy making and behavior.

Examining the Prescribing Influence Anomaly

The lack of correspondence between research evidence and common administrative practice is striking. This apparent anomaly raises some questions, beginning perhaps with whether we should accept the anomaly as real. Some have suggested that the research reviewed above is biased or flawed.

Is the Research Flawed?

The pharmaceutical industry has sponsored some of the studies showing adverse consequences of prescribing restrictions. Some commentators are accordingly skeptical of the results. For example, in reference to the Louisiana study mentioned above, Rucker and Morse advised, "Readers should proceed cautiously before accepting research sponsored or disseminated by interested parties."[40] Many writers have criticized the Horn et al.[29] study in particular for its funding source and for details of study design and method.

None of the studies reviewed above are definitive. They use before and after designs or correlational methods. Association does not show that formulary restrictiveness *causes* increases in utilization. There is no final proof that PrRs would generally be ineffective, e.g., as would be possible from a series of controlled clinical trials.

Formulary Terminology Is Vague

A related group of questions concerns the details of each PrR program. This would be related to the generalizability of the research reviewed above. It is possible that a variety of programs all sail under the same flag. For example, although many different programs may all be termed formularies, there are probably significant differences in both cost and effectiveness between (a) a formulary system operated as an educational tool in a hospital, in accordance with professional guidelines, and (b) a list of reimbursable drugs provided by a managed care network.

Likewise, there is a difference between a prior approval program that requires a consultation within a hospital and one that requires a telephone call to a nurse or a clerk in a benefits office. As mentioned above, some programs use DUE as a way of targeting educational programs, while others use DUE as a measure of compliance with guidelines. The exceptional PUD treatment policy studied by Cromwell et al., for example, placed few restrictions on choice of therapeutic agent, but emphasized restrictions on the manner of their use.[31]

Walser et al. have commented,

> Formulary decision making is an intrinsically difficult task. Patients often have complex requirements for pharmacotherapy, based on both medical and sociocultural needs, which physicians must address at an individual level.... Drug formularies are extremely complex instruments, especially in their regulatory incarnation.[41]

Effectiveness May Depend on Environment

PrR effectiveness may depend tremendously on specific circumstances, e.g., baseline prescribing quality, prescribers' range of competence, disease prevalence, and patient characteristics. For example, restrictive formularies or prior authorization may be more useful for improving extremely discrepant prescribing than for achieving incremental improvements in prescribing that is already reasonably appropriate.

Balance and Burden of Proof

If the evidence that PrRs sometimes have adverse consequences could be explained by ambiguities of terminology or study environment, then there should be countervailing evidence, and there would be a basis for scientific controversy. However, there is scarcely any countervailing evidence that prescribing restrictions improve outcome efficiency. The debate over the effectiveness of prescribing restrictions does not rise to the level of a scientific controversy, because nearly all of the published evidence is against prescribing restrictions, as they were actually used in the programs studied.

The case against them may be even stronger, because the overhead cost of operating prescribing restriction programs is often considerable; however, none of the studies reviewed above accounted for the cost of operating the prescribing restriction program. In this sense, these "negative" studies have at least some bias *in favor of* PrRs.

The burden of proof (or of accepting the risk of operating ineffective or dangerous programs) should be on those who wish to spend the resources necessary to operate an intervention, not on those who doubt its effectiveness. Certainly, this is the burden of anyone proposing a new drug for formulary inclusion. Certainly, this is the burden on anyone proposing to institute a pharmaceutical care system. Those opposed to the innovation are usually not obliged to prove that it is ineffective. So the rules for formulary inclusion seem to be reversed when it comes to the formulary program itself.

Suboptimality by Design?

This brings us to a second major question, "If PrRs may often be ineffective or even counterproductive, why are they commonly used?" One possibility is that overall cost-effectiveness is not actually the objective of PrR programs. Some other possible objectives and criteria might include minimizing drug product expenditures (net of manufacturers' rebates), including cost shifting within a payment program; and cost shifting to outside the program, including denial of service.

In their review, Kozma et al. advised that medical care services should not be viewed in isolation, but rather as a system of interrelated activities. Their view is certainly the medications use systems perspective of this book.

> Management with organizationally distinct benefit budgets which are controlled independently … may lead to suboptimal allocation of resources.[27]

Nonetheless, many PrR systems may be intended to control or minimize drug or "pharmacy benefit" cost rather than to achieve overall cost-effectiveness. Drug cost reductions were reported in many of the studies reviewed above. However, some PrRs may fail to achieve even this objective. Schweitzer et al. examined Medicaid drug programs in seven states from 1970 to 1980.[42] They concluded that restrictive formularies do not lower drug costs. Although total Medicaid costs were lower in states with more restrictive formularies, the authors found that restrictive formularies may not directly cause lower total costs, but happen to occur in states with other Medicaid cost-containment measures.*

The logic of drug cost minimization is *superficially* compelling. The argument must go as follows: if total cost is the sum of component costs, then reducing any component must reduce the total. This ignores the likely possibilities that (a) one component of health care can substitute for another, and (b) there may exist an optimal "input mix" at which efficiency is maximized. Changing the input mix to minimize selected input costs is well known as a way to *reduce* efficiency.

This situation is often described as being like squeezing a balloon, where reductions in one component cost simply cause equal inflation of another component. However, the research shows that this is not accurate. Often, the inflation in other cost components is substantially larger than the drug cost savings. This is understandable if prescribing restrictions (which save relatively small amounts per capita) also increase expensive physician office visits and hospitalizations. (See "Costs of Drug Therapy" in Chapter 5.) Drug therapy is a means, not an end. It can be evaluated properly only with reference to the outcomes of care.

Furthermore, the end point of minimizing component costs may become quite vague, if separated from the overall purpose. Drug therapy is intended to produce clinical outcomes that improve patients' quality of life. It should do that not only efficiently, but humanely. If drug cost reductions become self-referent, a PrR program might attempt to continue reducing drug cost year after year with targets that are not based on overall efficiency. The problem may not be with PrRs at all, but merely with their application beyond prescribing improvement into severe suboptimality. If this actually happens, the association between PrRs and total cost increases should be no surprise at all.

Promoting Products of a Favored Manufacturer

The objective of prescribing influence is to encourage the use of the most efficient therapeutic agents, not necessarily to assist in marketing the products of a favored manufacturer. Chapter 5 described a general method that is well recognized as a means of identifying cost-effective agents. How often a managed care organization actually uses these methods, however, may be unknown. The process of making such decisions is usually under the cloak of competitive business practices and therefore not publicly accessible.

Some PrR programs lose the objective even of getting their clients the best drug product for the dollar. According to *U.S. News & World Report*, PCS (a pharmacy benefit management company) invited pharmaceutical manufacturers to hire it to promote their drugs. Pfizer paid PCS $10 million

* The percentage of formulary approval of 120 new drug products approved by the FDA ranged from 19 to 73% in the seven states. The time from FDA approval to formulary adoption ranged from 15 to 72 months. (New York was an outlier with an average of 5 months.)

for that purpose. "What drug ends up on what formulary frequently depends on how lucrative a deal the P.B.M. [pharmacy benefit management company] has struck with a drug company" (Headden, S., "The Big Pill Push," *U.S. News & World Report*, September 1, 1997, p. 67). According to industry executives, this is a common practice for most PBMs and a growing source of revenue. This may be good business for a PBM, but it belies the stated goal of improving prescribing. Furthermore, the evidence against restrictive formularies seems so damning that this practice seems inconsistent with the stated quality goals of a health plan or the needs of its members. At the time of this writing, it is under criminal investigation.

Cost Shifting to Consumers

In addition to the objective of minimizing "pharmacy benefit" costs, which shifts costs among the components within a payer organization, some PrR programs may seek to shift costs to other payers, including the patient. Formularies can provide an indirect and covert means for denial of benefits, as in the West Virginia Medicaid example provided by Bloom and Jacobs.[30] This strategy seems actually to have been recommended by Dranove:

> Evidence ... suggests that neither an open nor a restrictive formulary generates optimal prescription practice.... Consider forcing recipients to absorb (internalize) some costs.[43]

If the person to whom the cost has been shifted can afford to purchase the medicine, then using prescribing restrictions may not interfere too much with drug therapy. However, unless a program has means tests, it may not know how much of a burden the shifted cost might be to the patient. When all of the patients are poor, as in Medicaid programs, cost shifting to the consumer would be close to outright denial of necessary benefits.

Summary: Toward Systematic Improvement of Prescribing

Prescribing is a necessary component of a safe and effective medications use system. Research studies suggest that much prescribing is inappropriate, especially in the elderly. Some literature directly links inappropriate prescribing with PDRM. Therefore, it is clear that prescribing improvement should receive a portion of efforts spent to improve the overall system. This chapter has outlined a systematic approach to improving the quality of prescribing.

Studies of the psychology of prescribing show that some prescribing involves active decision making based upon a prescriber's treatment objectives for a patient and his beliefs regarding effectiveness, safety, and other outcomes. In most studies, the great majority of prescribing can be correctly predicted on the basis of beliefs and objectives. Other prescribing is based on a prescriber's application of an informal, personal "policy" to a specific patient or skill-based habit.

Information relevant to prescribing decisions flows to prescribers through formal and informal social networks. Although commercial and other extra-professional channels may be useful for creating awareness of a new drug, professional channels, especially peer-to-peer relationships, seem the most important for valid information about appropriate use.

Inappropriate prescribing may occur because of an incomplete evoked set, incorrect beliefs, inappropriate treatment objectives (e.g., to cater unreasonably to patient demand), or inappropriate decision making, e.g., incorrect application of a prescribing policy. It is possible that some prescribing may be truly unreasoned, but there is little direct research evidence to support this.

Scientific studies of prescribing suggest educational approaches to prescribing improvement on theoretical grounds. There is confirmation of this theory with empirical results, mainly the good research support for face-to-face educational approaches.[9,21,23,44] Targeted education, consultation, and cooperation in practice are also effective. In other words, the most effective prescribing influence systems are directed at the decision-making process and beliefs. They do not attack prescribing behavior directly.

Two approaches to prescribing improvement seem especially promising, but require further development and evaluation. One is prescriber education, targeted on the basis of prescribing assessments. Routine drug regimen review is now mandated for nursing home patients and should be considered for other high-risk patients as well. This seems theoretically sound and may be quite efficient.

The second approach is to change the microsystems of care. For example, Chapter 9 describes a Danish asthma study that changed the relationship between physicians, pharmacists, and patients into a pharmaceutical care system. It was not directed at prescribing improvement per se, but that is what happened when physicians, pharmacists, and patients cooperated to improve patient outcomes. (See Chapter 9.) As part of a systems approach to improving outcomes, PDRM indicators (described in Chapters 2 and 3) could replace or supplement specific drug prescribing indicators.

The evidence of unintended consequences of prescribing restriction programs is believable from the perspective of medications use systems and is not surprising from the standpoint of the behavioral sciences. Prescribing restrictions may interfere with some decision processes, e.g., by blocking prescribing intention, without any real educational component. Most PrR efforts are based on unexamined and incorrect theoretical assumptions about the nature of prescribing and drug therapy.

Managed care organizations now should be able to anticipate that prescribing restrictions may produce unintended consequences. Given the literature, the term *unintended* seems a bit too euphemistic. Upon patients being injured by prescribing restrictions, we should be past the day when a pharmacy benefit manager can excuse his program by saying that drugs are expensive or that costs are rising, and that he meant no harm. In other industries, e.g., airline and automobile travel, this would not be an acceptable excuse. If, for example, airline passengers were injured by a known defect in an aircraft, which the airline chose to ignore, the airline could not excuse itself by saying that it did not intend those passengers to be injured.

The case of Donald Ashwell, described in Chapter 5, was doubly tragic because it demonstrated the persistence of a discredited prescribing restriction method. The official explanations of the Mississippi prescription cap demonstrated that prescribing restrictions seem to be sustained by a suboptimizing component cost-containment model. The cost of PDRM sometimes far exceeds the drug cost savings achievable through restrictions. It is clear that prescribing restrictions should lose all presumptions of effectiveness. Those already in place should be evaluated and, until proven, should operate much more flexibly than at present. New programs should be implemented only through an evaluated pilot phase.

Conclusion

This chapter has explored the place of prescribing in drug therapy, including prescribing quality or appropriateness and the proposition that changing prescribing quality can change patient outcomes. It argued that prescribing is meaningless (worthless or even dangerous), except as a part of a drug therapy and patient care process intended to improve people's lives. Accordingly, four domains of drug use quality were proposed, adaptations of the eight domains of health care quality listed in Chapter 5. These are timeliness, equitability, scientific appropriateness, and specificity to patient needs (TESS).

This chapter outlined a systematic approach to prescribing influence. This was described as three steps: data collection, assessment, and design of improvement activities. This is quite similar to the Shewhart quality improvement process that will be described in later chapters.

Psychological models and the sociology of diffusion provide two theoretical foundations for prescribing influence activities. Considerable research has been published about the psychology of prescribing. The sociology of diffusion has been well supported in other fields, but there is a lack of studies supporting its application to prescribing.

Common methods for prescribing influence divide broadly into indirect (educational) and direct (administrative) approaches. Research evidence supports indirect–educational approaches, while direct–administrative approaches appear to be worthless or actually counterproductive from the perspective of patient outcomes and total costs of care. Interestingly enough, however, administrative approaches seem by far the more commonly used, especially in managed ambulatory care networks.

In conclusion, attempts to study and improve prescribing may, in some ways, serve as a metaphor for understanding how to improve the outcomes of medications use. Prescribing is one step in the medications use process. Restrictions are a simple approach to prescribing improvement that do not work. Theoretically sound and systematic approaches are more complicated, but do (sometimes) improve outcomes with reduced total costs. Argument by analogy is risky, but maybe there is a useful lesson here. Perhaps simple approaches to improving outcomes of medications use, including overreliance on premarket drug product testing, prescribing improvements, and compliance improvements, may have their own unintended consequences. Perhaps they will disappoint just as prescribing restrictions have.

It happens, not by accident, that the material in this chapter intersects very well with overall system improvements. The best way to evaluate and improve prescribing influence is directly analogous to the best way to improve overall medications use, that is, to develop and implement patient-oriented indicators of drug therapy problems, drug-related morbidity, and desirable outcomes. Both drug therapy process and outcome indicators could provide the data needed for system improvements. These indicators are the subject of the next chapter.

References

1. Naish, J., Sturdy, P., and Toon, P., Appropriate prescribing in asthma and its related cost in east London, *BMJ*, 310, 97, 1995.
2. Gatens-Robinson, E., Clinical judgement and the rationality of the human sciences, *J. Med. Philos.*, 11, 167, 1986.
3. Thomasma, D.C., Philosophical reflections on a rational treatment plan, *J. Med. Philos.*, 11, 157, 1986.
4. Beers, M.H., Explicit criteria for determining potentially inappropriate medication use by the elderly, *Arch. Intern. Med.*, 157, 1531, 1997.
5. Samsa, G.P. et al., A summated score for the medication appropriateness index: development and assessment of clinimetric properties including content validity, *J. Clin. Epidemiol.*, 47, 891, 1994.
6. Hanlon, J.T. et al., A method for assessing drug therapy appropriateness, *J. Clin. Epidemiol.*, 45, 1045, 1992.
7. Fitzgerald, L.S. et al., Reliability of a modified medication appropriateness index in ambulatory older persons, *Ann. Pharmacother.*, 31, 543, 1997 (see comments).
8. Stolley, P.D. et al., The relationship between physician characteristics and prescribing appropriateness, *Med. Care*, 10, 17, 1972.
9. Schwartz, R.K., Soumerai, S.B., and Avorn, J., Physician motivations for nonscientific drug prescribing, *Soc. Sci. Med.*, 28, 577, 1989.
10. Denig, P. and Haaijer-Ruskamp, F.M., Therapeutic decision making of physicians, *Pharm. Weekbl.*, 14, 9, 1992.

11. Denig, P., *Drug Choice in Medical Practice: Rationales, Routines and Remedies*, Proefschrift Groningen, Groningen, Netherlands, 1994.
12. Denig, P. et al., Towards understanding treatment preferences of hospital physicians, *Soc. Sci. Med.*, 36, 915, 1993.
13. Lyon, R.A. and Norvell, M.J., Effect of a P & T committee newsletter on anti-infective prescribing habits, *Hosp. Formul.*, 20, 742, 1985.
14. Burt, R.S., Innovation as a structural interest: rethinking the impact of network position on innovation adoption, *Soc. Networks*, 1980.
15. Ekedahl, A. et al., Prescribing patterns and drug costs: effects of formulary recommendations and community pharmacists' information campaigns, *Int. J. Pharm. Pract.*, 2, 194, 1994.
16. Sagert, G. et al., Conformity with guidelines for antimicrobial prophylaxis against bacterial endocarditis, *Am. J. Hosp. Pharm.*, 51, 2403, 1994.
17. Blain, L. and OBrodovich, M.O., The effect of an education program on cefazolin prescribing, *Can. J. Hosp. Pharm.*, 42, 69, 1989.
18. Phillips, L. and Landsberg, K.F., Evaluation of a newsletter in altering physicians' prescribing patterns, *Can. J. Hosp. Pharm.*, 39, 102, 1986.
19. Avorn, J. and Soumerai, S.B., Improving drug-therapy decisions through educational outreach: a randomized controlled trial of academically based "detailing," *N. Engl. J. Med.*, 308, 1457, 1983.
20. Soumerai, S.B. and Avorn, J., Changing prescribing practices through individual continuing education, *JAMA*, 257, 487, 1987.
21. Gurwitz, J.H., Soumerai, S.B., and Avorn, J., Improving medication prescribing and utilization in the nursing home, *J. Am. Geriatr. Soc.*, 38, 542, 1990.
22. Soumerai, S.B. and Avorn, J., Principles of educational outreach ('academic detailing') to improve clinical decision making, *JAMA*, 263, 549, 1990.
23. Soumerai, S.B. and Avorn, J., Efficacy and cost-containment in hospital pharmacotherapy: state of the art and future directions, *Milbank Q.*, 62, 447, 1984.
24. Bloor, K. and Freemantle, N., Lessons from international experience in controlling pharmaceutical expenditure: II. Influencing doctors, *BMJ*, 312, 1525, 1996.
25. Ray, W.A., Schaffner, W., and Federspiel, C.F., Persistence of improvement in antibiotic prescribing in office practice, *JAMA*, 253, 1774, 1985.
26. Jang, R., Medicaid formularies: a critical review of the literature, *J. Pharm. Mark. Manage.*, 2, 39, 1988.
27. Kozma, C.M. et al., Economic impact of cost-containment strategies in third party programmes in the U.S. Part II, *Pharmacoeconomics*, 4, 187, 1993.
28. Horn, S.D., Unintended consequences of drug formularies, *Am. J. Health Syst. Pharm.*, 53, 2204, 1996.
29. Horn, S.D. et al., Intended and unintended consequences of HMO cost-containment strategies: results from the managed care outcomes project, *Am. J. Manag. Care*, 2, 253, 1996.
30. Bloom, B.S. and Jacobs, J., Cost effects of restricting cost-effective therapy, *Med. Care*, 23, 872, 1985.
31. Cromwell, D.M. et al., Can restrictions on reimbursement for anti-ulcer drugs decrease Medicaid pharmacy costs without increasing hospitalizations? *Health Serv. Res.*, 33, 1593, 1999.
32. Riffenburg, R.P. et al., Benchmark analysis of strategies hospitals use to control antimicrobial expenditures, *Am. J. Health Syst. Pharm.*, 53, 2054, 1996.
33. Sullivan, S.D. and Hazlet, T.K., Translog Cost Function Estimation of the Impact of Restrictive Hospital Drug Formularies on Hospital Drug Costs and Length of Stay, paper presented at APhA Annual Meeting, 142, 1995.

34. Sloan, F.A., Gordon, G.S., and Cocks, D.L., Hospital drug formularies and use of hospital services, *Med. Care*, 31, 851, 1993.
35. Hazlet, T.K. and Hu, T.-W., Association between formulary strategies and hospital drug expenditures, *Am. J. Health Syst. Pharm.*, 49, 2207, 1992.
36. Soumerai, S.B. et al., Effects of Medicaid drug-payment limits on admission to hospitals and nursing homes, *N. Engl. J. Med.*, 325, 1072, 1991.
37. Soumerai, S.B. et al., Effects of limiting Medicaid drug-reimbursement benefits on the use of psychotropic agents and acute mental health services by patients with schizophrenia, *N. Engl. J. Med.*, 331, 650, 1994.
38. MacKinnon, N.J. and Kumar, R., Prior authorization programs: critical review of the literature, *J. Manage. Care Pharm.*, 7, 297, 2001.
39. Sleath, B. et al., Effect of including both physicians and pharmacists in an asthma drug-use review intervention, *Am. J. Health Syst. Pharm.*, 54, 2197, 1997.
40. Rucker, T.D. and Morse, M.L., The Medicaid drug program in Louisiana: critique of the Hefner-Pracon study, *Am. J. Hosp. Pharm.*, 37, 1350, 1980.
41. Walser, B.L., Ross-Degnan, D., and Soumerai, S.B., Do open formularies increase access to clinically useful drugs? *Health Aff.*, 15, 95, 1996.
42. Schweitzer, S.O., Salehi, H., and Boling, N., The social drug lag: an examination of pharmaceutical approval delays in Medicaid formularies, *Soc. Sci. Med.*, 21, 1077, 1985.
43. Dranove, D., Medicaid drug formulary restrictions, *J. Law Econ.*, 32, 143, 1989.
44. Soumerai, S.B., McLaughlin, T.J., and Avorn, J., Improving drug prescribing in primary care: a critical analysis of the experimental literature, *Milbank Q.*, 67, 268, 1989.
45. Aparasu, R.R. and Fliginger, S.E., Inappropriate medication prescribing for the elderly by office-based physicians, *Ann. Pharmacother.*, 31, 823, 1997.
46. Beers, M.H. et al., Inappropriate medication prescribing in skilled-nursing facilities, *Ann. Intern. Med.*, 117, 684, 1992 (see comments).
47. Buetow, S.A. et al., Prevalence of potentially inappropriate long term prescribing in general practice in the United Kingdom, 1980–95: systematic literature review, *BMJ*, 313, 1371, 1996 (published erratum appears in *BMJ*, 314, 651, 1997).
48. Aronow, W.S., Prevalence of appropriate and inappropriate indications for use of digoxin in older patients at the time of admission to a nursing home, *J. Am. Geriatr. Soc.*, 44, 588, 1996.
49. Gregor, K.J. et al., Selective serotonin reuptake inhibitor dose titration in the naturalistic setting, *Clin. Ther.*, 16, 306, 1994.
50. O'Connell, H.M., Chance, S., and Bowman, L., Computerized drug-use evaluation, *Am. J. Hosp. Pharm.*, 51, 363, 1994.
51. Ray, W.A. et al., Psychotropic drug use and the risk of hip fracture, *N. Engl. J. Med.*, 316, 363, 1987.
52. Lindley, C.M. et al., Inappropriate medication is a major cause of adverse drug reactions in elderly patients, *Age Ageing*, 21, 294, 1992.
53. Hepler, C.D., Clyne, K.E., and Donta, S.T., Rationales expressed by empiric antibiotic prescribers, *Am. J. Hosp. Pharm.*, 39, 1647, 1982.
54. Menzel, H., Coleman, J., and Katz, E., Dimensions of being "modern" in medical practice, *J. Chron. Dis.*, 9, 20, 1959.
55. Coleman, J., Menzel, H., and Katz, E., Social processes in physicians' adoption of a new drug, *J. Chron. Dis.*, 8, 1, 1958.
56. Mapes, R.E.A., Physician's drug innovation and relinquishment, *Soc. Sci. Med.*, 11, 619, 1977.

Appendix: Examples of Prescribing Studies

The following examples were chosen to give an idea of the methods and findings of prescribing appropriateness studies.

Retrospective Study Using Explicit Drug Product Criteria

Aparasu and Fliginger estimated the prevalence of inappropriately prescribed medicines by analyzing 1992 data for patients aged 65 years and older from the National Ambulatory Medical Care Survey (NAMCS). The NAMCS is a nationwide cross-sectional survey of office visits by ambulatory patients. Prescribing appropriateness was measured as the prevalence of prescriptions for any of 20 medicines considered inappropriate for use in the elderly. Office-based physicians prescribed at least one inappropriate medication in about 8% of the elderly who received prescriptions.[45]

Prospective Cross-Sectional Studies with Explicit Drug Regimen Criteria

Beers et al. studied prescribing appropriateness in a prospective cohort study of 1106 residents of 12 nursing homes in the greater Los Angeles area. Prescribing appropriateness was evaluated using explicit criteria developed by 13 experts from the United States and Canada. The experts reached consensus about 19 drugs that should generally be avoided in the elderly and 11 doses, frequencies, or durations of use of specific drugs that generally should not be exceeded. Based on these criteria, 7% of all prescriptions were inappropriate: 40% of residents received at least one inappropriate medication order, while 10% received two or more concurrent inappropriate medication orders.[46]

Buetow et al. investigated the prevalence of potentially inappropriate long-term prescribing in general practice in the United Kingdom. Explicit criteria were developed through the review of 62 published studies of prescribing appropriateness. The proposed criteria were submitted to a panel of ten experts. The nominal group method was used to derive detailed criteria. The panel reached consensus for 19 indicators of inappropriate long-term prescribing representing five dimensions: indication, choice of drug, drug administration, communication, and review.[47]

Prevalence of potentially inappropriate prescribing varied by indicator and chronic condition. The lowest prevalence was found for inappropriate therapeutic drug choice (excluding drug cost). The highest was for inappropriate dosages. The authors concluded that the evidence of widespread inappropriate prescribing in general practice is unsound. Although inappropriate prescribing occurs, the magnitude of the problem could not be determined because of limitations in the literature associated with selection of a standard publication bias and uncertainty about the context of prescribing decisions. The authors concluded that indicators applicable to individual patients could yield evidence of prescribing appropriateness.

Prospective Cross-Sectional Medical Record Audit

Aronow carried out a prospective study of 500 consecutive admissions to a nursing home of patients aged 60 years. The objective was to estimate the prevalence of digoxin use and to evaluate indications for digoxin use at the time of admission. Ninety-six of the 500 patients (19%) were receiving digoxin at the time of admission to the nursing home. Fifty-one (53%) of the 96 patients receiving digoxin had an appropriate indication for digoxin use, and 45 (47%) had an inappropriate indication for digoxin use. Two of these 45 patients (5%) had evidence of digitalis toxicity on their admission electrocardiogram.[48]

Longitudinal Descriptive Study

Gregor et al. carried out a "naturalistic" study of selective serotonin reuptake inhibitors (SSRIs) using data from the Regenstrief Medical Record System. They analyzed the dosing of SSRIs in a cohort of 3350 outpatients of an urban teaching hospital. Of these, 2859 had received fluoxetine (Fx), 460 had received sertraline (St), and 31 had received paroxetine (Px). Mean daily doses were calculated for patients receiving Fx and St. A mean of 5.0% of all patients continuing Fx therapy had their daily dose increased with each prescription refill during the first nine prescriptions. A mean of 14.9% of all patients continuing St therapy had their daily dose increased with each prescription refill during the first nine prescriptions. The frequency of St dose increases was two to three times the rate for Fx. The authors used this information to compare the effectiveness of Fx and St for control of symptoms of depression during the initial stages of therapy.[49]

Comparison of Medical Record Audit and Computerized Screening

O'Connell et al. compared drug use evaluation of angiotensin converting enzyme (ACE) inhibitors by both medical record audit (MRA) and computerized methods. They developed consensus about six criteria for the use of ACE inhibitors. Fifty patients were randomly selected from 225 clinic outpatients who had begun taking an ACE inhibitor during a 6-month period. A pharmacist reviewed the clinic medical records of each of the patients to determine compliance with the DUE criteria. Criteria were also applied to electronic medical records of the same patients for the same time period. The MRA showed that ACE inhibitor therapy met two of the six criteria before exceptions (specific patient data) were considered and three criteria after exceptions were considered. Results of the computer evaluations were equivalent for only two criteria. The computer did not consider exceptions. Agreement between the MRA and computerized methods was good or excellent for four of the six criteria. Agreement was best for simpler criteria.[50]

Studies of Prescribing Outcomes

Ray et al. identified 1021 patients with hip fractures and matched case-controls. They concluded that the risk of hip fracture was approximately doubled for patients taking CNS agents with half-lives over 24 h (odds ratio (OR) = 1.8). For tricyclic antidepressants, OR = 1.9; for antipsychotics, OR = 2.0. The risk was dose related. "These data [show] that the sedative ... effects of psychotropic drugs increase the risk of falling and fractures in elderly persons."[51] (See Chapter 2.)

Lindley et al. studied 416 successive admissions of elderly patients to a teaching hospital. Of the 416, 26 (6.3%) were attributed to adverse drug reactions (ADRs). Thirteen of these 26 (50%) were due to inappropriate prescribing. Forty-eight patients (11.5%) had a total of 51 drugs with absolute contraindications (CIs) (3.8% of prescriptions). At admission, 175 unnecessary drugs were discontinued in 113 (27%) patients. A total of 103 patients (27.0% of those on medication) experienced 151 ADRs. Seventy-five of the 151 ADRs (49.7%) were due to unnecessary drugs or drugs with absolute CIs. This ADR rate was significantly higher than that observed for all prescriptions. The authors concluded, " ... much drug-related morbidity in the elderly population may be avoidable, as it is due to inappropriate prescribing."[52]

7

Medications Use System Performance Information

This chapter will describe the information used to manage a medications use system. Given a clear purpose, for example, "provide drug therapy intended to improve the quality of patients' lives in the most efficient manner," a manager needs four tools to manage patient care activities within a system:

- Performance *criteria* or guidelines
- A performance *database*
- Performance *indicators* (based on criteria or guidelines)
- A performance *standard*

Figure 7.1 shows how these are related in the operation of a performance management system. Chapter 11 will describe more about how this information is actually used.

The pharmaceutical care system (PCS) being managed is represented by the inner box. The management system is shown outside the box. (Details of a pharmaceutical care system are described in Chapter 10, and the parallels between the two systems are discussed in Chapter 11.)

The performance indicator data may reflect guidelines. Indicator data are sampled from a performance database and compared to standards, benchmarks from reference systems, or other expectations. If the comparison suggests that system performance is not acceptable, problem solving (e.g., root cause analysis) is carried out and actions are taken to correct the suboptimal performance. The effect of the corrective action is observed by means of the same indicators, and the process continues until the system is stable and consistent with standards.

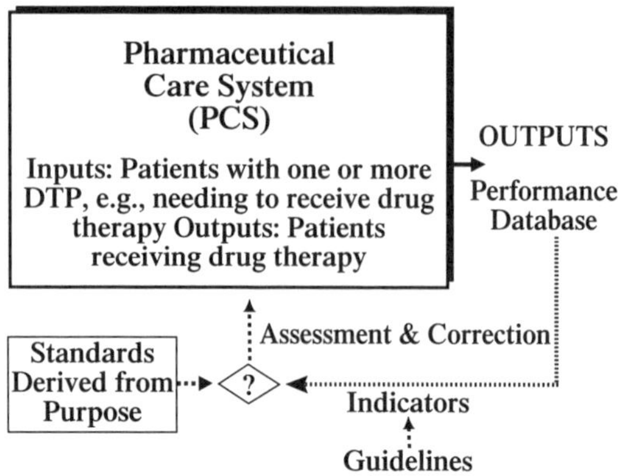

FIGURE 7.1
Relationships of system performance information.

Performance Database

A performance database is fundamental to quality management. The minimum requirement is merely a data source from which indicator data can be obtained. This source should contain reliable (accurate and consistent) information relevant to important clinical and support functions that affect patient outcomes (see below). There may actually be many databases in a performance evaluation system, for example, the dispensing records of various pharmacies, managed care organizations, or third-party payers. It is not unusual for prescription data to exist separately from other clinical data, e.g., diagnosis and laboratory results. However, separate databases must contain common information in a consistent format so that they can be linked if necessary and so that data from different sources are comparable. Liability claims data may provide a valuable source of sentinel indicators. (See "Types of Indicators," below.)

Performance Guidelines

Very simply, a *guideline* is a description of a desired care decision, action, or process. Guidelines can have almost any desired scope. For example, a disease management guideline would include recommendations for the diagnosis and treatment or management of a particular disease. Prescribing and medications use guidelines address just one aspect of disease management, but may include many treatments for many diseases.

The simplest examples are prescribing guidelines. The simplest of these is a formulary, which is, in effect, a set of general prescribing (drug choice) guidelines. Beers et al.[12,13] (see Chapter 6) developed, in effect, negative guidelines: lists of drug products and dosages that should usually be avoided in the elderly.

Prescribing guidelines can be more complex. Hanlon et al.[14] have developed ten drug regimen criteria for prescribing assessments that could also be used to develop prescribing guidelines:

1. Is there an indication for a drug?
2. Is the drug effective for the indication?
3. Is the dosage correct?
4. Is the duration correct?
5. Are the directions correct?
6. Are the directions practical?

7–9. Does the patient's drug regimen include clinically significant interactions (drug–drug, drug disease, therapeutic duplication)?

10. Is this drug the least expensive alternative?

A medications use guideline would refer not only to prescribing, but also to the use of medications over time. For example, a medications use guideline could include minimum and maximum dosages, durations of therapy, concomitant therapies, monitoring activities, and even outcomes. Later examples will make use of the following treatment guideline illustration.

A treatment guideline for bronchial asthma (given specific diagnostic details) might recommend combination therapy of regular daily inhalations of a preventer medicine like beclomethasone and occasional use of an inhaled "rescue" medicine like albuterol. (Albuterol is an adrenergic agonist, similar to epinephrine, that can open a constricted airway during an attack.) Increasing frequency of albuterol metered-dose inhaler (MDI) use may reflect either incorrect inhaler technique or worsening status of disease control. Patients with good inhaler technique who have to increase their frequency of rescue medicine use may need medical attention to find out why their asthma is going out of control. The maximum appropriate daily dosage of albuterol MDI is eight inhalations per day. An MDI containing 17 g of drug would contain enough for 200 inhalations. The minimum prescription refill interval that is consistent with that guideline would then be about 25 days.*

* This guideline is an example for illustration only. It was realistic at the time of writing but may not be reliable for actual clinical decisions.

Performance Indicator

"An indicator is a quantitative measure that can be used to monitor and evaluate the quality of important ... clinical and support functions that affect patient outcomes...."[1] A *performance indicator* is a quantitative criterion measurement that is related to a guideline, for example the percentage of prescriptions for a certain therapeutic objective that were written and used in accordance with guidelines. "An indicator is not a direct measure of quality. Rather it is a tool that can be used to assess performance and that can direct attention to ... issues that may require more intense review within an organization."[1] That is, in order to be useful, an indicator need not correctly identify every case, say as acceptable or unacceptable. It must, however, correctly classify enough cases to allow tracking of overall performance levels. This is the issue of indicator validity, explained further below.

An indicator can reflect either desirable or undesirable processes and outcomes of care. An example of the former is one that shows processes consistent with guidelines or a desired outcome.

A medication performance indicator is a measurement of one or more important aspects of the process or outcome of care in patients receiving drug therapy (or who have a valid indication for drug therapy). Performance indicators have five well-established uses:

1. To evaluate system performance
2. To identify specific process or outcome problems, quality variations, and trends in quality
3. To guide problem solving and system analysis
4. To track the effect of structural or process changes
5. To document quality to customers, regulators, and accreditors

Standards

Indicator data are obtained from an organized database and are usually statistically processed and compared to a standard. According to the Institute of Medicine, a *standard* is "a minimum level of acceptable performance or results; or excellent levels of performance; or the range of acceptable performance or results."[2] In customary usage, a standard represents minimum acceptable performance, e.g., the percentage of cases that follow a guideline. Inappropriate behavior may not be the only explanation for an indicator (see "Validity," below). Therefore, a standard might allow less than 100% conformity to a guideline.

Types of Indicators

Process and Outcome

Outcome indicators measure what resulted (or did not result) from care. They are, in principle, a necessary component of performance evaluations under outcome-oriented definitions of quality such as the OTA definition (see Chapter 5).

Process indicators measure definite activities that are a part of care. Although outcome indicators are preferable, process indicators help to link care activities to outcomes, especially where:[3,4]

1. The outcome lacks a valid or reliable measurement method.
2. Outcome measurement is not economically or logistically feasible.
3. The outcome is far removed from the process.
4. The process has a very strong, demonstrable link to outcome.
5. The processes (procedure, equipment, products) are of interest in themselves, e.g., very expensive.

Sentinel vs. Rate Based

A sentinel event indicator measures an important process or outcome event that rarely or never occurs when quality is adequate. The indicator itself (or its quality implication) is usually so significant that each event requires more detailed analysis. "Falls from bed by hospitalized patients" is a classic example of a sentinel nursing care quality indication. Certain dispensing errors and the use of certain contraindicated drugs in combination would be examples of sentinel events in medications use.

A rate-based indicator measures an event that is expected to occur in a certain proportion of cases even when quality is state-of-the-art. Further assessment is required if a threshold is crossed or a trend or pattern suggests an opportunity for improvement.

Baseline statistical data (incidence) is collected for a rate indicator. The process is investigated when nonrandom variation (a trend) is observed or when the rate crosses a predetermined threshold. (Chapter 11 includes an example of a control chart used for this purpose.)

Minimum Information Needed for an Indicator

To formally define a performance indicator, the following information is necessary:

Type: Sentinel or rate based.

Numerator: The numerator of a rate indicator (or the sentinel event itself) includes an operational definition of the event and the time period of observation, e.g., month. *Example:* Patient with asthma receiving more than (x) rescue inhalers in 1 month (where x is greater than 1). The numerator is the number of such events in a month.*

Denominator: Rate or ratio indicators require an adjustment for volume, often the sum of all desired and undesired events, e.g., total number of patients or courses of therapy. *Example:* The total number of patients refilling a prescription for a rescue inhaler.

Rationale: An indicator rationale is the connection between the event and quality of care. It is the basis for interpreting the indicator with respect to quality. The indicator should have, at least, a plausible relationship to either an outcome or an important aspect of process or structure. For example, a consensus guideline directly describes aspects of process and describes a means of achieving an outcome. Ideally, an indicator should also be empirically validated, although this remains a potential Achilles' heel for many indicators. Validity can be evaluated in many ways, as described below. Issues to address include the following:

1. Why indicator is useful
2. Value/harm of activity, event, or outcome to patient
3. Relationship of indicator to process or outcome
4. Usefulness in identifying issues that may require more intense review

Scope: Description of the system level and steps of process represented by the indicator. Related to rationale, scope describes the types of underlying factors that may explain variations in the indicator. Examples of system levels are as follows:

1. Patient factors
2. Practitioner factors
3. Organization factors
4. Environmental factors

Data source: Identification of data sources and procedure for collecting indicator data.

Examples of Medications Use Indicators

Corresponding to the guidelines discussed above, many indicators have been used to evaluate aspects of the medications use *process*. Drug use evaluation

* Indicators are usually quite specific. For example, an actual indicator would specify which specific drug products were included, usually by unique product code number. It would also describe how to calculate minimum refill time for different sizes of MDIs. For simplicity, the example assumes a 17-g inhaler.

(DUE) and other forms of prescribing assessment use simple indicators, often just drug name (identity), sometimes identity and dose, and rarely concurrent therapies. More sophisticated prescribing indicators have been developed.[5–7]

Medications use process indicators can also reflect such aspects as duplicate therapies, length of therapy, and doses received (as a proxy for doses consumed). Other indicators reflect aspects of medications use outcome, for example, adverse drug reactions (ADRs) or adverse drug events (see Chapter 3). Some examples of medication use indicators are:

Inappropriate asthma treatment

Type: Rate.

Numerator: Patient with asthma receiving more than two rescue inhalers and fewer than one preventer inhaler in 1 month.

Denominator: Number of patients with asthma receiving beta agonists by inhaler.

Rationale: High-rescue inhaler use and low preventer use both may predict emergencies and deaths in asthmatic patients. (Each additional MDI cannister doubles the risk of asthmatic crisis.[8,9])

Scope: Medications use process, including aspects of prescribing, patient behavior, and pharmacy behavior.

Data source: Pharmacy records, insurance (payment) records.

Asthma readmission

Type: Sentinel.

Numerator: A patient with asthma who was readmitted to hospital or who had emergency department visits within 15 days of last hospitalization.

Rationale: Frequent emergency care or hospital admission is inconsistent with appropriate management of asthma. (This indicator could also be written as a rate indicator if some such events were considered acceptable.)

Scope: Provider and practice group level; outcome of medications use process, quality of care, and other factors contributing to asthma control.

Data source: Insurance (payment) records.

Other examples of process indicators (numerators):

1. Apparently mistimed refills (MRs), i.e., inappropriate refill (repeat prescription) interval. MRs are prescription refills that are presented early or late relative to prescription instructions.
2. Apparent therapeutic duplication (TD). TD is defined as the occurrence of one or more refills of at least two drugs in the same therapeutic class, during the same time period. Examples of

specific drug classes that might be considered are oral antidiabetic agents (in particular, two sulfonylureas) and benzodiazepines.

3. Apparently inappropriate length of therapy (LT). LT is the duration from the earliest time of dispensing to the most recent, within a defined therapeutic class, where therapy was continuous. (Therapy was continuous if there was no interval longer than 2 weeks between theoretical refill dates and the next actual refill date.) An example is short length of therapy for selective serotonin reuptake inhibitor (SSRI) antidepressants. SSRIs may require many weeks to show therapeutic effect, and some patients may become discouraged and stop taking their medicine before it has time to work. Another example is long length of therapy for appetite suppressants, or cyclobenzaprine. These drugs lose their effectiveness after a certain period. Their behavioral side effects, possibly including habituation and dependency, would no longer be justified by their therapeutic effects.

The Joint Commission on Accreditation of Healthcare Organizations (JCAHO) has implemented five medications use indicators. The National Committee for Quality Assurance (NCQA) has developed HEDIS 3.0 (Health Plan Employer Data and Information Set), a database of performance measures for comparing the performance of managed care organizations. HEDIS consists of a set of performance measures that tell how well health plans perform in key areas: quality of care, access to care, and member satisfaction with the health plan and doctors. HEDIS requires health plans to collect data in a standardized way so that comparisons are fair and valid. Many HEDIS indicators are directly related to the use of medicines, for example:

- Treating children's ear infections
- Beta-blocker treatment after a heart attack
- Aspirin treatment after a heart attack
- Use of appropriate medications for asthmatic patients
- Antibiotics for HIV-related pneumonia

Medications use indicators have been used more in research than in routine management. Only DUE process indicators are used routinely for management. Also, most medications use indicators refer either to process or outcome, but not both. However, a new kind of medications management *performance indicator* is described below.

Criteria for Indicators

Like other measures, indicators must be tested for reliability and validity. *Reliability* reflects the precision of a measurement, while *validity* reflects the

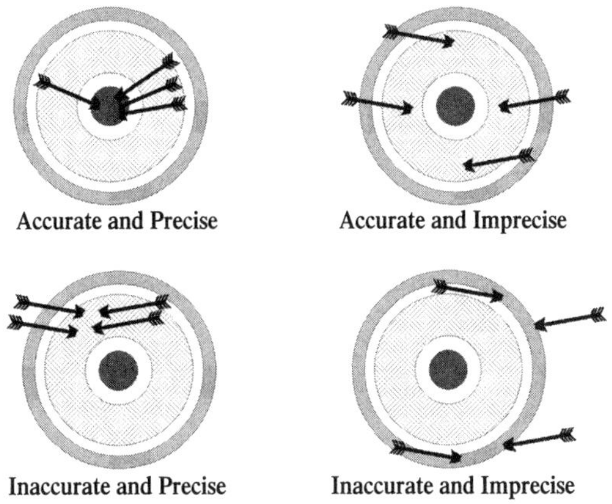

FIGURE 7.2
Target metaphor for precision (reliability) and accuracy (validity).

accuracy or representativeness of a measurement. In a well-known target-shooting metaphor, an archer aiming at a bull's-eye may shoot most of his arrows into the same small region of the target or scatter them all over the target (Figure 7.2). That is a matter of *precision* or reliability. The smaller the pattern, the more reliable the shooting. The nearer the pattern is to the bull's-eye, the more *accurate* (valid) the shooting is. Clearly, a tight pattern near the bull's-eye is both accurate and precise, i.e., valid and reliable.

Chapter 11 demonstrates the use of indicators in practice. It also includes some more technical discussions of indicator reliability and validity.

Reliability

The reliability of an indicator refers to consistency or reproducibility of measurement. It is a measurement of the ratio of true variation to total (observed) variation. Unfortunately, there is no way to observe true variation, but we can estimate it in a number of ways.

One way to measure reliability is to assess the correlation between two independent judgments of the same item. The correlation is the degree of measurement or classification agreement.

To make the notions of reliability quantitative, consider Table 7.1. Assume that two independent and equally qualified observers rate the same set of

TABLE 7.1
Indicator Reliability

	Observer A		
Observer B	**Yes**	**No**	**Total**
Yes	a	b	$a + b$
No	c	d	$c + d$
Total	$a + c$	$b + d$	n

objects as either "yes" or "no" concerning an attribute. The two observers can agree in two ways, if both vote yes or if both vote no. Therefore, a measure of reliability r_{xx} would be given by

$$r_{xx} = (a + d)/n$$

Another way to estimate reliability, useful with more than two observers, is to carry out a two-way analysis of variance (observers by indicators). Reliability is estimated by

$$1 - (MSE/MSO)$$

where MSO is the mean square for observers and MSE is the mean square for error (residual).

For numerical examples and further discussion of reliability, see Chapter 11.

Validity

Measurement validity addresses the fundamental issue of whether a measure reflects whatever it was intended to measure, including its accuracy or bias. Because measurement validity is such a fundamental topic, philosophers and researchers in many fields have thoroughly explored the idea. There are many approaches to validating a measurement. Some approaches lead to different facets of validity than do others. The most important thing to say about indicator validity is that it must be judged relative to the purpose for which it will be applied.

The application of quality indicators has a different purpose than the application of research measurements. Quality indicators are often used to identify cases for follow-up in formative assessments that precede problem solving and correction. In contrast, research measures are used to test theories and for summative measures, e.g., to characterize a population. It happens that although indicators are expected to have sound, evidence-based rationales, few have actually been formally validated, e.g., by comparison to medical record review. This would not matter much if the indicator were shown to lead to cases that actually had the important quality or performance issues predicted by the indicator. In general, quality indicators may be interpreted as *correlates* of quality rather than as direct quality measures.

Validity has a somewhat asymmetrical interpretation for sentinel event indicators. Sentinel events are (or should be) always followed up and evaluated. Therefore, false positives would tend to be recognized as such on follow-up. So nonspecific sentinel events might decrease efficiency, and perhaps lead to occasional resentment, but would not lead to errors of quality assessment. However, false negatives would not be investigated, and assessors would miss significant events. Therefore, insensitive sentinel indicators might lead to overestimation of quality.

This kind of misinterpretation may be commonplace in medications use. The usual (de facto) sentinel indicators for medications use tend to involve major errors in prescribing, dispensing, or administration, including noncompliance. However, these indicators are quite insensitive to many other kinds of quality failures, especially failure to monitor or respond to abnormal signs and symptoms in a patient. So, perhaps it is not surprising that we tend to overestimate the quality of drug use.

Face validity refers to how well an indicator reflects its rationale "on its face." Face validity is judged by a panel of experts who read the indicator description and decide if the language accurately represents the rationale.

Content validity reflects the scientific validity of the rationale and how completely an indicator or a set of indicators represents that rationale. For example, does the measure represent only a few examples or the whole domain? Consider the indicator above that refers to both asthma rescue and preventer medicine use. The content validity of this indicator is higher than it would be if it referred to only one or the other type of medicine, because it includes both of the two major epidemiological findings that connect asthma therapy with outcomes.

Finally, *criterion or concurrent validity* expresses the degree to which an indicator identifies situations or events in which quality can be improved. The criterion measure could be, for example, expert review of cases. This would lead to an array similar to that of Table 7.1.

In Table 7.2, however, instead of observer A, we have the reference standard or "gold" standard for the indicator. In place of observer B, we have the quality indicator or overall assessment being validated. Or a process indicator could be validated against an outcome. (There can be more than one rater for each measurement A and B. If the indicator or assessment is not reliable, this limits the possible validity.)

Now, the indicator is valid to the extent that (a + d) is larger than (c + b). This time, however, we should account for *false positives*, where the indicator is positive but the standard is negative, and *false negatives*, where the indicator is negative but the standard is positive. Three important validity measures are sensitivity, specificity, and positive predictive value.

Indicator sensitivity measures how many events that truly reflect quality problems (within the scope of the rationale) are detected by the indicator. *Sensitivity* is calculated as the proportion of reference positives (a + c) that are indicator positives: a/(a + c).

TABLE 7.2

Indicator Criterion Validity

Assessment Method Indicator	Reference Standard (S+)	(S–)	Total
Indicator Positive (I+)	a	b	a + b
Indicator Negative (I–)	c	d	c + d
Total	a + c	b + d	n

Indicator specificity measures the ability of the indicator to identify only cases in which there was a quality failure. *Specificity* is calculated as the proportion of reference negatives that are indicator negatives: d/(b + d). The *positive predictive value* of the indicator is given by the proportion of indicator positives that are true positives: a/(a + b). For numerical examples and further discussion of applications, see Chapter 11.

There is some debate about whether reliability is a prerequisite to validity. In the target-shooting example, the question is whether a dispersed pattern of arrows that happened to center on the bull's-eye would be accurate. On the one hand is a convincing theoretical argument that validity can be no higher than reliability. This also agrees with common sense, that if the judges cannot agree, the rating cannot be very valid. If no arrow hit the bull's-eye, shooting cannot be considered accurate, regardless of averages.

On the other hand, expert review is generally considered to be the gold standard for judging the validity of a quality measure. Paradoxically, peer review, e.g., medical record audit, has also been shown in many applications to be much less reliable than the indicator that it could be used to validate.

It is sometimes possible to increase reliability by repeated measures. That is, reliability can be improved by increasing the number of independent ratings. The average of measures will tend to be more reliable than individual measures. Therefore, a set of related indicators, taken together, may be more reliable than the individual indicators. In a classroom test, for example, many less reliable questions may add up to a much more reliable test score. According to the Spearman–Brown formula, doubling the number of raters, for example, would increase the reliability of the rating from r to [2r/(1 + r)].

Feasibility

The data needed for an indicator must be accessible at acceptable cost, relative to the indicator's management value. In other words, when indicators are used for routine management (rather than for research), the cost of collecting indicator data becomes a part of the cost of operating the system. Some trade-offs between the cost of information and the validity of indicators may be necessary. This must not, however, be seen to justify the status quo. A brief analogy may help. A financial accounting system, whether simple or elaborate, is an information system that produces many indicators — some are simple; some are more complicated. Financial accounting systems surely add to overhead. No single financial indicator, e.g., cash on hand, gives an accurate picture of the firm's financial status. Together, cash balance, accounts receivable, accounts payable, and other financial indicators are essential for management. A business would not last long without them.

The argument for medications use indicators is not quite as strong, but is essentially the same. Poor medications use systems waste lots of money in managed care organizations that have to pay for the consequences. The cost of medications management indicators should be evaluated in the context of improved efficiency and safety, i.e., the expenses saved by preventing preventable drug-related morbidity (PDRM). (See Chapter 2.) Furthermore, managing quality may increase customer satisfaction and reduce legal liability.

Medications Use System Performance Indicators

A new kind of indicator was introduced in Chapters 2 and 3 as a measurement of the prevalence of PDRM. This type of indicator, which contains both process and outcome elements, can also be routinely used as a performance indicator.

These indicators are based on the definition of preventable drug-related morbidity first given by Hepler and Strand in 1989 and described in Chapter 3.[10] A *preventable* DRM is one that was preceded by a *recognizable* drug therapy problem (DTP). Further, DTP must have the following three characteristics that constitute a *correctable* problem:

1. The possibility of the DRM must have been reasonably *foreseeable.*
2. The cause of the DTP and DRM must have been *identifiable.*
3. The cause must have been *controllable* within the scope of the therapeutic objective.

The outcomes used in the indicators are almost always either adverse outcomes or treatment failures. The performance indicators developed from this definition are then equivalent to PDRM indicators.

Indicator Development Process

The complete indicator development process comprises the following five steps:

1. *Literature review* — Published articles that associate an adverse outcome with a process of drug use or a treatment failure with nonuse of an indicated therapy.
2. *Draft (proposed) indicators* — Indicators in the outcome + process format are written based on the literature review.
3. *Delphi panel* — An expert panel reviews each proposed indicator according to the basic definition given above. The panel members may submit indicators of their own to a subsequent round. Acceptance by a majority of panelists is interpreted as face validation of each indicator and content validation of the set of indicators.
4. *Operationalization (coding)* — Indicator terms are translated into medical record codes for diseases, procedures, and drug products.
5. *Criterion validation* — After data collection, indicators are validated against patient data, e.g., medical records.

Examples of Indicators

The format of each indicator is patient outcome + process of drug therapy.

The following examples were developed in the MacKinnon[15] study, were revalidated in the Faris[16] study, and were the five most frequently found PDRMs in the latter study:

#45. A patient was admitted to hospital or emergency department (ED) with decompensated congestive heart failure (CHF) when he had a history of CHF and no record of angiotensin converting enzyme (ACE) inhibitor.

#33. A patient was admitted to hospital or ED with decompensated CHF or heart block when:
- He had a history of CHF or heart block or bradycardia.
- He had a recorded digoxin prescription and used it after diagnosis and prior to admission or visit.

#39. A patient was admitted to hospital or ED with gastritis or upper gastrointestinal (GI) bleeding or gastric ulcer or anemia and used two or more nonsteroidal anti-inflammatory drugs (NSAIDs) concurrently for 2 weeks or more.

#22. Hyperthyroidism + thyroid or antithyroid agent when T4/TSH not done within 6 weeks of initiation of therapy and at least every 12 months thereafter.

#48. A patient had status asthmaticus or an ED visit or hospitalization for asthma and:
- Had a history of asthma
- Used bronchodialators
- Did not use an inhaled steroid

Delphi Panel

MacKinnon[15] and Faris[16] used panels of seven experts. In order to accept an indicator, a panelist had to agree that the medications use process scenario described a *recognizable* drug therapy problem with a *foreseeable* adverse outcome and a probable cause in the medications use process that was both *identifiable* and *controllable* within the objectives of care. (See Chapter 3, under "Preventability.")

The amount of agreement among the seven panelists for the five examples after three rounds is shown in Table 7.3. These numbers reflect face validity (whether the proposed definitions represent valid medications use performance indicators). The overall agreement with the whole list by Delphi panelists represents content validity — whether the set of indicators reflects the concept of medications use system performance (as measured by system failures or PDRM). The range of agreement by Delphi panelists with the whole list was from 82 to 100%, with a mean of 92.7% agreement.

TABLE 7.3

Face and Content Validity of PDRM Indicators in Faris[16] and MacKinnon[15] Studies

Indicator (Outcome + Process)	Faris	MacKinnon
#45. CHF + no use of ACE inhibitor	6 (0.86)	6 (0.86)
#33. CHF, heart block, or bradycardia + digoxin	7 (1.0)	7 (1.0)
#39. GI bleeding + 2 NSAIDs	6 (0.86)	7 (1.0)
#22. Hyperthyroidism + no T4/TSH	7 (1.0)	6 (0.86)
#48. Asthma crisis + bronchodialator but no inhaled steroid	5 (0.71)	6 (0.86)

Data Collection and Results

Fifty-two operational definitions of PDRM in older adults received six or seven votes from MacKinnon's[15] Delphi panel. MacKinnon then used a combination of computer search (mainly for outcomes) and manual search of a computerized database describing the care of 3365 members of a Medicare managed care health plan. Ninety-seven patients had one or more PDRMs according to the definitions. The most frequently occurring PDRM, with 39 events, was

> a patient experiences a second myocardial infarction where there is no record of aspirin or a beta-blocker (e.g., metoprolol).

Faris[16] coded all of the diagnoses, procedures, and drug products used in his indicators and used completely automated search methods. He found an overall incidence of 6.25 per 100 patients per year.

The five most frequently occurring indicators accounted for 57% of all occurrences of PDRM (3.6% incidence per patient year). The top ten indicators accounted for 80% (5% incidence per patient year). Many indicators were not associated with any events. These results clearly suggest that substantial improvement in the performance of this medications management system could be achieved if relatively few recurring problems could be corrected.

Further Validation

The Delphi panel results provide information about reliability, face validity, and content validity (how well the set of indicators represents the domain of all possible PDRMs). Four additional procedures have been carried out to further investigate the validity of these indicators:

1. MacKinnon had a sufficient number of cases to carry out direct criterion-related validity for two of his indicators. These showed about 80% sensitivity and specificity against medical record review. (See Chapter 3.)
2. Both MacKinnon and Faris carried out risk factor studies that showed that the indicators have consistent, apparently stable rela-

TABLE 7.4

Correlation of Process and Outcome Elements in Five Indicators[16]

Indicator	P:O
#45. CHF + no ACE inhibitor	0.75
#33. CHF/heart block — digoxin	0.95
#39. GI bleed with duplicate NSAID	0.12
#22. Hyperthyroid + treatment, no T4/TSH	0.45
#48. Asthma — bronchodialator but no inhaled steroid	1.00

tionships with recognized patient characteristics associated with the risk of ADRs (number of drugs, number of diagnoses).

3. Faris submitted results from his leading indicators to an independent panel of physicians and pharmacists for root cause analysis. The panel members accepted the validity of the indicators that they were presented and were able to interpret the indicators constructively, to identify causes and propose solutions.
4. Faris studied the association of process and outcome within the indicators. This is summarized in Table 7.4. For example, 75% of the patients with CHF who did not receive ACE inhibitors decompensated during the observation period. All of the asthmatic patients receiving adrenergic agonists but not inhaled steroids had at least one asthmatic crisis.

It is particularly interesting that face validation and process:outcome (P:O) correlations do not completely agree. In particular, #48, the asthma indicator, received only five votes but had perfect positive predictive value in this sample.

Application

Performance indicators, used in a quality improvement program, should be validated for their usefulness in *formative* applications, i.e., problem identification and definition as steps in system performance improvement. Because a performance review team would review and follow up summative measures, the demands on their validity are less than for summative applications. For example, recall from Chapter 3 that this method is specific and identifies only those PDRMs that were defined.

Suppose that a set of performance indicators tends to underestimate the true prevalence of PDRM in a group of patients, in part because some kinds of PDRM are not represented in the set. For the sake of the example, also suppose that some indicators tend to miss a few cases of the type they were intended to detect. Many indicators include time periods for monitoring or for duration of therapy that could be too long or too short. Suppose that the set picks up only 90% of the total of true cases.

In a summative (research) application, a 10% underestimation might be a serious problem. In a performance improvement program it would be less so. An intervention that could correct the 90% that are detectable would improve some that were not detectable as well. Furthermore, the bias would apply to each measurement, so the changes in indicators with time would be accurate.

Pharmaceutical Care and Medications Use Management

Performance indicators such as the ones described above may accelerate acceptance of pharmaceutical care and medications management systems. They can be interpreted in two ways:

- As process-linked *outcome indicators* that can help to identify widespread problems in medications management
- As outcome-linked *process indicators* that can help pharmacists and physicians to identify patients who need better management

1. Their use would show whether a particular population (e.g., members of a managed care organization) has serious, recurring problems in medications use.
2. If problems were found with these indicators, the prevalence and association of unacceptable process and adverse outcome would show whether the outcomes resulted from system failures or from occasional bad luck.
3. The distribution of indicator positives could prioritize attention. Often, relatively few problems represent a large proportion of PDRMs in a particular population. Correcting relatively few recurring problems may improve outcomes for many patients.
4. The already-identified process failures should guide the root cause analysis to promising solutions. The statistical association of process and outcome elements would identify weaknesses in the pharmaceutical care system. Pharmacists (or others) could identify patients who are receiving processes of care associated with undesired outcomes, for example, patients with heart failure who are not receiving ACE inhibitors, or asthmatics who are not well controlled on inhaled adrenergic agonists and are not receiving inhaled steroids (either because none were prescribed or because they have chosen not to use them).
5. Quality assessors or third-party payers can evaluate the impact of system changes on outcomes. They can also use the process

component of the indicator to assess whether providers are actually providing appropriate care.

6. Standards of pharmacy practice could be developed that require managed care organizations and professional providers to operate a performance review program based on drug therapy problems and process indicators.[11]

Summary and Conclusion

This chapter has described medications use indicators, ranging from familiar, but incomplete, prescribing indicators to a more complete approach using sets of outcome–process indicators.

It seems clear that managed care and other health care programs do not take advantage of the potential value of the medications information that they possess. Considering (a) the magnitude of the problem, as described by research reports (Chapter 2), (b) the evidence that the causes are the inadequacies of medications use systems, (c) the availability of reliable and valid indicators, and (d) the ubiquity of computers and the low cost per gigabyte of storage and processing capacity, every provider and payer organization should be obliged to collect data relevant to the safety and effectiveness of the medications use systems under their influence.

Chapter 11 will provide an extended example of how performance information may be used to improve performance. If a health program were to implement medication performance indicators, it might discover a manageable and realistic pathway to the development (or improvement) of medications management systems. These indicators may help to coordinate care on both a system and a patient level and show a way to move from traditional practice to medications management.

References

1. Joint Commission on Accreditation of Healthcare Organization, *Primer on Indicator Development and Application*, Joint Commission on Accreditation of Healthcare Organization, Chicago, 1990.
2. Kohn, L.T., Corrigan, J.T., and Donaldson, M.S., *To Err Is Human: Building a Safer Health System*, National Academy Press, Washington, D.C., 2000.
3. Angaran, D.M., Quality assurance to quality improvement: measuring and monitoring pharmaceutical care, *Am. J. Hosp. Pharm.*, 48, 1901, 1991.
4. Angaran, D.M., Selecting, developing, and evaluating indicators, *Am. J. Hosp. Pharm.*, 48, 1931, 1991.

5. Anderson, G.M., Beers, M.H., and Kerluke, K. Auditing prescription practice using explicit criteria and computerized drug benefit claims data, *J. Eval. Clin. Pract.*, 3, 283, 1997.
6. Fitzgerald, L.S. et al., Reliability of a modified medication appropriateness index in ambulatory older persons, *Ann. Pharmacother.*, 31, 543, 1997 (see comments).
7. Samsa, G.P. et al., A summated score for the medication appropriateness index: development and assessment of clinimetric properties including content validity, *J. Clin. Epidemiol.*, 47, 891, 1994.
8. Ernst, P. et al., Risk of fatal and near-fatal asthma in relation to inhaled corticosteroid use, *JAMA*, 268, 3462, 1992.
9. Spitzer, W.O. et al., The use of beta-agonists and the risk of death and near death from asthma, *N. Engl. J. Med.*, 326, 501, 1992.
10. Hepler, C.D. and Strand, L.M., Opportunities and responsibilities in pharmaceutical care, *Am. J. Pharm. Educ.*, 53 (Suppl.), 7s, 1989.
11. Hepler, C.D., Regulating for outcomes as a systems response to the problem of drug-related morbidity, *J. Am. Pharm. Assoc.*, 41, 108, 2001.
12. Beers, M.H. et al., Explicit criteria for determining inappropriate medication use in nursing home residents, *Arch. Intern. Med.*, 151, 1825, 1991.
13. Beers, M.H., Explicit criteria for determining potentially inappropriate medication use by the elderly, *Arch. Intern. Med.*, 157, 1531, 1997.
14. Hanlon, J.T. et al., A method for assessing drug therapy appropriatness, *J. Clin. Epidemiol.*, 45, 1045, 1992.
15. MacKinnon, N.J., Risk Assessment of Preventable Drug-Related Morbidity in Older Persons (Elderly). Unpublished doctorial dissertation, University of Florida, Gainesville, 1999. Dissertation Abstracts International, 60, no. 06B (1999): p. 2633.
16. Faris, R.J., Explicit Definitions to Identify Preventable Drug-Related Morbidity in an Elderly Population and their Use as an Indicator of Quality in the Medication Use System. Unpublished doctoral dissertation, University of Florida, Gainesville, 2001. Dissertation Abstracts International, 62, no. 10B (2001): p. 4448.

8

Outline of a Medications Use System

> When our eyes see our hands doing the work of our hearts, the circle of Creation is completed inside us.
>
> **Michael Bridge**

Chapters 2 to 5 described medications use as a complex and potentially dangerous mode of care. The misuse of drug products causes preventable patient injury and death, even though those drug products have been demonstrated, by controlled clinical trials, to be safe and effective according to the food and drug law. This problem may well be endemic throughout the industrialized nations. The human and economic costs are staggering.

However, drug therapy is an essential part of health care. Clearly, underuse and nonuse of medications can be just as dangerous as adverse outcomes, so tightening safety requirements or avoiding medications use is not a reasonable alternative.

The complexity of the problem is demonstrated by the interplay of issues of access, cost, and quality, complicated by drug law and health insurance provisions. Medications use is further complicated by the interplay of clinical and personal values and the need for patients to cooperate in their own care. These are fundamental issues, part of the environment in which medications use takes place. They probably cannot be artificially simplified. The picture that emerges from Chapters 3 to 5 suggests that simple solutions may not be effective and, in fact, have not been shown to work.

If the "old" way is not satisfactory, what is the way forward? Obviously, drug therapy should receive more specific attention, both on the level of systems design and management and on the clinical level. Many patients (and many general practitioners) need specific professional assistance in managing drug therapy. This is approximately analogous to recognizing nursing care, dietetics, social work, and physical therapy as specific, yet integrated, parts of care.

The education and training of pharmacists is ideal preparation for this new professional role, as is their position in drug distribution. Specially trained clinical nurse practitioners could also provide the necessary clinical management services. Few pharmacists, nurses, or physicians have responded to this opportunity, so systems implementation is an open question. Simply adding another professional to the medications use process or changing professional roles may not be enough. A system of medications management should be designed at the clinical, practice, and program levels, and then managed. This virtually requires participation by government, health insurers, and managed care organizations.

This chapter will sketch the outlines of a safe and effective medications use system. *Medications use system* is a collective term for a *pharmaceutical care system* operated within a *medications management system*. Chapter 10 will describe a pharmaceutical care system in detail, and Chapter 11 will describe a medications management system in detail. The specific objectives of this chapter are fourfold:

- To introduce systems terminology, e.g., describe what is meant by terms like *a system* and *systems paradigm*
- To describe a generic system and to contrast it to a generic process
- To outline three models of an ideal pharmaceutical care system
- To describe how a medications management system contributes to improving the quality of a pharmaceutical care system

Pharmaceutical Care and Pharmaceutical Care System

Brodie et al. introduced the concept of *pharmaceutical care*, in its modern sense, in 1980:[1]

> Pharmaceutical care includes the determination of the drug needs for a given individual and the provision not only of the drug required but also the necessary services (before, during or after treatment) to assure optimally safe and effective therapy. It includes a feedback mechanism as a means of facilitating continuity of care by those who provide it.

Hepler described pharmaceutical care in 1987 as a covenantal relationship between a patient and a pharmacist. In that relationship, "the pharmacist performs drug use control functions … governed by awareness of and commitment to the patient's interests." Pharmacists should accept "as much responsibility for drug use control as [legal] authority will support."[2]

Hepler and Strand emphasized the importance of an orientation toward outcomes that had been implicit in the earlier definitions. They also addressed responsible relationships:

> Pharmaceutical care is the responsible provision of drug therapy for the purpose of achieving definite outcomes that improve a patient's quality of life.[3]

In these definitions, the word *care* was intended to invoke analogies to medical care and nursing care.[2]

To begin, we can define a *pharmaceutical care system* (PCS) as a set of elements (people, objects, decisions, and procedures) that directly interact *within a defined structure* to provide *pharmaceutical care* to individual patients (one patient at a time). We need this formal definition, but it is not very useful for introducing the important ideas of a PCS. To actually understand what a PCS is, we need to look at it in three mutually complementary ways: as principles of pharmaceutical care system design and operation, as relationships among the people who participate in it, and as systems flow diagrams. The three system models overlap, but emphasize different aspects of an ideal medications use system. All three are necessary to provide a complete outline. Later chapters will fill in some operational details.

Principles of Pharmaceutical Care

Weaknesses in the structure and process of medications use have been identified in the literature. Structural and environmental weaknesses that have been proposed as causes of preventable drug-related morbidity (PDRM) include:[4]

- Professionals' general knowledge and access to general information
- Time availability
- Interruptions
- Access to patient-specific data
- Professional understanding of practice roles
- Commercial concerns
- Economic and geographic barriers
- Inconsistent and ineffective prescribing influences (formularies, etc.)

Certain process failures and drug therapy problems (DTPs) repeatedly reappeared in the studies reviewed in Chapter 3. They were implicated as causes of PDRM:

- Inappropriate prescribing
- Patient noncompliance
- Overdose or underdose, either in general or for a specific patient
- Lack of a necessary drug therapy
- Failure to recognize symptoms of disease or early signs of adverse drug reactions, toxicity, treatment failure, etc.
- Delay in response, inadequate follow-up of clinical signs and symptoms
- Medication error

The next logical step would be to describe a system that could avoid or correct such process failures. This can be stated as five principles of pharmaceutical care system design and operation:

1. Patients need timely and accurate responses to signs and symptoms.

   This principle mainly refers to detection of, and response to, drug therapy problems. Pharmacist, patient, and physician each may have an essential part. This point is related to the cooperation principle, below.

   In addition, of course, patients need timely and accurate responses to their basic medical problems by the initiator (physician, nurse practitioner, etc.). Accurate assessment of medical problems (diagnosis) is prerequisite. The "right drug" for the wrong indication will not improve quality of life. Others involved in drug therapy often should defer to the physician's expertise. However, pharmacists, nurses, and patients may recognize problems related to undiagnosed disease or may see evidence that might change a diagnosis.

2. Patients need access to safe and cost-effective medications.

   There are at least five levels of access, as described in Chapter 5: national drug license laws; financial access, including insurance provisions and formulary inclusions; prescribing; inventory availability; and dispensing.

   - National drug licensing decisions (marketing controls) affect access. These are part of the *environment* of a medications use system and are beyond a professional's control in the treatment of a particular patient. (See Chapter 5.)
   - In the United States and other countries where patients are expected to share the cost of medications, some patients cannot afford the medications they need. An insurance program may discourage a patient's getting the medicine that the doctor would prefer. Financial access, in particular insurance provisions, is part of the environment of medications use, but a professional should recognize and resolve some problems involving formulary availability, prescription limits and exclusions, etc.
   - A prescriber must have responded to a patient problem before the patient can legally obtain prescription drugs and controlled substances. Underprescribing may be as important as overprescribing in influencing the overall cost and effectiveness of medications use. Appropriate prescribing should be responsive to the patient's needs. As obvious as this may seem, relatively few prescribing review programs are sensitive to problems such as failure to prescribe for a valid indication.

- A pharmacy must stock the medicine. This sounds obvious, but it is not. Some drug products are inconvenient, even dangerous to stock, because of their potential for theft. Others are expensive and slow moving.
- Dispensing and focused patient advice — correct dispensing requires more than a correctly filled prescription. In addition, when the patient or caregiver leaves the pharmacy, he should …

    Have received the medicine, with any necessary administration equipment, e.g., syringe and needles.

    Know how to use the medications and equipment properly.

    Know how to recognize key events relevant to DTPs (therapeutic success, therapeutic failure, emergence of adverse effects) and what to do if they appear (or fail to appear).

    Have consented to the therapy and accepted the necessity of cooperating in its use.

3. Patients need planned, professional follow-up.

This principle, closely related to the responsiveness principle, emphasizes the need for planned, continual monitoring throughout therapy. Systematic detection and response to drug therapy problems may be the most important area of possible improvement in medications use. Very briefly, pharmacists, nurses, or physicians should address the following questions for each new and repeat prescription:

- Is the patient actually getting the necessary medication? (This includes correct use of the product and associated devices.)
- Is the patient receiving the expected therapeutic effect in the expected or appropriate time interval?
- Is the patient experiencing any adverse effects such as toxicity, side effect, or adverse reaction?

Two levels of monitoring are necessary: facilitator (patient) and co-therapist (professional). Patient self-monitoring involves data or information. Sometimes the patient can correctly interpret information and correct therapy appropriately. An example of this would be "sliding scale" insulin dosage based on self-administered blood glucose determinations.

Monitoring drug therapy may often require professional judgment. For example, a patient may attribute dizziness to old age or fatigue when it may be a side effect that could develop into a DRM.[5]

Explicit therapeutic objectives should direct medications use. They are prerequisites to monitoring and patient participation in care. They provide the standard for judging the progress of therapy. Explicit objectives make these comparisons and judgments much more precise.

To be completely successful, monitoring should occur in the context of a system with the other four elements.

4. Patients need cooperation with and among health professionals.

   As with monitoring, two levels of cooperation can be discerned:

   Patient participation in care: Outcomes of drug therapy may be unpredictable and, in some cases, may depend on patients' beliefs, at least insofar as beliefs influence a patient's medication-taking behavior. Patients would often be in the best position to notice evidence that a therapy was or was not reaching the therapeutic objective. (See principle 3 above.) Therefore, professionals often need active cooperation by patients, especially for therapies that require close monitoring. The condition for full participation in care has been called *concordance,* which is, in effect, *informed consent to therapy,* the result of understanding the therapeutic objectives, negotiation, acceptance, and commitment to therapy.

   Interprofessional cooperation: The new roles in a pharmaceutical care system are not well recognized and may create ambiguity about who does what. Cooperation among professionals, especially when roles are not well established by tradition or accepted standards, can be facilitated by explicit (e.g., written) referrals. When referrals become frequent, they can be replaced by protocols and collaborative practice agreements so that the professionals who cooperate frequently know what to expect of each other.

   Cooperation among professional colleagues requires documentation and communication. Cooperating professionals must document decisions and actions to maintain coordination. Care given but not documented may sometimes harm the patient, e.g., if it leads to misdiagnosis or therapeutic duplication. The separate practice locations of community pharmacists and community physicians can be a problem, but it can be overcome by means of collaborative agreements and electronic communications.

5. Patients need medications use systems.

   The necessary processes of drug therapy should be organized into a system in which processes and interaction (cooperation) can occur consistently and predictably. These processes should be managed as a system. A medications use system comprises two subsystems: *pharmaceutical care systems* on the clinical level and *medications management systems* (MMSs) on the practice and program level.

   In a systems approach, many DRMs that do not seem preventable by simple solutions become preventable.[6,7] Some DRMs involve over-the-counter (OTC) medications, e.g., gastrointestinal bleeding from nonsteroidal anti-inflammatory drugs (NSAIDs), which underscores the importance of patient- rather than product-oriented care. Studies show that appropriate cooperative relationships between nurses, physicians, and pharmacists improve clinical outcomes, often at less total system cost. See, for example, the articles reviewed in Chapter 9. It also happens that most of the successful attempts to organize drug therapy systems have involved increased pharmacist–physician cooperation. Not enough is known about design details for a PCS, and it requires regular performance assessment through an MMS.

Relationships Diagram

A second way to describe a system is to show the relationships of the people within the system. (These were also described in Chapter 4.) The point of this exercise is to identify how the principles of pharmaceutical care (above) could be identified with existing professions, while avoiding the limitations of traditional roles. The principles suggest necessary functions, which can then be identified with professions that may be best suited to perform them effectively, safely, and efficiently. (See Figure 8.1.)

Initiators are professionals with legal authority to prescribe a needed regimen. Examples are general practice, primary care, and specialist physicians; physician's assistants; clinical nurse practitioners; dentists; podiatrists; and pharmacists, for OTC medications or who have prescribing authority.

Co-therapists are professionals who can cooperate with initiators and facilitators in providing and managing drug therapy after it has been initiated. Examples are pharmacists, physicians, clinical nurse practitioners, and physician's assistants. Pharmacists have the broadest legal authority to dispense and the best educational background for monitoring. Nurses may have the best training for patient communications.

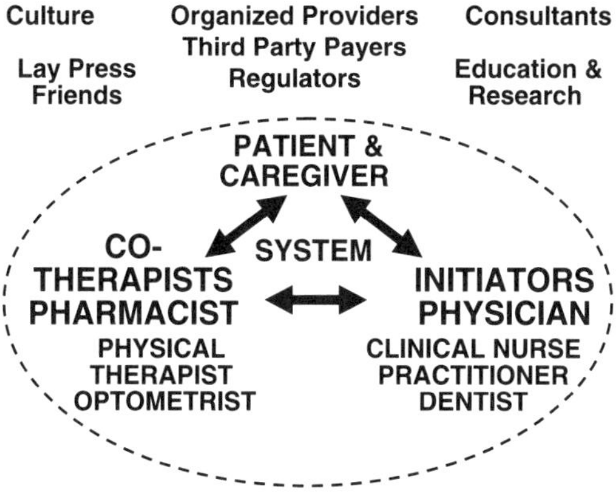

FIGURE 8.1
Relationships in a medications use system.

Facilitators assist with therapy. Most often this is the patient himself, if able and permitted to participate in his own care. Other examples include family caregivers, practical nurses, and nursing aides. In an institutional setting (where patients are usually not permitted to participate in their own care), a professional medication nurse might provide facilitation functions when administering medications and also perform as co-therapist when assessing outcomes.

Flow Diagrams: Pharmaceutical Care and Medications Management Systems

Having described principles of medications use and the basic functions of initiator, co-therapist, and facilitator, I will now describe how these functions may be organized into a system. To clarify how a pharmaceutical care system differs from a drug therapy *process*, and to clarify the contributions of both a pharmaceutical care system and a medications management system, consider three basic arrangements for providing drug therapy:

- A drug therapy process, in which we *hope* for the best
- A pharmaceutical care system, in which we *manage* for the best
- A medications management system, in which we improve or *maintain* the best

Drug Therapy Process

A *drug therapy process* is a set of elements (people, objects, decisions, and procedures) that directly interact to provide drug therapy to individual patients (Figure 8.2). This is familiar to almost everyone. It begins when a patient enters care. The *initiator* (physician, nurse practitioner) takes a history, reviews physiologic systems, assesses medical problems, and prescribes a treatment.*

The co-therapist (pharmacist, presumably) has minimal responsibilities — to dispense the medications and to advise the patient on their correct use.

The initiator may have a clear therapeutic objective, or not. A clear therapeutic objective is not essential to proceed in this process, because there will be no follow-up unless the patient initiates it. The pharmacist often does not recognize a need to know the purpose of the medication if he does not plan to initiate follow-up with the patient either. Patient advice about the use of

* A person who recognizes illness may consult a variety of people other than a physician, but for simplicity, this description is limited to prescription-only medications obtained after consultation with a physician or primary care nurse. Common variations, e.g., therapy with over-the-counter drugs obtained from pharmacies, are essentially similar and may have similar problems.

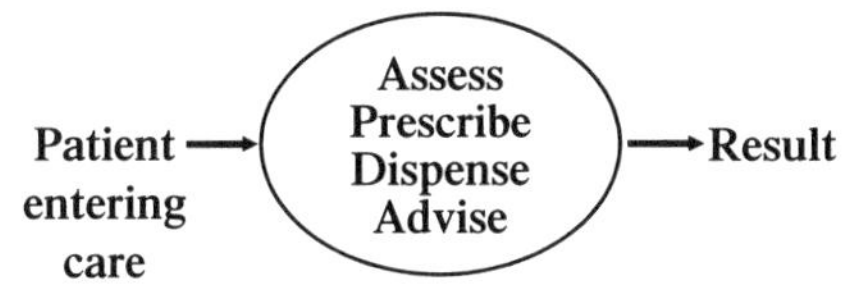

FIGURE 8.2
A drug therapy process (no feedback): hope for the best.

the medication is general, nonspecific, often as a standard leaflet describing the customary uses of the drug. The patient consumes the medicine, and we hope for the best.

Pharmaceutical Care System

Figure 8.3 outlines a systematic process of pharmaceutical care. Comparing Figures 8.2 and 8.3 will show the difference between a drug therapy process and a pharmaceutical care system.

A PCS is a patient-level system in which the initial steps are the same as those in a drug therapy process. In addition, feedback about patients is planned and carried out. To do that, therapeutic objectives are essential. Furthermore, the objectives have to be documented by the practitioners (so that they will not be forgotten) and communicated to the facilitators (patient and caregiver) and co-therapists (e.g., pharmacists).

As described by Hepler and Strand,[3] pharmaceutical care is a process for the systematic, cooperative management of medications use for individual patients. It includes monitoring of drug effects. In general terms, this may be understood as holistic patient assessment.

Pharmaceutical care should manage patient outcomes, not diseases. Within this holistic framework, however, the *responsible* provision of drug therapy for *definite outcomes* requires that periodic assessments include specific clinical indicators relevant to the management of drug therapy in that patient,

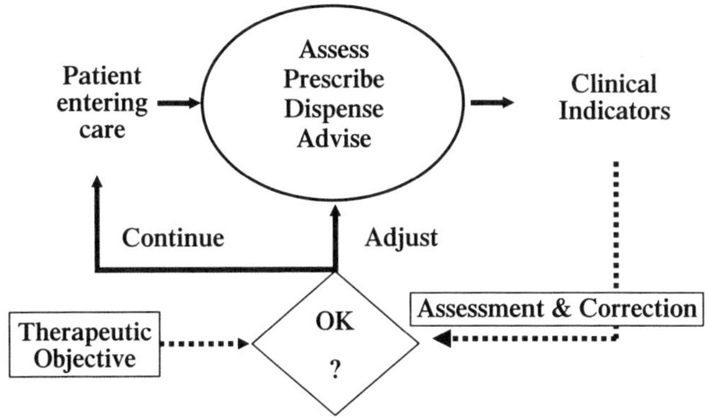

FIGURE 8.3
Systematic pharmaceutical care (with feedback): manage for the best.

for example, medications use, symptom status, and blood levels that fit the needs of the patient. Holistic care is consistent with concepts of quality of life, activities of daily living, and satisfaction with care (see Chapter 5). An indicator should never be taken to represent the whole picture. As the saying goes, we should manage therapy, not blood levels.

So, clinical indicators relevant to the therapeutic objective are selected for monitoring. These may be blood levels of drug, biochemical measurements like coagulation time, symptoms, quality of life, and activities of daily living.

A monitoring plan is formed for follow-up of the indicators at specific times, for example, improvement or remission of symptoms of asthma in 3 to 6 days following the initiation of inhaled steroids. If symptoms have not improved in 3 to 6 days, the cause has to be found and the therapy has to be corrected, or a therapeutic success may be impossible.

From the perspective of Chapter 3 (theory of DRM prevention), the objective of routine monitoring is to recognize drug therapy problems before they become DRM, and to resolve or refer them. Actually, this loop could be seen to describe an activity that would be carried out — with different emphases and levels of knowledge — by patients, pharmacists, physicians, and others.

For example, suppose a patient with asthma is not getting the customary effect from his beta-agonist metered-dose inhaler (MDI) and is using it more frequently. Two important possibilities are (1) the patient's inhaler technique has degraded and the patient is not getting the full dosage into his lungs; and (2) the patient's asthma is worsening, perhaps because of exposure to allergens. Possible resolutions of this problem would include: (1) assessing and correcting inhaler technique, (2) identifying and eliminating the new provocation from the patient's environment, or (3) initiating steroid therapy. Solution (1) is well within the pharmacist's province, solution (2) might benefit most from a visit by a nurse to the patient's home, and solution (3) requires a prescription from the patient's physician.

Medications Management System

Figures 8.2 and 8.3 should be familiar to most professionals as the "wrong" and the "right" way to provide drug therapy. They lay a foundation for Figure 8.4 and for what is to follow.

Figure 8.4 extends the idea of a pharmaceutical care system (which is a regular series of decisions and actions applied to one patient at a time) to a medications management system (which is applied to many pharmaceutical care systems at a time). Note that a pharmaceutical care system is drawn within the medications management system.

A *medications management system* is a controller for a group of drug use processes and pharmaceutical care systems. It indirectly controls the provision of drug therapy to many patients through many drug use processes and pharmaceutical care systems.

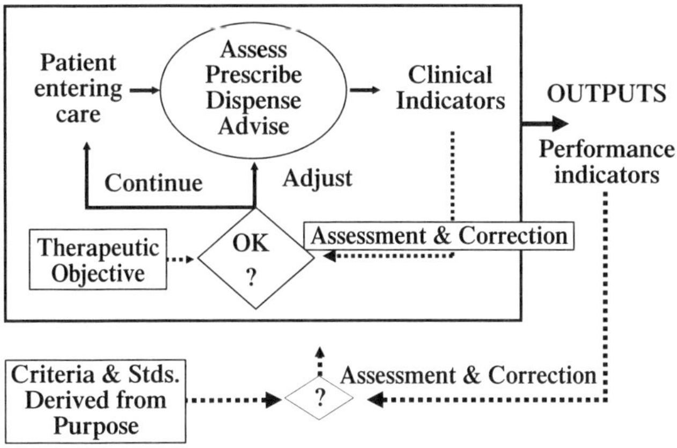

FIGURE 8.4
Medication management system (with performance feedback): maintain the best.

Note that pharmaceutical care (on a patient level) and medications management (on a practice or program level) are analogous activities. So, we can speak of *pharmaceutical care* within a *pharmaceutical care system* within a medications management system. The three activities are analogous, but not equivalent because they operate on different levels: patients, practices, and programs. An MMS uses performance indicators as pharmaceutical care uses clinical indicators. Furthering this analogy, a performance indicator is relevant to the performance of pharmaceutical care in many patients (perhaps in many practices) as a clinical indicator is relevant to the progress of drug therapy in a pharmaceutical care system.

The performance indicators are compared to benchmarks, standards, or other expectations. If the comparison suggests that system performance is not acceptable, problem solving (e.g., root cause analysis) is carried out and actions are taken to correct the suboptimal performance.

Performance Indicators

Just as pharmaceutical care should employ *clinical indicators,* which are observations of a patient's progress, medications management should employ *performance indicators,* which are observations of relevant aspects of system performance. (Performance indicators are described in detail in Chapters 5, 7, and 11.)

Chapter 7 described some performance indicators with the format of *patient outcome + process of drug therapy.* For example:

> A patient admitted to hospital or emergency department (ED) with decompensated congestive heart failure (CHF) when he/she had a history of CHF and no record of receiving an angiotensin converting enzyme (ACE) inhibitor.

Performance indicators in this format can link the MMS and the PCS. This is perhaps the most interesting application of these indicators. The MMS (Figure 8.4) is important for improving outcomes on a population level; however, the importance of the PCS (Figure 8.3) must also be stressed. General (program-level) problems shown by these indicators need not lead to imposition of general guidelines on the whole population. Individual patient assessment is still needed, and these indicators facilitate that.

Example

For example, in the Faris[18] study, described in Chapter 7, the positive predictive value of the process (no ACE inhibitor) for the outcome (cardiac decompensation) was about 75%. Not all heart failure patients without ACE inhibitors decompensated. So, on a population level, the indicator data tell us that many patients with decompensated heart failure did not receive a needed ACE inhibitor. They tell us that pharmacists and physicians should be more careful about that point in their patient assessments.

The population data do not address the possibility that other diseases, drugs, or patient problems may affect the decision to add an ACE inhibitor. They do not tell us which patients with heart failure who are not presently receiving an ACE inhibitor should receive one, or in what dose, or how they can be convinced to take the medicine, or how their side effects can be ameliorated while the therapeutic effect is optimized. The patients need pharmaceutical care for those decisions, preferably in a PCS, so that (a) all of the important issues will be addressed, and (b) all of the pharmacists they meet (at least in a given practice) will practice in a consistent pattern.

Summary

Proper medications use management requires three nested systems: a macrolevel MMS, a practice-level PCS, and patient-level pharmaceutical care, when possible with:

- Patient-specific *clinical indicators* that can help professionals follow the progress of therapy in a patient
- Outcome-linked *process indicators* that can help professionals identify patients who need better management
- Process-linked *outcome indicators* that can help identify widespread problems in medications management

Concepts in the Systems Paradigm

The detailed description of medications management systems is a specific application of systems thinking. It provides an opportunity to generalize the ideas. A generic system is defined simply as *an organized collection of potentially interacting elements capable of self-control toward common purposes.* System elements may include people, objects, equipment, decisions, techniques, and procedures. (This is a slight elaboration on the Institute of Medicine (IOM) definition given in Chapter 3.) The point of describing systems is to account for the interactions, control, and purpose — for example, to recognize necessary interactions and to make them more effective.

The word *system* also has colloquial meanings. For example, the health care "system" is widely recognized not to be a system at all, in part because its parts do not interact sufficiently and because it lacks self-control toward a common purpose. The language needed to clearly distinguish between colloquial almost-systems and technically ideal systems can be confusing and tedious. So, *systems paradigm* is used to denote the application of systems ideas to criticize a real process or to describe an *ideal* system. (See chapter appendix.)

System Model of Error Prevention

The importance of system structure, including communications (information flow), is shown by the following example. Suppose, for the sake of the example, that the steps in a *medications use process* comprise physician services, pharmacy services, and patient self-care (or family care), similar to the *process* shown in Figure 8.5.* The first three steps in Figure 8.5 (rectangles) are initiation functions. The physician assesses a patient's problem and writes a prescription. The patient takes the prescription to the pharmacist, who fills it. Then the patient takes it home and consumes it according to his interpretation of the label instructions and what he recalls of other directions for use. Now, suppose further that the risk of all drug therapy problems, including errors, is 1% at each step, and that there is very little communication between the steps in the process. To the extent that each person is unable to check on the progress of drug therapy, it is possible for the risk of DTPs at each step to accumulate, so the maximum risk of an unresolved DTP after one pass through the system is 3%. If some DTPs can recur over time, e.g., if the risk of a dispensing error recurs with each repeat prescription, the overall risk can increase with time.

In contrast, consider a PCS, such as in Figure 8.6. If each step has the information necessary to judge the correctness of the process up to that point, it can provide an independent check on the process. This would also require that the person performing each step take a critical attitude toward the workup to that point, and not assume that it is correct.

* Figures 8.5 and 8.6 show the same process and system as Figures 8.3 and 8.4, but they are less abstract and show more operational detail. Similarly, comparing them illustrates differences between a process and a system.

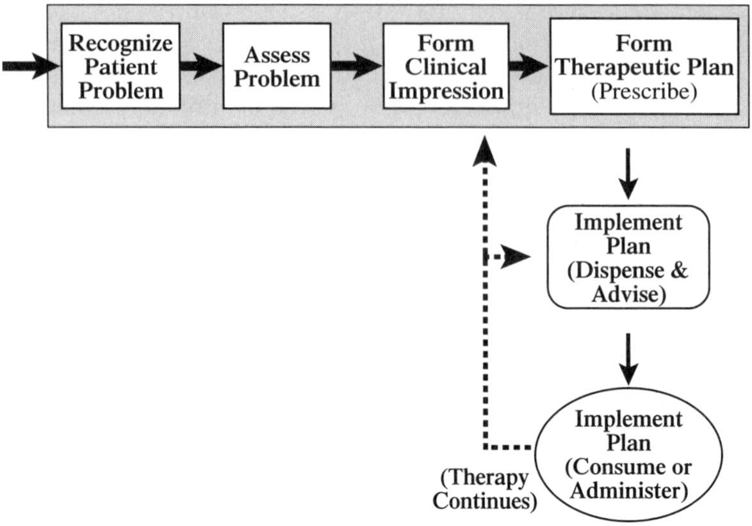

FIGURE 8.5
Another view of the medications use process (compare to Figure 8.6).

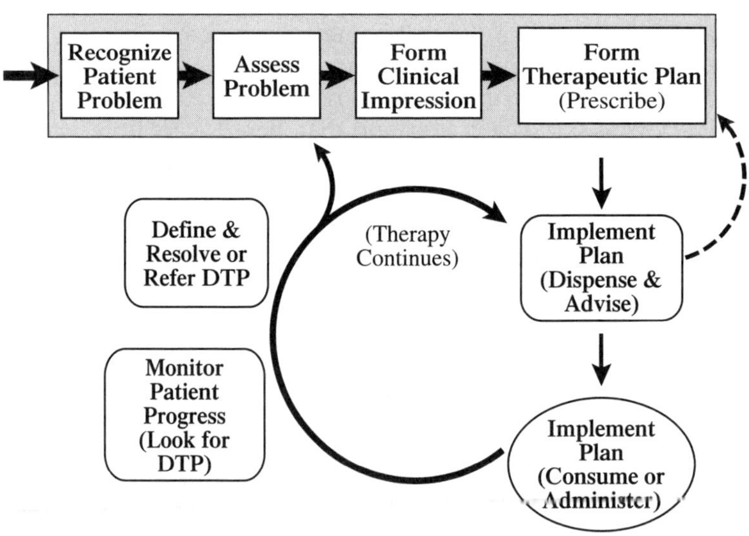

FIGURE 8.6
Another view of a pharmaceutical care system (compare to Figure 8.5).

Dispensing and advising, monitoring, and DTP recognition and resolution or referral (rounded rectangles) are co-therapist functions. The dotted line from *dispensing* back to *therapeutic plan* represents a feedback loop from pharmacist to prescriber. This is to illustrate the occasional need for a pharmacist to discuss therapy with the prescriber before filling a prescription.

Drug consumption or administration (ellipse) is a facilitating function. *Monitoring* should involve co-therapists and facilitators. The distinction between monitoring and managing care is important. It may be much easier to recognize a DTP than to resolve it. This essential step often does not require extensive physical assessment skills or theoretical knowledge, but it does require motive, opportunity, and systematic knowledge of what to look for and how to find it.

In contrast, the range of knowledge and skill required to interpret monitoring information, to define and resolve a problem, is much wider, and may require referral from pharmacist or nurse to physician, or from general practitioner to specialist. Furthermore, referral might be necessary when changes in therapy are required as part of a problem solution.

This is approximately the case of James Reason's[19] Swiss cheese model of error prevention (see Figure 8.7). In this model, an error at one point in a process may be stopped at a subsequent step in the process. In order to get to the patient, an error would have to escape detection and resolution at all subsequent steps. The arrows in Figure 8.7 are the latent injuries described in Chapter 3. The holes in the Swiss cheese are the latent failures. If the pharmacists and the patient are adequately informed and provide independent checks on the process, the risk of a prescribing error or DTP actually reaching the patient is the *product* of the three error probabilities, or .000001, 1 chance in 1 million. The risk of a pharmacist error reaching a patient is the product of two error probabilities, 1 chance in 10,000.

This model is an oversimplification, especially because it does not account for monitoring and feedback over extended periods (such as that shown in Figure 8.6). As the system continues to operate, the risk that an error will actually affect a patient may actually fall, from the same mechanism. A more detailed model will be described in the next chapter.

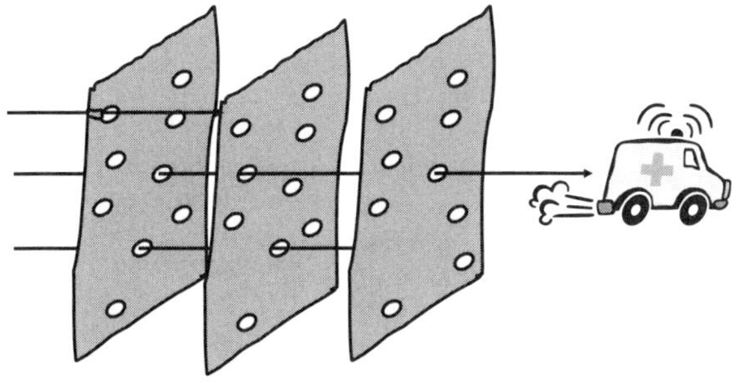

FIGURE 8.7
Swiss cheese (error filter) model (following James Reason).

The difference between 3 chances in 100 and 1 chance in 1 million provides a major theoretical argument for a cooperative pharmaceutical care system with adequate information flow.

Systems and Processes

One way to explain the systems paradigm is to contrast ideal systems and processes. Processes are more common than true systems, and so they are more familiar. Every system includes one or more processes, so one may see a process as an incomplete (or degenerate) system rather than as a fundamentally different structure.

A process more or less defines itself. For example, one follows a recipe by mixing ingredients in predetermined amounts and cooking by a predetermined method. In contrast, an ideal system is defined by six components: purpose, inputs, outputs, processes, control, and environment.

Systems tend to be seen in wholes, and interrelationships among parts are preserved. As a consequence, the systems paradigm simplifies by abstraction. Processes tend to be seen as component parts. The process or analytic paradigm attempts to simplify by specialization or analysis.

System Components

A generic system is shown in Figure 8.8. Note that a system comprises (a) a transformation (process), and (b) a control subsystem made up of a command signal, a comparator, and feedback.

A specific system is formally characterized by its purpose, inputs, outputs, processes, control (feedback, comparison, and correction), and environment. Purpose, control, and awareness of environment usually distinguish between processes and systems most clearly.

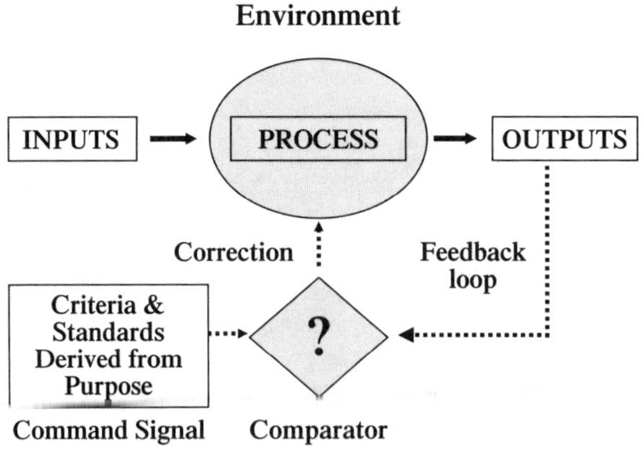

FIGURE 8.8
A generic system diagram showing components. Dotted line shows control information.

Inputs and Outputs

Both systems and processes convert inputs to outputs and are defined in part by means of those inputs and outputs. How one defines an input can influence the range of conceivable outputs, which in turn can limit the number of conceivable processes. The classic example is the difference between airlines and railroads. It has been said that railroads conceived of their output as a train ride. Airlines conceived of their output as transportation to a destination. This in turn influenced inputs (kinds of customers) and processes.

A medications use example is how the input to a pharmacy system is defined. If the input is understood as an unfilled prescription, the output will be a filled prescription. If the input is a patient with medications-related needs, the output may be a filled prescription and other actions designed to satisfy the patient's need.

Processes (Transformations)

Processes or transformations describe how a system converts inputs into outputs. In the process paradigm, the process is emphasized, indeed may be seen as defining the output. In the systems paradigm, the purpose or output (e.g., therapeutic objective) may define the process, but there is an assumption of *equifinality.* That is, in the systems paradigm, it is assumed that different processes can reach the same output.

This reduces reliance on defining process. For example, in a process view, there may be a specified drug of choice for a given therapeutic objective. In a systems view there may be many therapies available to achieve the same therapeutic objective.

In a process paradigm, the humans are expected to follow procedure. In a systems paradigm, humans allow a system to be teleological and provide flexibility (equifinality). This is explained further in the next section.

Purpose

Ideal systems are purposeful, in principle more purposeful and less procedural than processes. That is, systems tend to focus more on outputs than on procedural steps and more on the purpose or objective than "the book." Human systems, having purposes, are *teleological,* i.e., designed to seek one or more objectives consistent with a goal. Human systems are (or can be) *adaptive*; i.e., they can adapt to changing conditions by changing procedures and even by changing objectives (consistent with basic goals and values). In systems language, *first-order adaptation* involves managing processes to reach an external objective. *Second-order adaptation* involves changing processes (methods) to reach an external objective. *Third-order adaptation* is *reflective* — it involves changing the objectives themselves to reach a greater goal or changing goals to reach greater values.

It may seem odd to refer to a purpose as a component. This emphasizes the need for explicit (e.g., written) purpose, communicated to all actors in the system. One step in converting process-oriented management to system-oriented management is to make its purposes explicit and to communicate them, at least to all managers. Defining a purpose can be as simple as a detailed description of the intended output or as complicated as a general goal set.

For example, the management of a hamburger stand with minimally trained cooks may specify exactly how hot to make the griddle and how long to cook each side of a patty. The description of purpose, i.e., a palatable hamburger, might be merely implicit or ignored altogether. This makes the cooking process much simpler. However, if conditions are not as assumed by the instructions, e.g., if frozen patties were not thawed, the output from following the exact procedure would not be acceptable. By the way, this might not represent an *error* by the cook, who could explain that he "went by the book." Further, in a pure process, a recipe calls for specific ingredients to make a specific dish. If an ingredient is not available, the process may stop. If the hamburger recipe calls for Hamburger Bun XYZ from Vendor ABC, the process should stop if this bun is not available.

In an ideal system, a recipe is a means to an end, e.g., preparing hamburgers for sale, to make revenue and to satisfy customers. That purpose may take precedence over the recipe when necessary, and if an ingredient is not available, a substitute would be sought (e.g., buns from the market down the street). Of course, this book is not about hamburgers. The point of the example is standardization through procedure vs. standardization through defining outputs.

Control

The concept of *control* or cybernetics refers to how a system is regulated. Control of a system comprises a *feedback loop*, a *comparator*, and a *command signal*.

By definition, a procedure is not steered, although it may be subject to very exacting standards. Rather, a process is aimed and fired. Like a bullet (or a railroad train), a procedure runs in a particular direction regardless of whether it is actually approaching a particular goal. For example, a toaster may burn dry bread and undercook moist bread because it applies a certain amount of heat for a specific interval of time.

By definition, a system always contains provision for control, even if the system may not always remain in control.

A system may be controlled implicitly or explicitly. With *implicit* control, a system is designed to steer itself toward a goal and adapt to different conditions. It returns to the course automatically upon wandering off course. Corrections are small and immediate. An airplane (or cruise missile) autopilot is an example.

In contrast, with *explicit control*, an operator or manager outside the specific system gives orders to turn processes or components off and on. On the one hand, autopilots usually do a better job of flying an aircraft than a human pilot. On the other hand, they lack judgment and can fly into a mountain.

Feedback is information about outputs that is sent back to the processor through a logical unit (comparator). In systems design, positive and negative feedback have meanings different from their colloquial meanings. Positive feedback amplifies a part of the process, while negative feedback inhibits the process. Therefore, both are needed to maintain control of the system. However, because processes are set up to run, they often rely on negative feedback to keep them from running out of control. Too much positive feedback will overload a process and eventually destroy it unless stopped. The squeal heard when a microphone is held too close to a loudspeaker is an example.

A *comparator* compares the *command signal* (which is a standard or a description of what feedback from an in-control system should indicate) with the actual feedback. It or a human then decides if correction is needed — and if so, what correction is needed — and issues an instruction to the processor. (For example, think of an autopilot comparing apparent speed, position, and heading to preset values and then changing engine rpm or moving control surfaces.)

The *principle of requisite variety* states that unless a system has a response for every possible state that it can enter, it risks going out of control. Therefore, most complex systems are at some risk of going out of control. Generally, system design should include a means for recognizing when a system has entered a state from which it cannot return and a means of overriding the system. In computing, this is rebooting the computer. In health care, an example would be discontinuing all active orders when a patient enters intensive care and rewriting needed orders (i.e., restarting the system).

Environment

Inputs come from the environment, and outputs return to the environment. When designing or analyzing a system, the system boundary (between the system and the environment) can be drawn arbitrarily for convenient analysis. However, the environment should be taken into account. *Churchman's rule* defines a system environment as those things that can affect the system directly, but which the system cannot directly control. The list of possible environmental components is infinite, and naming them all is not necessary. However, the social, legal, and economic environment must always be considered when designing a system. For example, a health care finance program would be part of the environment of a health care provider. Its policies should be taken into account when designing or studying the provider's systems. (See Chapter 12.)

Connective Summary

This chapter presented five principles of pharmaceutical care, derived from the recurring problems described in Chapter 3. It also showed how the functions of pharmaceutical care can be organized into initiation, co-therapy, and facilitation. It sketched, in outline, an overall medications use system (MUS).

A patient is at the center of this sketch. The patient receives individualized pharmaceutical care, adapted from a general pharmaceutical care system model. The PCS is surrounded by one or more medications management systems. Each level controls (steers) some aspect of the level it surrounds by means of a therapeutic objective and specific data (indicators) from the inner level. Pharmaceutical care controls the therapy of the patient; the PCS controls the pharmaceutical care given to individual patients; the MMS controls the PCS.

Chapter 9 will continue the theoretical development of a MUS and will offer some empirical evidence in support of system theory. Chapters 10 and 11 will fill in detail to the sketch.

References

1. Brodie, D.C., Parish, P.A., and Poston, J.W., Societal needs for drugs and drug related services, *Am. J. Pharm. Educ.*, 44, 276, 1980.
2. Hepler, C.D., The third wave in pharmaceutical education: the clinical movement, *Am. J. Pharm. Educ.*, 51, 369, 1987.
3. Hepler, C.D. and Strand, L.M., Opportunities and responsibilities in pharmaceutical care, *Am. J. Pharm. Educ.*, 53 (Suppl.), 7s, 1989.
4. Hennessy, S., Potentially remediable features of the medication-use environment in the United States, *Am. J. Health Syst. Pharm.*, 57, 543, 2000.
5. Ray, W.A. et al., Psychotropic drug use and the risk of hip fracture, *N. Engl. J. Med.*, 316, 363, 1987.
6. Hallas, J. et al., Drug-related admissions to a department of medical gastroenterology: the role of self-medicated and prescribed drugs, *Scand. J. Gastroenterol.*, 26, 174, 1991.
7. Hallas, J. et al., Drug related events and drug utilization in patients admitted to a geriatric hospital department, *Dan. Med. Bull.*, 38, 417, 1991.
8. Herman, J., Beyond positivism: a metaphysical basis for clinical practice? *Med. Hypotheses*, 39, 63, 1992.
9. Jachuck, S.J. et al., The effect of hypotensive drugs on the quality of life, *J. R. Coll. Gen. Pract.*, 32, 103, 1982.
10. Eddy, D.M. and Billings, J., The quality of medical evidence: implications for quality and care, *Health Aff.*, 19, 1988.
11. Barr, D.P., Hazards of modern diagnosis and therapy: the price we pay, *JAMA*, 159, 1452, 1955.
12. Moser, R.H., Diseases of medical progress, *N. Engl. J. Med.*, 255, 606, 1956.
13. Porter, J. and Jick, H., Drug-related deaths among medical inpatients, *JAMA*, 237, 879, 1977.
14. Leape, L.L. et al., Systems analysis of adverse drug events: ADE Prevention Study Group, *JAMA*, 274, 35, 1995 (see comments).

15. Engel, G.L., How much longer must medicine's science be bound by a seventeenth century world view? in *The Task of Medicine: Dialogue at Wickenburg*, White, K.L., Ed., Henry J. Kaiser Family Foundation, Menlo Park, CA, 1988, p. 113.
16. Engel, G.L., The need for a new medical model: a challenge for biomedicine, *Science*, 196, 129, 1977.
17. Hepler, C.D. and Strand, L.M., Opportunities and responsibilities in pharmaceutical care, *Am. J. Hosp. Pharm.*, 47, 533, 1990.
18. Faris, R.J., Explicit Definitions to Identify Preventable Drug-Related Morbidity in an Elderly Population and their Use as an Indicator of Quality in the Medication Use System. Unpublished doctoral dissertation, University of Florida, Gainesville, 2001. Dissertation Abstracts International, 62, no. 10B (2001): p. 4448.
19. Reason, J., *Human Error*, Cambridge University Press, Cambridge, England, 1990.
20. Kuhn, T.S., *The Structure of Scientific Revolutions*, 3rd ed., University of Chicago Press, Chicago, IL, 1996.

Appendix: Medications Use Paradigms: Product, Process, or System

The manner or framework within which we happen to think about a scientific topic is an artifact of human intelligence rather than a "fact" of nature. This may be inconvenient, for example, when it makes knowledge less certain to someone who is looking for certainty. Regardless of such difficulties, however, it would be as big a mistake to suppose that there is one way to organize knowledge as it would be to believe in any other demonstrably false thing. It is necessary to discuss the framework of knowledge, especially because the conventional (and perhaps unexamined) manner of thinking about medications use is no longer as useful as it once seemed.

Paradigms

Thomas Kuhn[20] pointed out in his groundbreaking book, *The Structure of Scientific Revolutions*, that scientific research and thought are defined by paradigms, or conceptual worldviews, comprising formal theories based upon accepted experimental results and methods. He suggested that despite all efforts at objectivity, scientists typically accept a prevailing paradigm. Kuhn argued that the paradigm determines the kinds of experiments scientists perform, the types of questions they ask, the way they interpret results, and the problems they consider important. Eventually, efforts to extend knowledge within a paradigm may generate insoluble theoretical problems or experimental anomalies that expose a paradigm's inadequacies or contradict it altogether. This accumulation of difficulties triggers a crisis that can only be resolved by a "scientific revolution" in which a new paradigm, once disdained and doubted, replaces the old one.

A shift in the paradigm alters the fundamental concepts underlying research and inspires new standards of evidence, new research techniques, and new pathways of theory and experiment that are radically discontinuous with the old ones. A recent example of a paradigm shift was the "physics earthquake" that led to reinterpretation of Newtonian mechanics and its partial replacement by quantum physics and general relativity.

Academic Disciplines

Within paradigms, scientific knowledge is customarily organized into classic academic disciplines, e.g., physics, chemistry, biochemistry, physiology, pharmacology. Such disciplines are usually thought of as hierarchical. In this example, we would recognize that pharmacology rests on physiology and biochemistry, which rest on chemistry and physics. There are hierarchies within disciplines as well.

TABLE 8.1

Three Medication Use Paradigms

Paradigm	Product Paradigm	Process Paradigm	System Paradigm
Dimension			
Model of drug therapy	Prescribing and consuming drug products	Discrete ordered steps; each step assigned to an occupation or institution; little interaction	Interdependent functions that may cross occupational boundaries; interaction (e.g., feedback)
Scientific bases	Simple biomedical (clinical pharmacology)	Biomedical (clinical pharmacology) + mass communications	Biopsychosocial (biomedical + social psychology)
Objective of therapy	Simpler; objectively measurable	(Transitional)	Complex, objective and subjective; e.g., quality of life
Issues in quality	Safety, efficacy, product cost	(Transitional)	Risk, effectiveness, total system cost
Representative term for an adverse drug event	ADR	(Preventable) adverse drug events	PDRM
Cause of adverse events	Disease of medical progress; intrinsic product characteristics	Negligence, error; failure of a person, occupation, or institution	System failure; malfunction of multiple system components
Likely response to adverse event	Identify product causing ADR; remove product or change labeling, e.g., chloramphenicol	Identify person responsible; remove or punish person, e.g., change practice privileges	Find root cause and correct system deficiency; follow up correction and modify further as necessary
This view is the philosophical basis of …	Drug licensing law, product liability, adverse drug reaction reporting programs	Professional regulation; quality assurance	Quality improvement
Research approach	Phase III controlled clinical trial of drug product	Epidemiology, postmarketing surveillance of drug product	Prospective clinical trial of system arrangements
Independent variable	Drug or therapeutic class	Patient, provider	System, patient

Specialization and reductionism are hugely effective and successful ways to organize knowledge. However, there are severe limits to learning more and more about less and less. Attempts to resynthesize such knowledge leave gaps in understanding, just as attempts to build a creature out of body parts result in a nonfunctioning collection of sewed-together parts rather than an intact organism. Herman has called life "a temporary suspension of the Second Law of Thermodynamics."[8] Physics does not quite explain chemistry, chemistry does not quite explain biology, biology does not quite explain pharmacology and psychology, and so on.

Paradigms of Medications Use

Attempts to describe how drug therapy works, including the phenomenon of adverse outcomes of drug therapy, seem to fall into three categories, each with its own (implicit or explicit) paradigms and disciplines. (See Table 8.1.) Perhaps ways of thinking about drug therapy do not rise to the level of Kuhn's paradigms, but they span the boundary between the biomedical model and the biopsychosocial model, which probably is a legitimate paradigm shift that is occurring in our time. Further, there do seem to be underlying perspectives and frameworks in understanding medications management, they do seem to influence what questions are asked and how evidence is interpreted, and they do seem to replace one another, just as Kuhn described.

Three such paradigms are summarized in Table 8.1 and described below, in order of increasing complexity, and approximately from oldest to newest. There is hardly any published philosophical discourse about the first two paradigms, so I have tried to describe them based on my interpretation of how people write about drug therapy and descriptions of programs intended to improve it.

Product Paradigm

This view of drug therapy focuses on the drug product. It tends to disregard both patient-specific details and the environment in which medications are used. It is consistent with the biomedical model of physical and biological science, approximately the content of "clinical pharmacology," i.e., the interaction of the drug molecule (as formulated into a drug product) and a *typical* human. In this paradigm, therapeutic objectives emphasize objectively observable consequences such as physiologic response to therapy, e.g., concentration of drug in blood or serum, anatomical or biochemical data. An example of an outcome in this paradigm would be a patient's diastolic blood pressure response to antihypertensive therapy.[9] An example from the surgical literature in this paradigm would be to define the outcome of angioplasty based on whether the artery remained open.[10] (Compare to outcomes in system paradigm, below.) Familiar terms consistent with this paradigm are *disease management, therapeutic drug monitoring* (TDM), and *physical assessment*.

The value of a drug product is defined, in this view, in terms of safety and efficacy (i.e., clinical effect compared to placebo in a controlled clinical trial). Quality is defined in this paradigm as a function of value per unit of product cost. Chapter 3 described some aspects of this view, which sees drugs as two-edged swords and adverse outcomes as unavoidable, unintended "diseases of medical progress"[11,12] *In other words, the product paradigm sees adverse drug reactions (ADRs) as the largely unavoidable imperfections of the drug itself.* The product paradigm was prevalent in the late 1950s and early 1960s, although it survives as the philosophical basis of drug law, product liability litigation, and most ADR reporting programs. Typical studies in the product paradigm are controlled clinical trials of drug products. They tend to report ADRs by drug or by therapeutic class. They find relatively few preventable adverse outcomes.[13] In this view, patient assessments are mostly physical assessments for diagnostic purposes.

Process Paradigm

In this view, drug therapy is seen to occur through a series of steps, for example, manufacturing, licensing, promoting, prescribing, dispensing, advising, and administering or consuming drug products. This paradigm adds behavioral sciences, especially those related to mass communications, to the "clinical pharmacology" emphasis of the product paradigm. The justification for people's attempts to improve steps in the medications use process seems to come from within a process viewpoint; i.e., an assumption that improving one step in the medications use process should improve the outcome. Perhaps if every step were carried out correctly, a successful result would be likely, if not certain. Accordingly, the process paradigm tends to treat professions and other occupations as having clearly distinct functions based on relatively specialized knowledge. People who observe medications use from this view, e.g., for outcome studies or for performance evaluations, tend to see PDRM as the result, in part, of an error or failure in a component step in the process (but they seldom see failures involving interactions among components). Components mentioned most often as the causes of PDRM are drug product regulation (e.g., new drug approval), prescribing, administration and patient compliance. Consistent with an occupational view of professional competence, there is a tendency to identify error at a particular step in the drug use process and to fix responsibility for failure on the person, profession, or institution in charge of that step.

This may be the prevailing contemporary view. The process paradigm is the implicit basis of professional licensure, competence standards, most malpractice litigation, and the currently popular medical error literature, such as the IOM report. The approach is occupationally distinct. For example, each profession has standards for professional competence. However, from this perspective, standards for the *process itself* are not necessary. For example, if a profession attempted to establish standards for many steps in the drug use process, say prescribing, dispensing, and consuming, it might appear as professional encroachment. There would be no enforcement mechanism. Studies within the process paradigm tend to use epidemiological approaches, e.g., postmarketing surveillance applied to drug products. Patient assessments in the process paradigm emphasize physical measures. Their rationale is principally diagnosis and therapeutics, e.g., therapeutic drug monitoring of blood levels and to check on the performance of previous steps.

System Paradigm

This paradigm may be the future for our understanding of medications use. In this view, drug therapy occurs through a dynamic and goal-oriented drug therapy system in which the components may interact with each other.[3,14] The scientific framework of the system paradigm is the biopsychosocial model.[15,16] In comparison to the process paradigm, the system paradigm deemphasizes mass communications and emphasizes individual and small group behavioral sciences. Also, the systems paradigm may emphasize specific functions more than general occupations. In the *biopsychosocial* paradigm, therapeutic objectives include functional assessments and subjective evaluations by the patient. For example, in the biopsychosocial paradigm, outcomes of antihypertensive therapy would include quality of life; outcomes of angioplasty would include measures of pain and activities of daily living, e.g., ability to walk.[10] Terms consistent with the biopsychosocial paradigm are therapeutic outcomes monitoring, patient assessment, activities of daily living, and quality of life.

Value is defined in terms of effectiveness in actual use (rather than under a clinical research protocol) in comparison to other therapeutically active agents (rather than placebo). Quality is defined as value per dollar of total cost of providing therapy. Studies using a systems model find that adverse outcomes are often preventable because they are caused in part by the failure of more than one component step or by inadequate communication of information among system components. There is less of a tendency to find error or to fix responsibility on an individual, and more interest in identifying and correcting root causes.

This paradigm is familiar in manufacturing industries and appears to be increasing in popularity in health care. It seems to be the philosophical basis of the family practice movement and some health care accreditation programs, e.g., the Agenda for Change of the Joint Commission on Accreditation of Healthcare Organizations (JCAHO). Studies tend to use quasi-experimental approaches in which systems rather than drug products are compared.

Pharmaceutical care is based on the systems paradigm. The goal of pharmaceutical care is to narrow the range of actual patient outcomes and to move that range "upward" in the scale of beneficence, reducing harm and increasing good. Its objective has been stated as drug therapy to achieve definite outcomes intended to improve a patient's quality of life.[17]

The distinction between illness (or sickness) and disease is related to the distinction between the biomedical and biopsychosocial paradigms. *Illness* is often used to denote a patient's subjective experience of being or feeling sick. *Disease* is used to refer to an objective, biologically recognizable abnormality. The biomedical model is concerned with diseases. (See Chapter 4.)

In contrast, the biopsychosocial model sees illness as the primary experience, while disease is the label that professionals give to the inferred cause of an illness. It is obvious (but sometimes ignored) that diseases are inferences, not direct experience. Patients can feel ill when they have no identifiable disease, and they can have a disease without feeling ill. Therefore, health-related quality of life can depend more in the short term on the experience of illness than on the presence of disease. Finally, many patients may use health care resources (and evaluate quality) based at least as much on how they feel (illness) as on biomedical criteria (scientific management of disease).

9

Effect of Pharmaceutical Care Systems on Outcomes and Costs

The eye sees only what the mind is prepared to comprehend.

Henri Bergson

Chapter 8 presented a simple theoretical argument in support of expanded pharmacist and patient responsibility in medications use. The argument was based on the Swiss cheese metaphor. It showed that safer and more effective drug therapy might be possible if (a) essential information were regularly communicated from step to step in the medications use process, and (b) pharmacists and patients were responsible for evaluating selected aspects of therapy.

It showed that if people at successive steps in the medications use process can detect and resolve drug therapy problems, the risk to the patient is geometrically reduced. The example showed that a 1% rate of prescribing drug therapy problems (DTPs) and errors could theoretically be reduced to a 1 in 1 million chance of affecting a patient. A 1% dispensing error rate could theoretically be reduced to a 1 in 10,000 risk to the patient.

This chapter will first develop a somewhat more elaborate model in which each step can create as well as detect DTPs (including, but not limited to, errors). This model will be used as the basis of a simulation of medications use over an extended time period, because many of the medicines known to cause drug-related morbidity (DRM) do so over time. The second part of the chapter will review some studies that compared medications use systems (MUSs) to the traditional drug use process. These studies do not prove the superiority of medications use systems, but they add empirical support to the theory developed here. The theory and evidence are sufficient to guide and encourage projects to develop safer and more effective medications use systems.

Simulation Model of Medications Use

Simulation is a technique of mathematical modeling, the use of a numerical model to represent a dynamic process. Given initial conditions, parameters, and exogenous variables, a simulation is run (almost always on a computer) to represent selected aspects of the behavior of a real system over a period of time. This simulation is like an experiment in which a real system can be studied and manipulated, except in a simulation we manipulate and study a numerical representation of the system. This allows us to study a system that is impossible to study in reality. Computer and video games are familiar examples of simulations.

Simulations are useful for developing hypotheses, especially when the reality is impractical to create for study purposes (e.g., too complex or expensive, too dangerous to manipulate, etc.). For example, engineers commonly simulate the behavior of structures (bridges, buildings, etc.) in a variety of weather conditions.

An ideal pharmaceutical care system would be such a system (expensive to construct for an experiment and dangerous to manipulate for study). Therefore, simulation can be used to study the behavior of such a system before one is actually constructed. Some simulation models can be thoroughly validated against the real systems they were designed to represent. Such simulations can sometimes be used to predict real behavior. Other simulations are more heuristic, used only to explore possibilities and to direct the design of real systems. Our simulation falls into the latter group. It will be adjusted by comparing it to some real-world data and then tested by comparing it to other real-world studies of pharmaceutical care systems.

The simulation model described in this chapter is intended to simulate the safety and effectiveness of a pharmaceutical care system like the ones shown in Figures 3.2, 8.3, and 8.6. The model has two main parts, corresponding to (a) start-up — the beginning of drug therapy (initial prescribing, dispensing, and drug taking), and (b) maintenance — medications use by patients over time, with return visits to the physician and pharmacist.

The events of interest in the model are drug therapy problems. The model simulates their origination and extinction.* Part (a) is simulated by one pass through a deterministic model. Part (b) takes the results from part (a) and calculates outcomes with a Markov simulation.

The model is built up from a very simple basic unit, as shown in Figure 9.1. A patient enters care with one DTP, for example, an untreated indication for drug therapy. The physician then corrects the DTP (probability pc1) or does not correct it (probability 1-pc1), and either creates a new DTP or not (with probabilities pdtp and 1-pdtp).

* Within the formalism of the birth and death of DTPs, patient assessment and clinical impression (diagnosis) appear only in terms of DTP, e.g., an unrecognized, untreated indication.

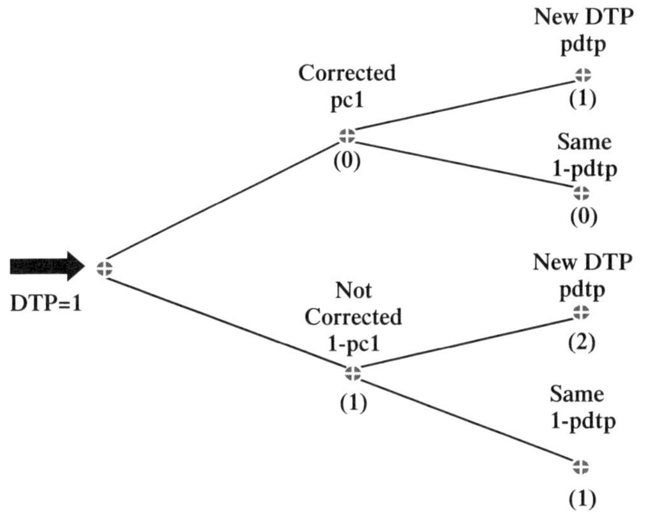

FIGURE 9.1
The basic tree structure used in simulation part 1.

For example, a patient enters care with untreated pain. The probability pc1 that the initiator will diagnose and treat the pain is arbitrarily set at 99%, so the complementary probability (that he will not diagnose and treat the pain) is 1%. If he treats it (top branch), the probability pdtp that he will treat it with an appropriate regimen is (arbitrarily) 99%, and the probability is 1% that he will not. If he does not treat the pain (lower branch), he may still create another DTP, for example, by prescribing a drug for which there is no valid indication. There are three *terminal states* after the assessment and prescribing phase: 0, 1, and 2, corresponding to a patient's leaving the encounter with zero, one, or two DTPs.

In developing the model for the part 1 (start-up) simulation, the basic unit was repeated for the dispensing and advising phase. In effect, the tree of Figure 9.1 was replicated at each of the four nodes, so there were 16 terminal nodes after the second phase. The tree of Figure 9.1 was then replicated for each of the 16 terminal nodes, producing 64 terminal nodes to represent system states after the patient has picked up the medicine, returned home, and begun to consume it.

The output of the start-up simulation is a probability distribution of DTPs. (The model ignores the probability that a patient may develop a DRM immediately after consuming the medicine, e.g., have a severe allergic reaction.)

Figure 9.2 shows an example of the output of a start-up (part 1) simulation. In this example, 63% of patients will have no DTP shortly after they begin to take a new prescription, 32% will have one DTP, and about 5% will have two DTPs. A very few (0.1%) may leave this part with three DTPs. The probabilities of creating and correcting DTPs in the simulation were based on realistic data, and the mean of the distribution in Figure 9.2 agrees with reported data from Cipolle et al.[1]

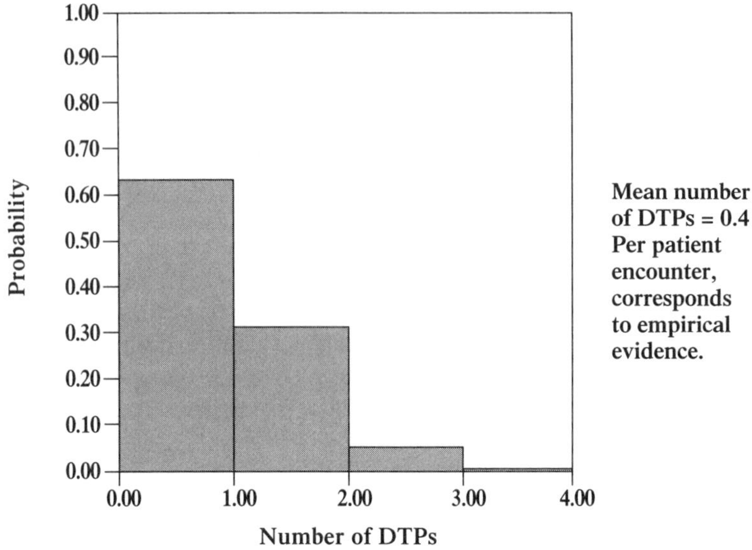

FIGURE 9.2
Distribution of DTP output from simulation part 1.

Part 2 of the simulation (maintenance) represented medication-taking behavior over an extended time. A population of patients is assumed to have the distribution of DTPs created in the start-up simulation (Figure 9.2). The patient is assumed to visit his physician and pharmacist each month. At each visit, a probability was set that any existing DTP would be corrected, and another probability was set that a new DTP could be created, by the physician, pharmacist, and patient.

The logic of the maintenance simulation was similar to the basic logic for the start-up, shown in Figure 9.1: in each time period, a patient can have a DTP corrected (or not) and have a new DTP created (or not). The probability of developing a new DTP is set at 13%, to correspond to data reported by Cipolle et al.[1] The probability of correcting a DTP was varied, as will be explained below.

The maintenance simulation does not end after one pass. Rather, a new "month" begins. Each patient's state at the end of the previous month (his number of DTPs) and a transition probability table determine whether he will develop a DRM. Table 9.1 shows the probabilities of a DRM, given a patient's state at the end of a month. For example, if a patient has a DTP, his risk of a DRM is 20%, but if he has four DTPs, his risk is 100%. If a patient has a DRM, it is counted and his state is reset to zero DTPs, as if he had received a thorough, expert drug therapy review. Nobody in this model is allowed to be permanently injured from a DRM or to die (unlike a video game). Figure 9.3 shows part of the tree. (States for zero and one DTP are not shown but are similar to the states shown. The DRM state jumps only to the zero DTP state.)

TABLE 9.1

Probabilities of Developing a DRM, Given Number of DTPs[a]

Number of DTPs	Probability of DRM
0	0
1	.2
2	.45
3	.75
4	1

[a] Assumption for a Markov simulation.

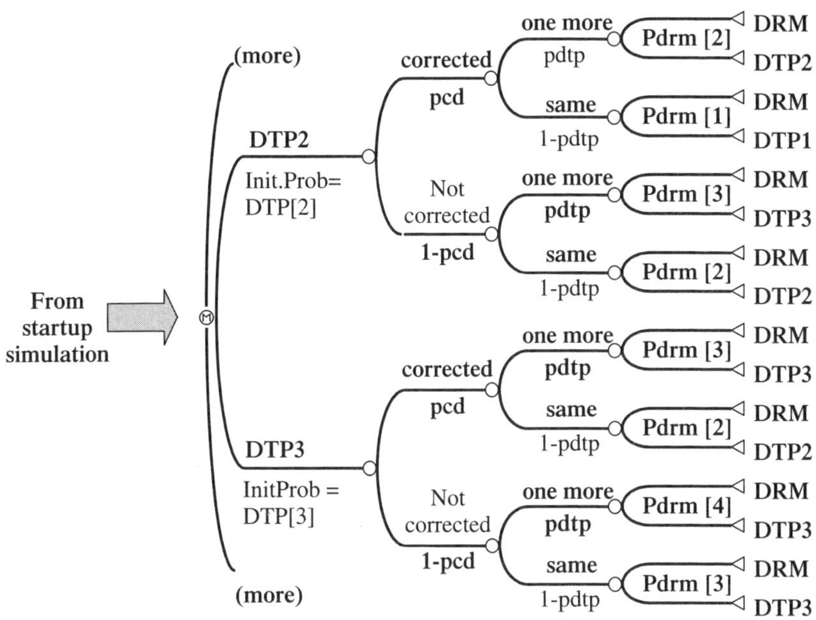

FIGURE 9.3
Markov simulation tree used in simulation part 2.

The simulation was run for 6 "months" of simulated time. The result of the simulation was a number (or percentage) of simulated patients who developed DRMs. In addition, a total cost function could be derived.

Simulation Results: Total Cost Function and Risk of DRM

Figure 9.4 shows the output of the simulation, when pcd = 0.80 (80% chance of resolving a DTP). Ten percent of the simulated population had one DRM in 6 months and 1% had two. The average number of DRMs per patient in 6 months was therefore 0.12, with a standard deviation of 0.35. This average may be somewhat higher than empirical studies have shown, but it is not so discrepant as to invalidate the simulation for the purposes that follow.

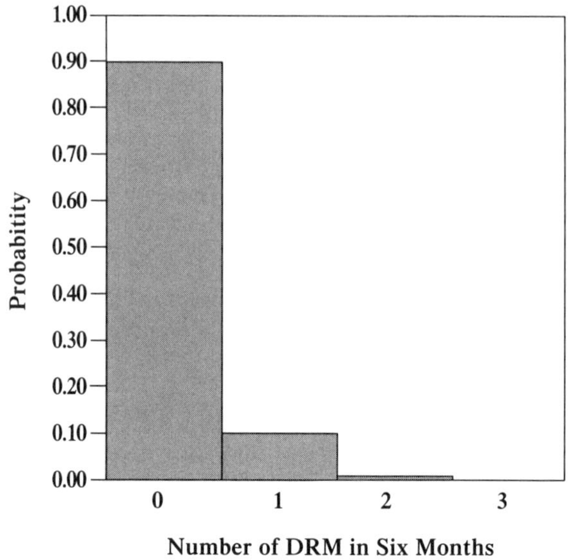

FIGURE 9.4
Distribution of DRM output from simulation part 2.

For example, Faris[17] found a preventable DRM (PDRM) rate of about 6% per year for the 52 indicators they studied. PDRMs are typically about half of all DRMs, so the comparable prevalence is 12% per year. The PDRMs in the Faris and Hepler study were severe, requiring emergency department visits or hospitalizations. Additional DRM types that were not represented by one of their indicators and some less severe DRMs would reduce the discrepancy even further.

In the simulation, the risk of DRM would depend on three probabilities:

- The probability that a new DTP will develop in a time period — pdtp
- The probabilities of developing a DRM from a DTP (as given in Table 9.1)
- The probability of resolving a DTP during a time period — pcd

The value of pdtp used in the simulation leading to Figure 9.4 approximates reported data. A "typical" risk of developing a DRM from a DTP is not known, and the data in Table 9.1 are assumed. The probability of resolving a DTP would depend to a great extent on system design, but a rate of 0.8 was arbitrarily chosen to produce Figure 9.4. (The value of pcd will be varied in the next section.)

The relationship between risk of DRM and pcd would be important in designing a system. The value of pcd was varied from 0 to 1 and was plotted against the risk of DRM. This is the curved, dashed line in Figure 9.5. As expected, the risk of DRM is highly sensitive to the probability of resolving

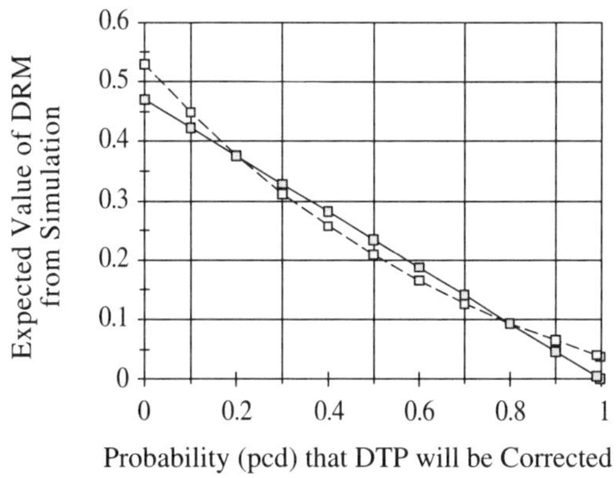

FIGURE 9.5
Mean risk of DRM vs. probability of correcting a DTP.

DTPs. When very few DTPs are resolved, a bit more than half of all patients will have a DRM in 6 months.

To describe the relationship further, a straight line was fit to the data. The intercept of the fitted line, 0.48, corresponds to the risk of DRM when no DTPs are corrected. The slope of the fitted line shows the approximate rate of reduction in DRM risk as the percentage of corrected DTPs increases. (The straight line is a reasonable fit — it underestimates the simulated risk of DRM by about 5% at the extremes.) Given the assumptions of the model, the risk of DRM is approximately related to pcd by the following equation:

$$\text{risk of DRM} = R(\text{pcd}) = 0.48 - 0.47 * \text{pcd}$$

In words, the risk of DRM when no DTPs are being resolved during care is about 50% and is reduced by about half a percent for each 1% increase in the rate of resolving DTPs.

Total Cost of Care

To study the relationship between pharmaceutical care and the total cost of care, it is necessary to construct an equation that shows the contribution to total cost of care that was due to medications use. This would be given by the sum of three components: (1) the cost of drugs and dispensing, (2) the cost of correcting DRM, and (3) the cost of preventing DRM (recognizing and resolving DTPs). The cost of drugs and dispensing is largely independent of the other two costs and would not affect the value of the optimal expenditure on DRM prevention. So, we can write the cost function (excluding cost of drug products and distribution) as

$$\begin{aligned} C' &= \text{cost of correcting DRM} + \text{cost of preventing DRM} \\ &= C_1\,[R(\text{pcd})] + C_2(\text{pcd}) \end{aligned}$$

where C' is the cost of medications use exclusive of drug product and dispensing cost; C_1 is the cost of correcting a DRM; C_2 is the cost of resolving all DTPs for 6 months; R(pcd) is the risk of DRM, expressed as a function of pcd (the relationship for this simulation example is given above as approximately 0.48 – 0.47 * pcd); and pcd is the probability that a DTP will be resolved.

C_2(pcd) involves a simplifying linear assumption. Given that an intervention to identify and resolve DTP costs C_2, C_2 (1) is the cost of resolving all DTPs, C_2 (0.5) is the cost of resolving half of all DTPs, C_2 (0) is a zero cost for resolving no DTP, and so on. This assumes, in effect, that the costs of detecting and resolving one DTP is the same whether 10 or 90% of DTPs are detected and resolved.

The cost of correcting DRM should *decrease* as pcd increases. The cost of preventing DRM should *increase* with increasing values of pcd. Therefore, a plot of C' vs. pcd should have a shape somewhat like the letter U, with a minimum cost corresponding to the optimum expenditure to prevent DRM. The exact shape and location of the minimum cost point should depend on the values of C_1 and C_2.

Figure 9.6 shows an example for C_1 = \$1000 and five different values for C_2 (\$180, \$240, …). The C' values corresponding to pcd = 0 estimate the total cost contribution when no DTPs are resolved. This corresponds to a complete neglect of DTPs, i.e., ineffective monthly follow-up visits to the physician, clinical nurse, or physician's assistant; no monitoring from the pharmacist when prescriptions are refilled; and ill-informed or uncooperative patients or other facilitators. The C' values corresponding to pcd = 1 estimate total costs when all DTPs are resolved by a co-therapist or facilitator, costing the full value of C_2 for 6 months.

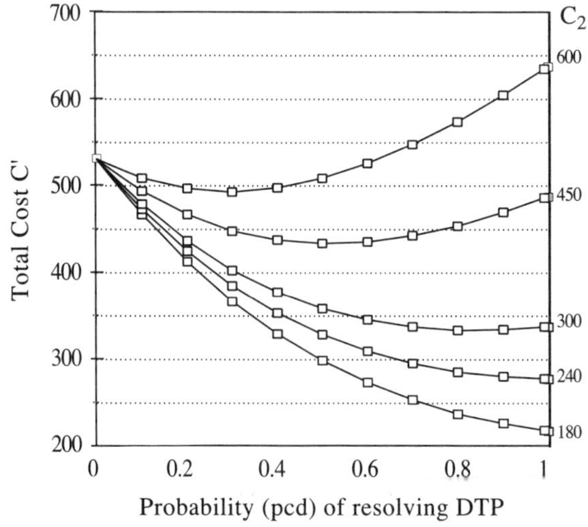

FIGURE 9.6
Total cost function C' vs. probability of resolving DTPs.

The analysis shows that constructing a medications use system can increase cost efficiency, while improving outcomes, over a rather wide range of possible expenditures. For example, if a completely effective monitoring program could be established and operated for $300 or less ($50 per patient per month), it would be cost-effective to resolve all DTPs. If a completely effective monitoring program could be established and operated for $450 (about $75 per patient per month) or less, it would be cost-effective, compared to no monitoring, to resolve all DTPs.

If a completely effective monitoring program would cost more than $300 (or if the average cost of correcting a DRM were less than $1000 per event), then the cost curve would have a minimum at pdtp < 1. In other words, resolving some DTPs would decrease total costs, but resolving more than that would increase total costs. This analysis allows us to estimate the incremental cost of improving monitoring beyond the optimal point. It is the incremental cost, not average cost that should be used in decision making. Intentionally designing systems that were not fully effective might make financial sense, but it would be highly questionable from an ethical standpoint.

This analysis ultimately depends on the structure and assumptions that went into the simulation. Nonetheless, the model and the analysis do appear robust enough at least to establish the need for more inquiry into effective medication system design and operations.

Summary

This simulation tested a model representing a pharmaceutical care system. The logic of the model was straightforward. The assumptions used for costs and probabilities were made as realistic as possible. The basic results of the simulation (distribution of DRM) seem to be high, but not entirely inconsistent with research findings. The simulation underscores two important points. First, it supports the monitoring principle (Chapter 8). The risk of DRM is inversely related to the probability that DTPs will be detected and resolved over the entire duration of therapy.

Second, optimization and incremental cost analyses may justify policies that are counterintuitive to some people today. At least managed care policies consistent with this analysis are rare, in my experience. The model is robust enough, despite its limitations and simplifying assumptions, to demonstrate that money spent on resolving DTPs and preventing DRM may be money well spent.

Review of Research Evidence

The simulation described above explored the theoretical relationship between design, outcomes, and costs in a pharmaceutical care system. This section will present examples of studies that changed the medications use process in ways that are consistent with systems theory (see Tables 9.2 and 9.3). These studies were often evaluations of system changes initiated by the investigators. They were often minimally funded, and many have one or more design weaknesses. The generalizability of any study may be questionable. However, they do provide empirical evidence relating medications use systems to improved patient outcomes and reduced total costs of care.

Sleath et al. described a Medicaid drug utilization review project that evaluated the impact of sending a communication about suboptimal therapy to physicians and pharmacists.[2] The study identified 80 patients, aged 24 to 93 years, who were receiving more than four short-acting beta-agonist inhalers or more than two long-acting beta-agonist inhalers in a 2-month period. Letters and fact sheets were sent to the physicians of the 45 patients in the control group (C) and to both the physician and the pharmacy of the 35 patients in the intervention group (I). There were no significant differences in preintervention costs between the two groups. The total cost of care fell significantly for patients in the I group, while it rose in the C group. A reasonable explanation of the results is that informing pharmacists about patterns of medications use improves system performance. (See also Chapter 6.)

Lipton et al. studied clinical pharmacists' consultations in a prospective, randomized controlled trial. Patients aged 65 years and over, discharged on three or more medications for chronic conditions from a 450-bed community hospital, were assigned at random to intervention (I) and control (C) groups. In the I group, pharmacists consulted with patients and their physicians at hospital discharge and periodically for 3 months after discharge. Using a standardized method, a blinded panel evaluated the appropriateness of prescribing for a random sample of 236 patients. Eighty-eight percent had at least one or more clinically significant drug problem, and 22% had at least one potentially serious and life-threatening problem. Experimental patients were less likely to have prescribing problems in any category ($P = .05$). A summary score, measuring the appropriateness of the patients' total drug regimen, indicated that I patients' regimens were more appropriate than those of controls ($P = .01$). "Results of this trial reveal that clinical pharmacists can improve the appropriateness of geriatric drug prescribing in outpatient settings."[3]

Borgsdorf et al.[18] studied the effect of a pharmacy consultation clinic on DTPs and use of health care resources, using a before–after design. Physicians referred 836 patients to the pharmacy clinic for assessment of therapy and medication consultation. The investigators compared health care costs from the year before the clinic was founded to those the year after, based on an audit of a random subsample of 91 patients. The average reduction in total cost of health care services was $644 per patient year. Savings due to reductions in physician visits, emergency room use, and hospitalizations for the 91 patients was $46,320, almost four times greater than the $12,064 savings in drug cost.

TABLE 9.2

Examples of Community Practice and Ambulatory Care Outcomes Studies

Author, Year (reference no.)	Setting	Design	Sample	Intervention	Results
Feedback on Medicines Use					
Sleath et al., 1997 (2)	Community practice	Controlled trial	35 I 45 C	Mailed information about patient drug use I — pharmacist and physician C — physician only	In I, total cost of care/patient/month reduced by $30, including asthma drug cost reduced by $21 In C, total cost of care/patient/month increased by $123 in C group, while asthma drug cost was reduced by $19
Referral					
Lipton et al., 1992 (3)		Randomized controlled trial	n = 236	I — pharmacy consultations C — no consultations	Patients of physicians receiving pharmacy consultations had improved prescribing and significantly fewer drug-related problems
Borgsdorf et al., 1994 (18)	Clinic	Before–after design	n = 836 patients	Referral of patient to pharmacy clinic for medication consultation	Average cost savings of $644/patient year after patients were referred to pharmacy for assessment of therapy; savings mostly through reductions in physician visits, emergency room use, and hospitalization

(continued)

TABLE 9.2 (CONTINUED)

Examples of Community Practice and Ambulatory Care Outcomes Studies

Author, Year (reference no.)	Setting	Design	Sample	Intervention	Results
Cooperative Drug Therapy Management					
Wilt et al., 1995 (4)	Family practice clinic	Cohort-control	n = 112 patients receiving oral anticoagulants	I — pharmacist and physician cooperation C — physician-only management	I patients had 1/20 risk of adverse events from oral anticoagulants; cost savings of $4073/ patient year
Herborg et al., 2001 (6,7)	Community practice	Controlled	n = 413 asthmatic patients attending 16 I and 15 C pharmacies distributed throughout Denmark	I — cooperative pharmaceutical care (Therapeutic Outcome Monitoring) C — usual ambulatory care in Danish community practice	Asthma patients receiving pharmaceutical care had fewer MD visits, higher drug costs, fewer sick days, higher symptom control, improved quality of life, and asthma prescribing closer to guidelines

TABLE 9.3

Examples of Inpatient Care Outcomes Studies

Author, Year (reference no.)	Setting	Design	Sample	Intervention	Results, Design
Cooper, 1985 (8)	LTCF	Time series	72 beds, 5 observations over 3 years	Consultant pharmacist reviewed medication orders	Pharmaceutical consultations reduce numbers of prescriptions and costs of drugs
Clapham et al., 1988 (9)	Hospital	Controlled design	n = 168 admissions of medical-surgical inpatients admitted over 5 months	I — rounding team included pharmacist C — team without pharmacist	Patients on I teams had average LOS of 1.5 days less (cost savings of $1200 per admission) after correcting for diagnostic and age differences
Bjornson et al., 1993 (10)	Hospital	Controlled design	n = 3081 general medical-surgical patients admitted over a 1-year period	I — clinical pharmacist participation in health care teams (2/5 medical, 1/2 surgical) C — team without pharmacist	I patients had a shorter average LOS than C patients; the average cost savings for I teams was $377 per inpatient admission; the benefit-to-cost ratio was 6.03:1
Leape et al., 1999 (19)	Hospital ICU	Mixed	n = 120	I — rounding team included pharmacist C — team without pharmacist	Preventable prescribing ADEs decreased from 10.4/1000 patient days *before* to 3.5 *after* (66% reduction); in C, the rate was essentially unchanged, 362/366 (99%); pharmacist recommendations related to drug ordering were accepted by physicians

Note: LTCF = long-term-care facility.

Wilt and Gums carried out a cohort-control study of a pharmacist-managed anticoagulant management service.[4] Their intervention (I) group was a convenience sample of 68 patients referred to the service over 1 year. The control group (C) had 44 patients, comprising 28 person years. Results for the C group showed:

- 17 major + 2 minor adverse events
- Total cost of care = $5040/patient year

The I group had:

- 2 minor adverse events (1/20 the risk of adverse events compared to controls)
- Total cost/patient year of $967 ($4073 less than C)

The authors concluded that a pharmacist-managed anticoagulant management service can result in improved outcomes for patients receiving warfarin and is cost-effective.

Herborg et al. studied the effect of pharmaceutical care for asthma patients on process and outcome measures. Intervention pharmacies were trained to provide Therapeutic Outcomes Monitoring (TOM), a model of pharmaceutical care for community pharmacists.[5] Their sample comprised 16 intervention (I) and 15 control (C) Danish community pharmacies throughout the country (1 I and 1 C pharmacy in 15 counties, and an additional I pharmacy in the county including Copenhagen). The final sample comprised 413 asthma patients (204 I, 209 C). The control was community pharmacy as usual in Denmark. Compared to C patients, I patients showed evidence of improved asthma management:

- Improved symptom status
- Improved health-related quality of life (HQOL)
- Improved knowledge of asthma
- Improved patient satisfaction (at 6 months only)
- Fewer inhaler errors
- Fewer days of sickness 0.6 vs. 0.3

Medical resource utilization included some evidence of decreased general practitioner (GP) and specialist visits and increased telephone calls to GP (per patient per month) at 12 months. The pattern of GP visits over the duration of the study showed an initial rise and then an average 15% rate of decline from the fourth month until the end of the study. Pharmacists may have tended to refer patients more often early in the study, either because of anxiety about their new role or because they found many unresolved problems that required a referral. Drug cost was slightly higher in the I group than in the C group (U.S. $45.90 vs. $46.95 ($P$ = .15)).

In addition, asthma prescribing and drug use patterns shifted among I physicians (compared to C physicians) toward national consensus guidelines, for example:

- Combination therapy of inhaled steroids with inhaled beta-agonist increased.
- Monotherapy with inhaled beta-agonist decreased.
- Monotherapy with theophylline decreased.

From a theoretical perspective, these prescribing changes are very interesting. Prescribing changes among I physicians were compared to changes among C physicians, so the TOM intervention is the most reasonable explanation. However, the TOM protocol used by the I pharmacists was focused exclusively on managing the care of individual patients. It did not include any activities directed at changing general prescribing behavior. Systems theory would predict that cooperative patient management within a system, with frequent feedback and consultation, has wide-ranging effects. These results are consistent with that prediction.

Herborg et al. concluded that beneficial effects were found for asthma symptom status, global and asthma-specific QOL, days of sickness, knowledge of asthma medications, and inhaler technique. Prescribing changed toward compliance with recommended guidelines.[6,7]

Table 9.3 summarizes studies of systems changes in hospitals and a long-term-care facility.

Cooper studied the effect of consultant clinical pharmacist services in a 72-bed geriatric long-term-care facility. He used a time series design with five observations: at initiation, termination, and reinitiation of consulting service (drug regimen review and physician communication on patient drug use) and at 3 months and 3 years after reinitiation.

Following both initiations of service, drug use was reduced (to 46.1 and 42.7% of the previous level, respectively). The number of recorded diagnoses per patient was essentially unchanged at each observation time. After the consultants' services were terminated, drug use rose to approximately original levels. Cooper concluded that "the consultant clinical pharmacist has an impact on drug cost in long-term care facilities that is reversed when drug regimen review is removed and renewed when services are reinitiated."[8]

Clapham et al. studied the effect of adding a pharmacist to the medical care team in a teaching hospital.[9] Both groups received drug distribution through a centralized unit dose system. The control (C) group received usual care (no pharmacist on the patient care units). Length of stay (LOS), total cost per admission (TCA), and drug cost per admission (DCA) were collected prospectively for 496 medical-surgical patients admitted to a teaching hospital during a 5-month experimental interval. Data were corrected for age and diagnostic group before main effects were compared. The authors concluded that adding a pharmacist to the rounding team yielded, on the average, 1.5 days shorter LOS, $1293 lower TCA, and $155 lower DCA than the control system. Large differences among months were evident, probably because different pharmacists were used in different months.

Bjornson et al. studied the effects of clinical pharmacist participation in a sample of 3081 patients admitted over a year to a hospital's general medicine and general surgical units. Two of five general medical teams and one of two surgical teams included a pharmacist. Health care teams that included a pharmacist had a shorter length of stay and lower drug costs per admission. The investigators found no difference in mortality rates. The average cost savings for intervention (I) teams was $377 per inpatient admission, and the benefit-to-cost ratio was 6.03:1. The authors concluded that adding pharmacists to hospital care teams was cost-effective.[10]

Leape et al. studied the effect of pharmacist participation in an intensive care unit (ICU). The study was carried out as a before–after comparison, with additional comparison of "after" data to a control group. They randomly selected 75 patients. In addition, 50 patients were randomly selected from the control unit during the baseline period. In the intervention (I) group, a pharmacist rounded with the ICU team, remained for consultation in the morning, and was on call throughout the day. In the control (C) group, care was provided under the usual arrangements (no pharmacist). In summary, the results showed that preventable prescribing adverse drug events (ADEs) decreased by 66% from 10.4 per 1000 patient days *before* to 3.5 *after*. In the control unit, the rate was essentially unchanged during the same time periods: 10.9 and 12.4. The pharmacist made 366 recommendations related to drug ordering, of which 362 (99%) were accepted by physicians. The investigators concluded that the presence of a pharmacist on rounds as a full member of the patient care team in a medical ICU was associated with a substantially lower rate of ADEs caused by prescribing errors.[19]

Connective Summary

Chapter 2 reviewed published evidence that preventable drug-related morbidity constitutes a serious problem in the delivery of drug therapy in both ambulatory care and inpatient care. Chapter 3 reviewed researchers' attributions of DRM to causes within the medications use process. It developed a theoretical explanation of how DRMs come into existence. According to this theory, DRMs begin as errors and other events. Some may occur at random or for unknowable reasons. *Preventable* DRMs then manifest themselves as drug therapy problems that are both recognizable and correctable, but which were not corrected. Failures to correct DTPs are not random events, but rather reflect weaknesses in system design or failures of system operation. PDRMs, therefore, are evidence of system failure. Systems that are known to fail frequently are unpredictable and therefore unsafe.

Chapter 8 developed and explored a model of a pharmaceutical care system. This chapter used simulations using this model to demonstrate and partially confirm that model. The simulations show (a) that the risk of DRM is highly sensitive to the system's ability to detect and to resolve DTPs, and (b) that the true contribution of drug therapy to total health care costs, which includes both the cost of correcting DRM and the cost of preventing DRM, may be lowered by appropriate levels of therapeutic outcomes monitoring.

Finally, some studies that changed medications use processes toward the theoretical model were reviewed. These studies show that changing the medications use system by introducing feedback and monitoring may result in improved outcomes, lower total cost, or both. Many studies clearly confirm the theory developed earlier: pharmaceutical care systems lower total costs *by means of* improving patient outcomes. Reviews and critiques of many more such studies are available in the literature.[11–16]

Chapters 10 and 11 will fill in some details about the composition of a MUS. Chapters 12 and 13 will describe the variety of managed care organizations that exist. Chapters 14 and 15 will propose a way forward.

Every study is limited by its sample, methods, and environment. There may never be enough studies, with "perfect" designs and completely generalizable samples, to "prove" that medications use systems are safer and more cost-effective than the processes that they would replace. Each process and system contains some unique elements or exists in a unique environment. Understanding of medications use systems is still incomplete, so acceptance of studies as generalizable might be difficult. Furthermore, as Chapter 14 will describe, resistance to change is a common human trait.

Two points are true, nonetheless. The combination of theory and evidence, along with the availability of indicators as described in Chapter 7, should mandate further development and testing of pharmaceutical care systems by managed care organizations, including governmental programs. Furthermore, the evidence seems strong enough to mandate that every health care delivery system evaluate its own performance, preferably against benchmarks established in experimental systems.

Health care managers and policy makers should not wait for the definitive research study before they address the problem among their own patients. A few research projects will not be accepted to guide a wide variety of applications. Instead policy (and standards) should encourage (require) that health care programs use a quality improvement approach, in which each system studies itself and finds ways to improve its own performance. Then, better system theory can be developed from studying the common elements among successful programs.

References

1. Cipolle, R.J., Strand, L.M., and Morley, P.C., *Pharmaceutical Care Practice*, McGraw-Hill, New York, 1998, p. 1.

2. Sleath, B. et al., Effect of including both physicians and pharmacists in an asthma drug-use review intervention, *Am. J. Health Syst. Pharm.*, 54, 2197, 1997.
3. Lipton, H.L. et al., The impact of clinical pharmacists' consultations on physicians' geriatric drug prescribing: a randomized controlled trial, *Med. Care*, 30, 646, 1992.
4. Wilt, V.M. et al., Outcome analysis of a pharmacist-managed anticoagulation service, *Pharmacotherapy*, 15, 732, 1995.
5. Grainger-Rousseau, T.J. et al., Therapeutic outcomes monitoring: application of pharmaceutical care guidelines to community pharmacy, *J. Am. Pharm. Assoc.*, NS37, 647, 1997.
6. Herborg, H. et al., Improving drug therapy for patients with asthma: Part 2: use of antiasthma medications, *J. Am. Pharm. Assoc.*, 41, 551, 2001.
7. Herborg, H. et al., Improving drug therapy for patients with asthma: Part 1: patient outcomes, *J. Am. Pharm. Assoc.*, 41, 539, 2001.
8. Cooper, J.W., Effect of initiation, termination, and reinitiation of consultant clinical pharmacist services in a geriatric long-term care facility, *Med. Care*, 23, 84, 1985.
9. Clapham, C.E. et al., Economic consequences of two drug-use control systems in a teaching hospital, *Am. J. Hosp. Pharm.*, 45, 2329, 1988.
10. Bjornson, D.C. et al., Effect of pharmacists on health care outcomes in hospitalized patients, *Am. J. Hosp. Pharm.*, 50, 1875, 1993.
11. Hatoum, H.T. et al., An eleven-year review of the pharmacy literature: documentation of the value and acceptance of clinical pharmacy, *Ann. Pharmacother.*, 20, 33, 1986.
12. Hatoum, H.T. et al., Evaluation of the contribution of clinical pharmacists: inpatient care and cost reduction, *Drug Intell. Clin. Pharm.*, 22, 252, 1988.
13. Hatoum, H.T. and Akhras, K., 1993 bibliography: a 32-year literature review on the value and acceptance of ambulatory care provided by pharmacists, *Ann. Pharmacother.*, 27, 1106, 1993.
14. Willett, M.S. et al., Prospectus on the economic value of clinical pharmacy services: a position statement of the American College of Clinical Pharmacy, *Pharmacotherapy*, 9, 45, 1989.
15. McKenney, J.M. and Wasserman, A.J., Effect of advanced pharmaceutical services on the incidence of adverse drug reactions, *Am. J. Hosp. Pharm.*, 36, 1691, 1979.
16. Kennie, N.R., Schuster, B.G., and Einarson, T.R., Critical analysis of the pharmaceutical care research literature, *Ann. Pharmacother.*, 32, 17, 1998 (erratum appears in *Ann. Pharmacother.*, 32, 612, 1998).
17. Faris, R.J., Explicit Definitions to Identify Preventable Drug-Related Morbidity in an Elderly Population and their Use as an Indicator of Quality in the Medication Use System. Unpublished doctoral dissertation, University of Florida, Gainesville, 2001. Dissertation Abstracts International, 62, no. 10B (2001): p. 4448.
18. Borgsdorf, L.R., Knapp, K.K., and Miano, J.S., Pharmacist-managed medication review in a managed care system, *Am. J. Hosp. Pharm.*, 51, 772, 1994.
19. Leape, L.L. et al., Pharmacist participation on physician rounds and adverse drug events in the intensive care unit, *JAMA*, 282, 267, 1999.

10

A Pharmaceutical Care System

Ah! Malpractice cure!

(Anagram of *pharmaceutical care*)

Effective drug therapy requires three overlapping functions: *initiation*, which is prescribing based on medical problem assessment; professional *supervision* of therapy by the prescriber or a co-therapist (e.g., pharmacist, nurse, or physician's assistant); and *facilitation* or actual administration of therapy, e.g., by the patient himself, a family caregiver, nurse, etc. (See Chapters 4 and 8.)

This chapter describes the functions of a professional co-therapist in a pharmaceutical care system, namely, cooperation with facilitator (patient or caregiver) and initiator (e.g., physician) in supervising the progress of drug therapy. Nurses, physicians, and physician's assistants all can function as co-therapists. However, pharmacists are the best educated in pharmacology, and therapeutics and are well placed in medications use processes. This is the pharmacist's greatest potential contribution in a pharmaceutical care system, and it seems to us, most pharmacists' brightest prospect for the future.

There are at least two prerequisites for a co-therapist to function effectively:

1. *A cooperative relationship among all participants.* Cooperation requires shared goals, trust, respect, and communication. At least, each participant should understand the cooperative intent and overall goal of the pharmacist's involvement. The most direct ways for a pharmacist to obtain this is to offer his services to both patients and physicians. This approach is seen most clearly as a patient referral or cooperative practice agreement.

   Some pharmacists seem to prefer a more informal approach, "stealth" pharmacy, in which they may simply begin a new practice. However, when patients or physicians notice that the pharmacist is doing some new activities, they may misunderstand what the pharmacist is doing and why. For example, a patient may interpret the pharmacist's unusual interest as a sign that something is wrong with his prescriptions. A physician may become defensive because the pharmacist is asking so many new questions.

2. *Basic information about the patient.* In cooperating practices, patient information may be available through shared medical records or computer linkages. Otherwise, the main source may be a patient history taken within the pharmacy practice.

Need for a Consistent Process

In the early development of a new practice, each practitioner may need to develop his or her own process of care. Many pharmacists completed their educations without having learned a consistent process. Some have developed their own process, which they naturally would prefer to others. There is no convincing research showing that one process is better than another. It is reasonable to ask why each pharmacist cannot be left to practice in his or her own way.

Within a practice group, such as a community pharmacy, too much variety in process has major disadvantages from the standpoints of both the practice and practice management. These are easily explained by reference to the ideal of pharmaceutical care:

> Responsible, cooperative provision of drug therapy for the purpose of achieving definite outcomes intended to improve a patient's quality of life

1. A consistent process is easier to document correctly. Whichever process is used should promote cooperation, assignment of responsibility for a part of process, and shared responsibility for outcomes. These in turn require documentation. Documentation also improves efficiency by allowing each person to see what has already been accomplished and to add to it, rather than repeating work already done. Efficient documentation is much easier if the process is consistent among the providers.
2. Consistency allows patients and physicians to develop expectations about a practice and then confidence that the practice will meet those expectations. This may be necessary before they will increase their level of cooperation and trust the pharmacists with more responsibility.
3. A practice is much easier to manage if the pharmacists all are following a consistent process of patient care and documentation. Consistency allows the manager to develop standards and

performance indicators relevant to those standards. This simplifies the job of detecting quality problems in the practice.
4. Patients and third parties may be much more likely to pay for care that consistently meets a standard.

Figure 10.1 shows detail of a co-therapist's functions in a pharmaceutical care system. These functions are described in detail below. The practice model in Figure 10.1 is based on the Therapeutic Outcomes Monitoring (TOM) project developed at the University of Florida.[1,2] It is presented below as eight steps, in order to emphasize certain activities during the beginning of therapy and other activities during its continuation. This model is a cycle in which information is repeatedly acquired, analyzed, and used as the basis of decisions and actions. Cipolle et al. have described another, similar model in more detail.[3]

The steps can be carried out by a pharmacist or by a physician–pharmacist–nurse team, with assistance from aides, etc. Who carries out each step is less important than ensuring that all eight steps are done, in order, during each cycle of care.

Although the steps of care should be carried out in order, the process of patient assessment requires professional dialog, as described below. Dialog with a patient cannot be strictly stepwise. The dialog may cycle back to an earlier step based on new information. For example, it may happen that a pharmacist learns about a new drug therapy problem (DTP) at step 5, while advising a patient. Naturally, she would cycle back through steps 1 to 4 to work up this new problem, before completing step 5.

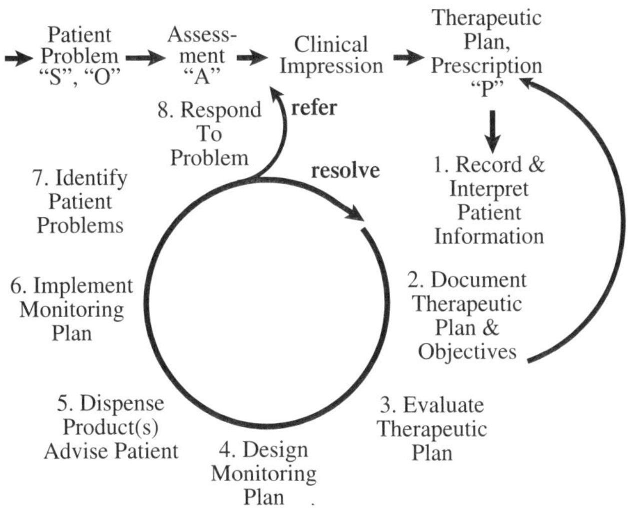

FIGURE 10.1
The Therapeutic Outcomes Monitoring model.

Also, she might spend a different amount of time on a given step, depending on the stage of care. For example, step 1 would require significantly more time for a new patient than for a continuing patient, and more time for a new regimen than for continuation of a stable regimen. However, at least a brief review of each step is necessary at each cycle. This is described further below, under "Documentation."

1. Record and interpret relevant patient information.

   What do we need to know about this patient?

   The objective of this step is to have a problem list, including allergies and major events involving medicines. In cooperating practices, or when a patient requests it, the problem list can be obtained from the patient's primary physician. Also, the patient or family caregiver can often provide basic information by completing a questionnaire. The pharmacy's prescription profile is also a necessary part of this record, but it may require updating with information about over-the-counter (OTC) medicines and prescription medicines that were purchased elsewhere. The pharmacist may need to go further into some questions depending on circumstances.

   In particular, the patient's medical and psychosocial status and current medication profile can provide a clinical impression of past and present medications use and may suggest the need for additional information about the patient. This may lead to finding some untreated indications and some unnecessary medications.

   The emphasis of pharmaceutical care on patient outcomes starts here. One of the first things to find out is what the patient wants to achieve through care or treatment. In contrast, a drug-oriented profile review, even though it may seem similar in function, lacks the orientation to patient outcome and may miss untreated medical problems.

   The co-therapist should understand systems on the level of individual patients. This sounds difficult, but it can actually be quite straightforward. A health professional can understand a patient's care system as easily as she can understand a patient's physiological system, if she knows what to look for and how to organize her thinking. A good way to understand a patient's specific system of care would be to review the five principles of medications use described in Chapter 8.
2. Document therapeutic plan and desired therapeutic objectives for the patient.

   What do we intend to achieve with this therapy in this patient?

   Explicit clinical and quality-of-life objectives of each drug in the regimen will be necessary as a partial basis for evaluating patient progress. Evaluate the therapeutic objectives, because to be useful they must be clear and attainable. Sometimes, therapeutic objectives will be obvious. For example, symptom remission would be the immediate therapeutic objective of an antibiotic prescribed for a urinary tract infection (UTI) (an intermediate objective on the way to curing the infection). At other times, the pharmacist may need to ask the prescriber about clinical objectives and ask the patient about psychosocial objectives. However, even seemingly obvious objectives may be vague. For example, when the pharmacist is developing a monitoring plan (step 4), she may need to decide a specific time period, e.g., 36 h, within which she should expect UTI symptoms to resolve, if therapy is ultimately to achieve a cure.

3. Evaluate therapeutic plan.

   Is this an acceptable plan to achieve those objectives for this patient?

   This step gets particular attention during review of new therapy. For therapy in progress, the questions in step 6 may be more useful. The objective is to reconcile the therapeutic plan with the therapeutic objectives, rather than to produce a standard therapeutic plan or to conform with drugs of choice.

   3.1. Review potential drug therapy problems.

   A systematic and useful means for evaluating a new prescription or other change in a therapeutic plan is to consider categories of potential drug therapy problems. See Tables 10.1 and 10.2.

   3.1.1. Is there legitimate medical or psychosocial justification for the regimen? Is the therapeutic objective sufficiently clear?

   From a patient-oriented perspective, it is logically impossible to judge the suitability of a regimen without reference to the indication (problem list) and therapeutic objective. Also, a clear therapeutic objective will facilitate managing therapy.

   3.1.2. Is the medicine appropriate for the patient's clinical and psychosocial objectives and psychosocial circumstances?

   - Has an appropriate medicine been prescribed in a potentially inappropriate dosage, frequency, route, or regimen?
   - Is there reason to believe the patient may experience a drug interaction or drug–food incompatibility, or that the regimen may interfere with an essential laboratory test?
   - Is there reason to believe that the patient may not actually receive the therapy for economic, psychological, or other reasons? For example, perhaps the patient may be unable to afford it, unable to use necessary administration

TABLE 10.1

Examples of Clinical Indicators

Basis	Assessment or Question
Therapeutic Agents	
Nonsteroidal anti-inflammatories	Test[a] for occult fecal blood or hematocrit?
Theophylline	Rapid pulse rate, nausea, agitation?
Sedating drugs, especially in elderly	Morning confusion, dizziness?
Digoxin	Slow pulse rate, episodes of nausea, visual disturbances?
Oral anticoagulants	INR,[a] bruises, nosebleeds, "pink toothbrush," fecal blood?
Antidepressants	Mood, sexual dysfunction
Patient circumstances	
Infection	Prompt symptom resolution?
Caregiver administers medicines	Problems in administration, e.g., to a baby?
Administration devices	
Metered-dose inhalers	Refill or dosage frequency, inhaler technique?
Syringes	Injection technique, injection sites?

[a] Questions about test results are shorthand for whether test was done, when, and the results.

equipment, unable to remember the regimen, or unwilling to begin or continue the regimen.

3.1.3. According to the problem list, does the patient have an as-yet-untreated indication? Might he need additional drug therapy or other forms of therapy or information (e.g., diet)?

3.2. Judge the likelihood that the patient would develop one or more DTPs when following the therapeutic plan and the probable severity of those DTPs.

Estimating probable severity would depend in part on how readily a potential DTP would be detected and controlled if it were actually to develop. Moreover, for these judgments to be realistic, they should be made in the context of the severity of the medical problem and specific therapeutic alternatives.

3.3. Decide whether it is necessary to modify the regimen, and if so, make a recommendation to the prescriber.

3.4. Document major concerns and recommendations.

Comment: Patients should receive regimens with high likelihood of reaching therapeutic objectives and low likelihood of allergy, hypersensitivity, or other drug therapy problems. Before the patient has begun the therapy, there is some room for discussion about what therapy would be ideal. Research may favor some agents in general over others within a given therapeutic class, so-called drugs of choice. Experts sometimes

TABLE 10.2

Classification of Drug Therapy Problems

Access	Effectiveness	Safety
1. The patient has a medical problem that requires drug therapy (a drug indication) but is *not receiving*[a] a drug for that indication. Potential causes: a. A prescription drug has not been ordered. b. The patient cannot —Afford it —Accept it —Obtain it —Use administration devices correctly	2. **Wrong drug:** The patient has a drug indication but is taking an *ineffective drug* for that indication or has a *drug interaction* that diminishes therapeutic effectiveness. 3. **Wrong dose:** The patient is being treated with *too little* of the correct drug. Potential causes: —Dose ordered is insufficient for patient's actual need —Low drug bioavailability —Drug–drug or drug–food interactions —Dispensing or administration error, including patient or caregiver nonadherence	4. **Wrong drug:** The patient is taking an absolutely or relatively *contraindicated drug*, including a drug that ***interacts*** with another to create an adverse reaction, side effect, or toxicity. 5. The patient is having an *adverse drug reaction or side effect* to the correct drug. 6. **Wrong dose:** The patient has a problem resulting from *too much* of the correct drug (toxicity). Potential causes: —Dose ordered is excessive for patient's actual need —Excess drug bioavailability —Drug–drug or drug–food interactions —Dispensing or administration error, including patient or caregiver nonadherence 7. The patient is taking a drug for *no medically valid indication* (including inappropriate duplicate therapy). 8. The patient has a problem resulting from a *drug–laboratory interaction* (a real problem obscured or a merely apparent problem).

[a] Various verb tenses: may not receive, did not receive, etc.

have stronger opinions about this than the evidence really warrants, because drug of choice is a matter of conjecture for any patient before therapy has begun. This is a very common example of a theoretical DTP without an actual problem being observable in the patient (see below).

The minimum outcome of steps 1 to 3 should be a list of the patient's medical problems, an idea of how his current medications address those problems, and the therapeutic objective for each therapy, including what the patient wants to get from therapy.

4. Design a monitoring plan.

   What evidence will we need to assess progress of therapy?

   The objective is to develop a simple, written plan to collect necessary information at some future time. The information would be used to evaluate patient progress toward therapeutic objectives.

   4.1. Decide what information to collect about the progress of the patient's drug therapy and when and how to collect it.

   The evaluation of therapy carried out in step 3 is one basis for these decisions. Another useful basis is a standard protocol for managing a particular disease state or drug therapy, especially clinical indicators of the status of therapy.

   4.2. If necessary, arrange for a follow-up visit or telephone call (see also step 5.3, below).

   4.3. Document the monitoring plan in the patient's record and on a calendar.

5. Dispense drug products and advise patient.

   Can this patient (or family caregiver, etc.) now make the best use of this medicine?

   5.1. Decide to whom, when, and how you will dispense the medicine.

   In some cases, e.g., new prescriptions requiring use of administration devices, an educational dialog with the patient may be necessary. This requires that the patient be willing and able to have that dialog. If the patient is tired or in a hurry (or the pharmacist is pressed for time), it may be necessary to arrange a more favorable time.

   5.2. Provide effective patient education.

   Patient advising should be done with the objective of recruiting and empowering a therapeutic partner. That is, the patient ideally should be able to address four points:

   - How he will use the medicine; demonstrate the use of administration devices, when appropriate.
   - How he will recognize when therapy is succeeding.
   - How he will recognize major problems.
   - What he will do if they occur.

   5.3. Discuss roles and responsibilities.

   In pharmaceutical care, the responsibilities of the pharmacist and patient may differ from those to which the patient is accustomed. Overall, patient and pharmacist responsibilities increase. For example, the patient should actively cooperate in his own care, and the pharmacist monitors outcomes more carefully. This step should include, when appropriate, some discussion of what the patient and pharmacist should expect each other to do, for example, when the pharmacist will call the patient according to the monitoring plan and what she will want to know, and when the patient should call the pharmacist or physician for help.

5.4. Document the discussion.

6. Implement the monitoring plan.

   What evidence do I need to assist in evaluating this patient's progress?

   Information about actual problems is needed in three general areas:

   6.1. Access and adherence: Is the patient actually receiving the medicine as intended? Does the patient intend to continue? Can the patient describe how she takes the medicines? Can she demonstrate the use of administration devices?

   6.2. Effectiveness: Is there evidence that the medicine is having the desired effect relative to the original therapeutic objective? Does the patient feel better? Is the patient able to function better?

   6.3. Safety: Is there evidence that the medicine is causing a new medical problem or interfering with necessary or desired activities of life, e.g., morning drowsiness from CNS drugs.

   Comment: Implementing the monitoring plan can be as simple as telephoning a patient. It may require the patient's visiting the pharmacy for a more extensive interview. Some of the information obtained should be based on the specific regimen, therapeutic objectives, or patient circumstances. Assessments should include *clinical indicators* (ideally, chosen earlier, in step 4) and should focus on pertinent patient activities, data from therapeutic diaries, demonstrations (e.g., of metered-dose inhaler technique), and specific physical assessments as necessary. (See Table 10.1 for some examples.) It should also include general information, e.g., feelings of comfort or well-being and activities of daily living. The process should be carried out as a dialog that results in a series of clinical impressions to be evaluated in the next step.

7. Identify possible drug therapy problems.

   Is this patient progressing toward therapeutic objectives? Are there indicators of drug therapy problems?

   The pharmacist may have begun this step while interpreting responses to his follow-up questions in step 6. For some of the actual problems identified in step 6, the pharmacist needs to consider potential DTPs as the possible root causes (see Table 10.2).

So, to finish the analysis and interpretation of the clinical impressions after the follow-up interview or examination, review the access, effectiveness, and safety questions in turn. Then consider possible causes of problems identified. These could be analyzed using the logic of DTP categories. (See step 3 and Cipolle et al.[3])

8. Respond to problems.

   What action should I take now?

   The disposition of any identified drug therapy problem depends, among other things, on the nature of the problem and the pharmacist's competence and professional relationships.

   8.1. Refer.

      8.1.1. Refer without recommendation. The pharmacist can call the evidence of a problem to the patient's or prescriber's attention. This might be a good choice if the pharmacist has noted a serious medical problem without a potential DTP or if the pharmacist is simply not confident in making a recommendation.

      8.1.2. Refer with recommendation. When possible, the pharmacist should recommend specific alternative solutions to the prescriber.

   8.2. Resolve. The pharmacist could recommend to the patient safer or more effective ways to take the medicine (e.g., improving inhaler use, taking medicine with food). Depending on the circumstances, this may need to be discussed with the prescriber in advance, or the pharmacist may simply notify the prescriber of the recommendation.

      Whether or not therapy was changed, the pharmacist would continue to monitor patient progress, revise her monitoring plan, and report patient progress to the prescriber. This is essentially a return to step 1.

To summarize, drug therapy management comprises eight fundamental steps performed in a cycle. Steps 1 and 2 lay a foundation for therapy. Step 3 is a preliminary assessment of the therapeutic plan in the context of therapeutic objectives. In step 5, the co-therapist provides the necessities of therapy (drug products and information) to the patient. Steps 4 and 6 require assessment of progress toward therapeutic objectives and recognizing evidence that something may be interfering with achieving them, i.e., a drug therapy problem. In step 7, the co-therapist decides whether the patient is making acceptable progress and, if not, defines the basic cause of the problem. In step 8, she identifies, evaluates, and chooses among alternative solutions and carries them out (essentially resolves or refers the problem). She may continue the cycle with steps 1 to 3, perhaps briefly considering whether more information is needed and reconsidering the therapeutic plan. Then monitoring (steps 6 to 8) recurs.

TABLE 10.3

Minimum Follow-Up Questions in Pharmaceutical Care

	Access	Effectiveness	Safety
6. Is there an actual DTP or a DRM?			
7. Is there a potential DTP?			
8. How can we resolve it?			

Describing this process presents a dilemma. On the one hand, it should be presented as completely and unambiguously as possible. On the other hand, presenting it in this way makes it seem more complicated than it really is. (Try to give detailed instructions on how to walk, and you will see how a detailed explanation can make a common skill seem too complicated to learn.) After one learns the basics, the practice is really straightforward. For many patients who are continuing therapy, steps 1 to 4 take little time, and the cycle is essentially the three steps shown in Table 10.3.

Drug Therapy Problems

As defined in Chapter 3, a *drug therapy problem* is a patient- and time-specific circumstance that, according to professional judgment, may be inconsistent with an optimum outcome from drug therapy. (DTPs are also commonly known as *drug-related problems*.)

A DTP is an intermediate result of therapy, but it is part of the *process* of care. The detection, assessment, and resolution of DTPs comprise the central activity of the eight steps described above.

Some patients receiving drug therapy do not develop a DTP. Others have one or more DTPs, for example, side effects that never become severe. In Chapter 3, these were called latent precursors and resident pathogens because they can erupt unexpectedly into drug-related morbidity (DRM). For example, a patient may go for years with somewhat undertreated asthma or may live with a side effect. Some DTPs develop rather quickly into drug-related morbidities.

Classification of DTPs

A systematic classification of theoretical DTPs is a useful checklist during profile review, to evaluate therapy before it has begun. It is also useful to assist us in considering possible causes of actual DTPs during therapy. Several classification systems for DTPs have been proposed over the years. For example, Cipolle et al. have developed an exhaustive categorization of DTPs and have discussed them at length.[3] See Table 10.2. The basic eight classes have been retabulated into three groups: access, effectiveness, and safety.

Some DTPs are virtually clinical indicators for managing some patients, diseases, or therapies. They are well known and recognized as causes of DRM in certain patients. Clinicians should routinely monitor such clinical indicators, including questions asked of the patient (see Table 10.1). For example, perhaps every patient getting a refill of an oral anticoagulant should be asked when he last had a prothrombin time determination (or when his doctor last drew blood), and asked about bruising, nosebleeds, or prolonged bleeding after brushing teeth, etc., regardless of whether the warfarin use appears to be correct.

Theoretical and Actual DTPs

To use the concept of a DTP clinically, it is necessary to distinguish between *manifest patient problems* and *theoretical problems*. A manifest patient problem (patient problem, for short) is one that is observable (manifest) in a patient — usually an unexpected sign or symptom or the absence of an expected response. Examples include frequent wheezing or shortness of breath, coughing, or sleep interruptions reported by a patient with asthma.

A theoretical DTP refers to a theoretical discrepancy in the patient's drug regimen. Inadequate use of inhaled steroids, as shown by inappropriately long refill intervals, is an example. Some very common examples are potential drug interactions, perhaps flagged by a computer program, when a patient has been taking the combination for a long time without problems. A theroetical DTP exists independantly of an individual patient. An actual DTP is the conjunction of a theoretical DTP and a patient problem (quadrant (a) in Table 10.4).

The starting point for problem resolution is recognizing a connection between a patient problem such as "trouble breathing" and a theoretical DTP such as inadequate use of inhaled steroids. Table 10.4 summarizes the practical significance of these ideas. A pharmacist may first notice an actual DTP as either a theoretical DTP or a patient problem. That is, a theoretical DTP may cause the pharmacist to interview a patient to discover an actual problem, recommend a laboratory test, etc. Conversely, a patient problem may

TABLE 10.4

Definition of Actual and Potential DTPs in Terms of Theoretical DTP and Manifest Patient Problem

Patient (Manifest) Problem	Theoretical DTP	
	Yes	**No**
Yes	a. **Actual DTP or DRM:** Requires manifest problem and plausible explanation involving a theoretical DTP	c. **Not drug-related:** Consider referring problem for further diagnosis
No	b. **Potential DTP:** Correct or monitor for later development of an actual problem	d. No further action

send the pharmacist to review the patient's use of medicines, looking for one or more theoretical DTPs that might be causing the problem.

For example, suppose a pharmacist notices that an asthmatic patient uses his steroid "preventer" inhaler substantially less often than directed by the doctor. This theoretical DTP suggests the possibility that the patient's asthma is out of control. (There are other nonclinical explanations as well.) The pharmacist should look for evidence regarding the patient's asthma status, e.g., coughing, wheezing, waking up at night, problems with normal activities caused by breathing, pulmonary function tests, frequent attacks, or frequent use of the "rescue" inhaler. Conversely, the presence of actual problems such as coughing, wheezing, etc., may cause the pharmacist to ask more carefully about medications use. (If a patient problem associated with a theoretical DTP caused disability, were permanent, or required substantial professional care to resolve, we would call it a DRM.)

So, an actual DTP (or a DRM) requires both an observable event and a plausible explanation involving drug therapy. (Plausible in this case means that the actual problem should have a known relationship to the DTP and that the DTP should have preceded the problem or should exist concomitantly.) The steps taken to resolve the problem should reflect the perceived strength of the connection.

A *potential DTP* is one in which the patient has a theoretical DTP but no manifest problem to match it (quadrant (b) in Table 10.4). That is, a potential DTP is a theoretical DTP in the context of an individual patient. Whether to correct a potential DTP that is having no evident effect on a patient is a matter of professional judgment. It depends on how likely, severe, and correctable one expects the patient problem would be. The potential DTP could be a latent precursor to a sudden and severe DRM.

For example, the possibly poorly controlled asthma patient could suddenly experience a life-threatening attack. It might be reasonable for a pharmacist to treat such a potential DTP as if it were actual. Some potential "wrong drug" DTPs are so likely to cause severe problems that the problem must be resolved before therapy has begun. Suppose an elderly patient has been receiving a long-acting benzodiazepine in a moderate dose, with no apparent toxic effect. Since these drugs often accumulate slowly in elderly patients, and since their use is associated with severe falls, the problem should probably be corrected immediately. Failing that, it would be important to warn the patient and to make a note to monitor him regularly for as long he is taking that drug. For other potential "wrong drug" DTPs, the actual problem, if it happens, might be detectable before it causes any real harm.

In some drug-of-choice disagreements, if the pharmacist is unsuccessful in changing initial therapy, she should note the DTP in the record, include it in her monitoring plan, and wait until the patient has begun the therapy. If actual problems develop, the recommendation to use another agent would have a basis in reality, a sounder basis than drug of choice. Sometimes, the pharmacist will have seen the patient more recently than the physician and have essential information on therapeutic effectiveness or developing side effects.

Documentation: Problem-Oriented Medical Records and SOAP Notes

Documentation of care is necessary for reasons of efficiency, coordination, cooperation, and quality management. Documentation captures information and allows the members of a practice to share it. Without documentation, each pharmacist in the practice group may need to repeat patient interviews and other processes of care. This may render care extremely inefficient and may block all but the simplest kinds of care.

For example, therapeutic objectives are necessary for therapeutic monitoring. If objectives are not documented, they cannot be used reliably, and the same information would have to be collected in each patient encounter. Documented information can be communicated to other professionals in a care team, e.g., physicians. Patient care records are essential for quality assessments, including those that occur as part of accreditation reviews and malpractice litigation.

The problem-oriented medical record (POMR) is an accepted and effective way to organize pharmacists' clinical notes. In this system, documentation is organized according to a problem list. The initial problem list may consist of patient complaints, e.g., headaches. As time passes, some problems will be permanently resolved, while others will become more refined categories, such as clinical diagnoses.

Drug therapy problems should be linked to medical problems through drug indications and therapeutic objectives. (See steps 2 and 3 of the pharmaceutical care plan, above.) For example, suppose a pharmacist notices that a patient has been taking a nonsteroidal anti-inflammatory drug (NSAID) for arthritis. This therapy is known to cause gastrointestinal bleeding in some patients. Suppose that the patient has not been followed with regular hematocrits, tests for occult fecal blood, etc. The clinical note describing the need for follow-up should be entered under arthritis in the problem list, as a part of the plan that includes NSAID therapy.

If a patient mentions, or the pharmacist detects, a problem without a clear medical cause, the pharmacist can list it as a new problem until it is understood better, and then move it where it belongs. Also, pharmacists often discover new and untreated medical problems.

SOAP Notes

Clinical notes on each problem may be organized in the so-called SOAP format. SOAP is an acronym for *subjective* and *objective* data acquisition, data *assessment* or *analysis*, and therapeutic *plan*. The POMR-SOAP format keeps the practitioner focused on the patient and facilitates cooperation if many people use the record.

SOAP is such an easy mnemonic that some of the original ideas proposed by Lawrence Weed, the originator of the concept, may be forgotten. To avoid this, some modified acronyms have been proposed. Although they are unpronounceable, they increase attention to two important details. For example, some would suggest SOATP-F to reemphasize that the clinician should establish and record *therapeutic objectives* before developing a *therapeutic plan,* and that the plan should include *follow-up*:

Therapeutic objective is an observable event that is relevant to the assessment, e.g., cure, control of disease, relief of symptoms, improvement of quality of life.

Subjective data include the patient's illness experience: patient complaints and descriptions of problems, as well as some observations by a health professional, e.g., "patient appears agitated." *Objective data* include vital signs, laboratory values, medical history, physical examination, and results of other diagnostic procedures. Current medications would be listed under objective data.[4,5]

Assessment is a written appraisal of patient data for diagnostic or therapeutic purposes. These purposes include continuing, modifying, or terminating diagnosis or therapy and referral to another practitioner.

A *therapeutic plan* is a means to achieve the therapeutic objective. It should include a scheduled *follow-up* to assess whether the plan is succeeding.

Documenting the Eight Steps

The eight-step pharmaceutical care model should be documented in the SOAP (SOATP-F) format, although the order of steps may be different for the co-therapist than for the initiator. When the co-therapist sees the patient, the therapeutic plan might be clear from the prescription profile, but the therapeutic objective might often be unclear. (See Table 10.5.)

TABLE 10.5

Documenting the Eight Steps of Pharmaceutical Care

Pharmaceutical Care Process	Documentation
1. Get patient information	S, O
2. Establish or learn therapeutic objectives	T
3. Evaluate therapy	A
4. Design monitoring plan	P-F
5. Dispense and advise	P-F
6. Monitor	S, O
7. Identify DTP	A
8. Resolve DTP	P-F

Professional Dialog

In addition to describing a useful format for clinical notes, SOAP comes close to describing a useful process for a patient workup (as distinguished from documenting that workup). The expression "SOAP-ing a patient" is used to mean "carrying out the process that leads to a SOAP note." However, pharmacists who take the SOAP process too literally may tend to collect too much information. Furthermore, experienced professionals rarely work this way, although they may say that they do.

For example, according to one paper, "Once *all pertinent data* ... have been collected, this information must be assimilated to formulate a treatment plan ... or to obtain additional needed information"[6] (emphasis added). The quotation contains a contradiction. Does one collect "all pertinent data" and then assess it, or collect some data, assess it, and collect more data? Logically, one would not know what data to collect in advance of the assessment. One might even need additional data while formulating the therapeutic plan.

The initial workup, beginning with questions about what the patient hopes to accomplish through therapy and subsequent patient follow-up, does not follow a linear S, O, A process, even if it is useful to record data that way. Rather, it is more like a purposeful conversation or dialog, as diagrammed in Figure 10.2. Professional dialog is a form of active listening in which the professional asks questions that progressively focus the discussion to a conclusion.[7,8]

Dialog begins with data, which may come from a uniform history form, set of oral questions, an informal patient interview, or even a casual comment. The professional interprets and integrates the data in the context of his knowledge, values, and beliefs to form a preliminary impression, a mental model of some aspect of the patient's status. Then the professional decides

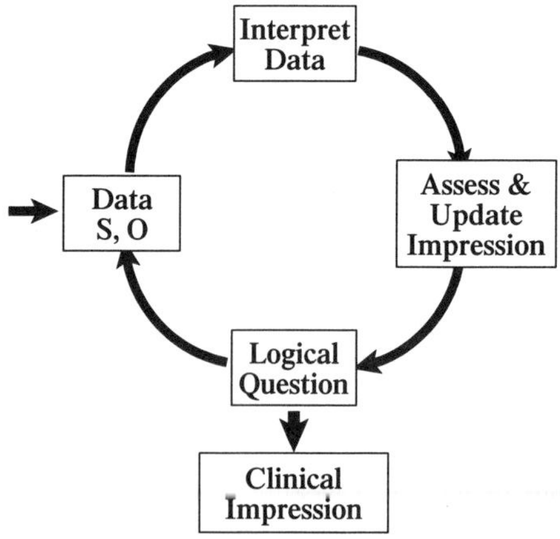

FIGURE 10.2
Diagram of professional dialog.

what additional information he needs (logical question or proposition) and how to get it. A skillful interviewer can find significant and discriminating questions based on that impression, and can ask them in a way that increases the chance of an accurate response. The professional would interpret the patient's responses in light of that impression.

He might also revise the impression, e.g., from "a patient who is using too much albuterol" to "a patient who does not know how to use a metered-dose inhaler" to "a patient who needs a spacer for his MDI." The process continues until the professional has formed a stable clinical impression, e.g., responses to questions seem consistent with the (revised) impression.

Two important technical points concern the validity and the reliability of information collected through dialog. A clinician can assess validity to some extent according to the diagnostic discriminations that can be made from the questions and their compatibility with objective data such as laboratory data (from outside the dialog per se). In other words, we might accept information as valid when it fits an interpretable pattern (a clinical impression). A clinician can assess the reliability of the data according to the consistency of the responses to similar questions. Perhaps we would not even call the result of dialog a clinical impression until we were satisfied with the validity (interpretability) and reliability of the data.

Example

The following case is an example of how patient assessment would fit into pharmaceutical care in a community pharmacy setting. The point of this case is to illustrate the process of patient assessment and the logic of clinical dialog, rather than the therapeutics of asthma. Consensus about appropriate therapy may change with time and may vary from one professional to another.

Background

Katherine LaDichosa is a 13-year-old white female. She is evidently well nourished and within normal limits for physical, mental, and social development. She has a history of the usual childhood diseases but is healthy except for chronic bronchial asthma. According to her parents, K.D. has had asthma "since she was a baby." She is currently in the care of Dr. L. Michael. She has been admitted to the hospital on five occasions over the past 10 years with status asthmaticus. (Note the similarity to Katherine LaStima. Ms. LaDichosa represents our chance to demonstrate the care that might have saved Katherine LaStima.)

K.D.'s recent history of doctor visits and prescription purchases from the Belchertown Oaks Pharmacy is as shown in Table 10.6. Her mother usually picks up her prescriptions. Although the pharmacist has been at Belchertown Oaks Pharmacy for some years, she is not usually present when the LaDichosa's come in. Today is July 10. Mrs. LaDichosa has returned to the pharmacy for a refill of K.D.'s albuterol.

TABLE 10.6

Pharmacy Record for Katherine LaDichosa

Visit or Prescription	Dates
Visit to Dr. L.M.	4/13, 4/20, 4/27, 5/18, 6/15
R albuterol inhaler, use as needed	3/30, 4/27, 5/25, 6/8, 6/21, 6/29
R SR-Theo 300 mg #60, 2 twice a day	3/30, 4/27
N triamcinolone tablets 8 mg #40, 5 daily, refill _1	4/13
N triamcinolone tablets 8 mg #10, 3 daily for 2 days, then 1 daily for 2 days, then 1 every other day until gone, NR	4/20
N triamcinolone inhaler, use 4 times daily as directed, refill 6 months	4/27

Note: R = refill; N = new prescription; NR = nonrefillable prescription. The albuterol and triamcinolone MDI each contain a 30-day supply.

The first step in clinical dialog is collecting relevant subjective and objective information. The prescription record is an important source, but it requires interpretation. The following is an example of an interpretation of the information in Table 10.6:

1. K.D. apparently had an acute exacerbation of her asthma around April 13, which was treated with short, intensive triamcinolone. Her condition evidently improved. (Make a note to confirm this with Mrs. LaDichosa.)
2. On April 20, she returned to Dr. L.M., presumably for a scheduled visit. He seems to have seen improvement because he changed her therapy to taper the oral steroid. She did not use the refill of the 40 mg/day triamcinolone, evidently because Dr. L.M. changed her dose.
3. She evidently continued to improve because 7 days later (April 27) she returned to Dr. L.M., and he prescribed triamcinolone by metered-dose inhaler (TMDI), which she obtained from the pharmacy, along with refills of her albuterol MDI and theophylline.
4. Since April 27, she has been using albuterol, and possibly using TMDI and theophylline. She visited the pharmacy on April 27 and saw Dr. L.M. again about 3 weeks later, on May 18, and then a month after that (June 15). Meanwhile, her medications use emphasized beta-agonists, especially albuterol, and deemphasized steroids. Her last three albuterol refills were 14, 13, and 8 days apart. She has not refilled the TMDI.
5. Clinical impression: This pattern of use is inconsistent with the therapeutic objective of controlling K.D.'s asthma. Relative risk of asthmatic crisis doubles for each beta-agonist inhaler over one per month and is reduced tenfold by regular use of inhaled steroids.[9]

Table 10.7 illustrates a dialog with Mrs. LaDichosa and Katherine, based on the review of her record. The logic proceeds from left to right, proposition, question, response, and interpretation (assessment). (See Figure 10.2.) It concludes with a treatment plan.

Commentary

The scenarios of both Katherine LaStima and Katherine LaDichosa are somewhat fictionalized versions of the death of Jennifer C. (See preface and Chapter 1.) Jennifer/Katherine LaStima died, in status asthmaticus, one day after visiting a county fair. Her pharmacist apparently did no patient assessments like the ones described above. He continued to refill her rescue medicines (albuterol metered-dose inhalers) at frequent intervals. She evidently did not use preventers (steroids) appropriately, and there is no evidence that the pharmacist tried to encourage their use. Possibly, her already worsening asthma, concealed by overuse of rescue medicines, was pushed into status asthmaticus by exposure to additional allergens. The long-standing misuse of medications in the actual case illustrates the proposition that preventable drug-related morbidity and mortality may result from systems failure rather than from failure of a single component or participant.

Summary

This chapter has described a systematic approach to providing and documenting pharmaceutical care one patient at a time. There may be many ways to accomplish that. However, a given practice may have many pharmacists, many patients, and many repeat visits. A consistent and uniform sequence of care within a practice is important for reasons of safety and effectiveness, as described above. The eight-step process is, however, somewhat arbitrary. Other models may be used, but one model should be adopted as the basic template for a practice. Also, the needs of a patient may differ from visit to visit. While a pharmacist should consider each of the eight steps, in order, professional judgment and common sense may show that one step can be minimized while another must be emphasized.

Documentation of care may be a major difference from a dispensing practice. Documentation is essential for reasons of safety and effectiveness. The SOAP format, with minor modification for the co-therapist function, is recommended.

Although SOAP is an effective means for organizing clinical notes, it is not, literally, an algorithm for conducting a patient interview. The process of clinical dialog consists of four active-listening steps, organized in a cycle.

A consistent and predictable pharmaceutical care system is a necessary, but not sufficient, part of a medications use system. The other major component is a medications management system, as described in Chapter 11.

TABLE 10.7

Example of an Assessment Dialog between Pharmacist and Mrs. LaDichosa

Co-therapist's Objective of Question (Proposition)	Co-therapist's Question[a]	Response	Interpretation
Confirm medical history.	Did K.D. have a flare-up of her asthma back in April?	Yes, she did.	Interpretation of prescription record confirmed. It has not been that long since April. Perhaps the basic cause is still present in K.D.'s environment. Make a note to follow this up later.
	Did it get better in a few weeks?	Yes, Dr. L.M. gave her steroids and that seemed to work. Thank God she didn't have to go to the hospital again.	
Rule out other (nonclinical) explanations for TMDI underuse.	Is K.D. using TMDI, e.g., from another supply?	No	Confirms underuse of TMDI
K.D. may be misusing rather than overusing albuterol MDI.	K.D., please show me how you use your albuterol MDI.	K.D. demonstrates correct use.	Consistent with overuse of albuterol; increases likelihood she is beginning another exacerbation
Any objective evidence?	Does K.D. use a peak flow meter and keep a diary?	No	Note to discuss with Dr. L.M.

	Is K.D. coughing a lot, waking up at night, having trouble catching her breath on exertion?	Yes	Exacerbation; acute problem is coming. She may need intervention.
Telephone discussion with Dr. L.M.		He says, "Ask Mrs. L. to watch K.D. carefully. K.D. must use TMDI. Mrs. L. should call me if K.D. has to use more than 4 puffs/day of albuterol" (unhappy about recent albuterol refill history).	
How can I convince K.D. to use TMDI?	K.D., why don't you like to use both inhalers the way the doctor said to?	TMDI tastes terrible and does not help me breathe. It doesn't fit in my pocket with the other MDI.	Consider changing brands of TMDI.
How can I encourage Mrs. L. to reinforce and supervise K.D. to use her TMDI?	Did the doctor tell you why the TMDI is important?	I don't remember. K.D. has to take so many medicines for her asthma. The [albuterol MDI] seems to be the only one that really helps her.	Mrs. L. may not appreciate the value of TMDI. She may not connect that medicine to the tablets that helped resolve K.D.'s last exacerbation. Priorities for treatment plan: 1. Supervision of K.D.'s asthma status and information about what to do 2. Get her to use TMDI 3. Discuss diary, etc.

[a] This column is intended to show the purpose of the question. An actual patient interview would require that a therapeutic relationship already exist or that one be established. Many questions would require more skill than is shown by these somewhat bluntly worded questions. The question about whether K.D. gets TMDI from another source especially might require more tact than is shown here.

References

1. Herborg, H. et al., Improving drug therapy for patients with asthma: Part 1: patient outcomes, *J. Am. Pharm. Assoc.*, 41, 539, 2001.
2. Grainger-Rousseau, T.J. et al., Therapeutic outcomes monitoring: application of pharmaceutical care guidelines to community pharmacy, *J. Am. Pharm. Assoc.*, NS37, 647, 1997.
3. Cipolle, R.J., Strand, L.M., and Morley, P.C., *Pharmaceutical Care Practice*, McGraw-Hill, New York, 1998, p. 1.
4. Wallace, C. and Franson, K.L., Incorporation of ability-based outcome education into pharmacotherapies using an expanded S.O.A.P. format, *Am. J. Pharm. Educ.*, 60, 87, 1996.
5. Weed, L.L., Medical records that guide and teach, *N. Engl. J. Med.*, 278, 652, 1968.
6. Pauley, T., Marcrom, R., and Randolph, R., Physical assessment in the community pharmacy, *Am. Pharm.*, NS35, 40, 1995.
7. Hepler, C.D., Philosophical issues raised by pharmaceutical care, *J. Pharm. Teaching*, 5, 19, 1996.
8. Zaner, R.M., Medicine and dialogue, *J. Med. Philos.*, 15, 303, 1990.
9. Spitzer, W.O. et al., The use of beta-agonists and the risk of death and near death from asthma, *N. Engl. J. Med.*, 326, 501, 1992.

11

Medications Management System

> In its current form, habits, and environment, American health care is incapable of providing the public with the quality health care it expects and deserves.
>
> **IOM Committee on the Quality of Health Care in America**

Earlier chapters, especially Chapters 9 and 10, show that the quality of drug therapy can be improved on the patient and provider levels, perhaps with no increase in overall expenditures for care. The theoretical and empirical evidence show an economically feasible way to improve the quality of drug therapy. Establishing pharmaceutical care systems, however feasible, will not be simple. The bright picture of systematically managed drug therapy for individual patients, described in Chapter 10, is incomplete.

Drug therapy is an intimate part of health care delivery. It is probably unlikely that the "second drug problem" can be ameliorated without far-reaching changes in health care delivery, at all four of the levels enumerated by the Institute of Medicine: patient, provider, organization, and environment.[5] It is possible, however, that slow development of medications management systems could retard, or at the least lag behind, development of safer and more effective health care delivery systems.

Medications management is quality improvement and control for pharmaceutical care and other activities that go on at the patient and provider levels. Managed care, including, for example, government programs, health insurance, and comprehensive prepaid provider networks, is ideally placed to create systems. Creating such systems will require voluntary action by managed care organizations, perhaps with a push from the environment of laws, regulations, and standards. (The reasons for concern about managed care's responsiveness are described in Chapter 6.) The fourth level of the system, environment, is discussed in Chapter 14.

This chapter will describe a medications management system (MMS). An MMS evaluates quality of medications use in a patient group, e.g., all patients in a practice or an insurance program; identifies root causes, e.g., system weaknesses or failures thought to explain low quality in the patient group; devises improvements in structure and process; and implements

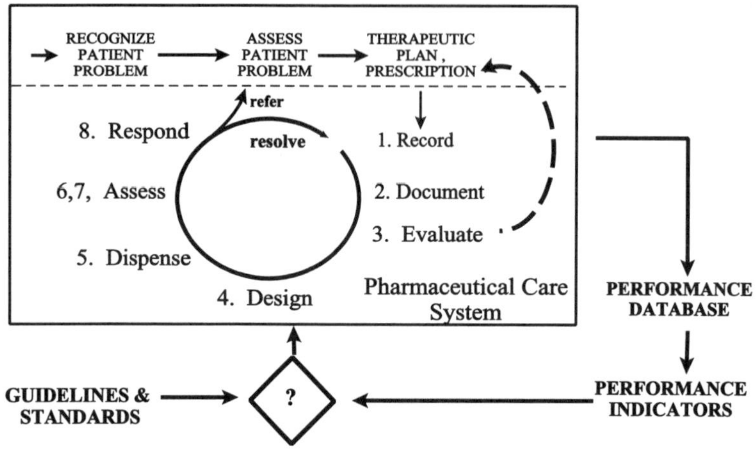

FIGURE 11.1
Medications management system with nested PCS.

improvements and evaluates their effect. It is an application to medications use of activities that may be familiar under other names, for example, performance management, performance-based evaluation, quality control, quality improvement (QI), and clinical governance.

This chapter will provide practical details of how to apply ideas about systems and their control information that were presented in Chapters 7 and 8. Figure 11.1 reviews the basic structure of a medications management system. A rectangle has been drawn around a simplified diagram of the pharmaceutical care system (PCS) (Chapter 10). (The underlined activities are initiation activities, and the arc from "evaluate" back to "plan" diagrams a feedback loop for a co-therapist's discussion of initial therapy with the initiator.)

The feedback loop at the lower right of Figure 11.1 shows an ongoing sequence of data collection, organization, and assessment according to criteria. The diamond with a question mark within it represents comparison of indicator data to guidelines and standards for the purpose of problem detection. Then, when necessary, a quality leader (system manager) renews or changes parts of the structure and process of the patient care system.

Note, however, that the vertical arrow does not extend into the rectangle representing the PCS. That is to demonstrate that an MMS is intended to change the PCS as a whole, but not to become directly involved in the management of individual patients. The professionals in the PCS are assumed (should be expected) to be competent to care for their patients. Furthermore, they should be involved in many aspects of decision making about quality. This allows a quality manager to supervise a PCS effectively, without necessarily being a superior clinical practitioner.

The process of measurement, evaluation, and change continues, and the manager can observe the effects of the changes, make further corrections, etc.

Pharmaceutical Care and Medications Management

Pharmaceutical care and medications management systems are complementary and analogous. Both require similar processes of decisions and actions, one on a patient level and the other on a practice or program (multipatient) level. Both a PCS and an MMS involve (1) assessing progress toward objectives and recognizing evidence that something may be interfering with achieving them; (2) defining the basic cause of the problem or deciding that the situation is normal; (3) identifying, evaluating, and choosing alternative solutions; (4) recommending or implementing an intervention; and (5) following up the intervention (which is actually a return to step 1). This point is significant for two reasons. First, an understanding of both a PCS and an MMS may be deepened by seeing their similarities. Second, pharmaceutical care and medications management are mutually supportive. Professionals might discover the need to construct an MMS from experience operating a PCS. Likewise, quality managers in an MMS might discover the need for a PCS as the result of root cause analysis.

Pharmaceutical care was initially presented, a decade or more ago, as an abstract system. Then various writers and researchers described it more concretely, developed demonstrations, and explored its effects on outcomes and efficiency. Clearly this approach has produced some change, but the change is incomplete. Perhaps pharmaceutical care has been understood mainly as a pharmacy project, perhaps as an occupational strategy. Approaching pharmaceutical care from the medications management perspective, through process and outcome indicators, might make it more obvious that pharmaceutical care is most important as a system idea about patients, more than an occupational strategy.

Elements of Systematic Improvement in the Quality of Medications Use

Developing a medications management system parallels the quality improvement process. First, we must specify three elements: goals, tools, and processes. The *goal* of QI is to optimize structure and process with respect to outcomes and (usually) efficiency. The goal of medications management is specifically to optimize the contribution of drug therapy to patient outcomes. The basic *tools* of QI were presented in Chapter 7. They are performance indicators, practice guidelines and standards, and a performance database.[1] A well-known *process* for improving quality of health care services is the so-called FOCUS-PDCA cycle, described in examples below.

Medications management is usually needed on two levels. One level is the *program* level, comprising many practice groups. In American managed care, it would be a health maintenance organization (HMO), e.g., a state Medicaid agency or a defined part of one, such as a regional division. In the British National Health Service (NHS), this would be the level of a regional health authority, and perhaps the level of larger primary care trusts. A program would have access to large amounts of data and resources to identify recurrent quality problems. It could carry out analyses and recommend improvements to the practice level.

The second level is the *practice* level, the level at which health professionals cooperate to provide care to patients. A useful illustrative example is an independent practice association (IPA) in U.S. managed care (see Chapter 12). In the NHS, an example of a practice-level organization is a primary care group (PCG). The practice level is the so-called "sharp end" where patient and professionals interact. Practices may need to adapt general recommendations to local circumstances, and would need to follow up (locally) to assess their impact.

Virtually infinite numbers of specific variations are possible. The examples below are intended to explain the ideas in fairly concrete terms, but not to describe the only, or even the best, realization of a medications management system.

Example of Medications Management on the Program and Practice Levels

Introductory Note

The description and discussion of an MMS that follows is presented as a case study of a fictional managed care organization. This device is intended to complement the material already presented more conventionally in Chapters 7 and 8. The example is based on actual data and a real managed care organization, but it goes beyond them. It is extensive, and somewhat visionary, designed to present a coherent picture of many practical topics in quality improvement, including some that are not widely used today.

Perhaps a single real program would not need all of the aspects described. The example may, therefore, seem utopian, and in a sense it is. Like a utopia, perhaps, the example is intended to show the possibilities that medications use can be made better, to illustrate at least one way that MMSs could be constructed and operated. If aspects of the example seem unfamiliar, these would be the very aspects in which contemporary systems might need improving.

Acme Zenith Health Plan

Dr. Elizabeth Theriz, the pharmacy benefit manager of the Acme Zenith Health Plan (AZHP),* has recognized that a significant number of AZHP members may experience significant and costly preventable drug-related morbidity (PDRM). To assess the possible magnitude of the problem, she cooperated with a team of researchers from a nearby university, who implemented a set of indicators such as the medications use system performance indicators described in Chapter 7. Dr. Theriz chose AZHP's Medicare managed care program (for people over age 65) for the study.

The format of each indicator is *patient outcome + process of drug therapy*. Many indicators produced positives, but to keep the example simple, we will consider the five most frequent positives. Table 11.1 summarizes the results of the investigation.

TABLE 11.1

Medications Use System Performance Indicators

	Indicator	N	Prev.	P:O	FV
45	The patient was admitted to a hospital or emergency department (ED) with decompensated CHF when he had a history of CHF and no record of ACE inhibitor.	270	18	0.75	0.86
33	The patient was admitted to a hospital or ED with decompensated CHF or heart block and had (a) a history of CHF or heart block or bradycardia, and (b) recorded digoxin prescription and use after diagnosis and prior to admission or visit.	184	12	0.95	1.0
39	The patient was admitted to a hospital or ED with gastritis or upper gastrointestinal bleeding or gastric ulcer or anemia and used 2 or more NSAIDs concurrently for 2 weeks or more.	129	8.6	0.12	0.86
22	The patient had hyperthyroidism while being treated with thyroid or antithyroid agent when T4/TSH was not done within 6 weeks after initiation of therapy and at least every 12 months thereafter.	103	6.9	0.45	1.0
48	The patient had status asthmaticus or an ED visit or hospitalization for asthma and (a) had a history of asthma, (b) used bronchodialators, and (c) did not use an inhaled steroid.	89	5.9	1.00	0.71

Note: N = number of indicator positives in 12,000 patient records; Prev. = prevalence per 1000 patient years (N/15,000); P:O = positive predicted value of process part of indicator for outcome; FV = face validity proportion of 7 judges accepting definition a priori.

* AZHP is a fictional American managed care organization. The major points of the example would apply to other programs, e.g., the British NHS, although details would vary. The data are loosely based on results from the studies by MacKinnon and Faris (see Chapters 2 and 7).

The overall prevalence of PDRM as measured by 50 indicators was 66 per 1000 patient years. The five indicators in Table 11.1 accounted for about 60% of all such events. Patients with one or more indicator positives cost AZHP, on average, $12,400 annually, compared to $2600 for patients without a positive. Some, but probably not all, of the extra expenditures were to correct or ameliorate the effects of the PDRM.

Separating out specific consequences of each presumed PDRM required audit of actual medical records. Dr. Theriz ordered this expensive procedure on a small sample of patients and concluded that the events represented by the indicators might cost AZHP, on average, $500 per member year. It was obvious to her that AZHP had serious financial and quality problems with medications use. She decided that AZHP should consider a medications management system.

Goals and Objectives of Medications Management

The objectives of a medications use QI program are to modify existing processes (or design new processes) and to systematically monitor, analyze, and improve performance, for the goal of improving the outcomes of drug therapy.* Performance improvements are selected and evaluated on the basis of data. Improvement may comprise both improvement in average quality and reduction in quality variation.

This is based on the philosophy that value in health care requires desired outcomes, resulting from an appropriate balance of care and support services. In order to add value to the care and services provided, a health care organization must understand the relation between (a) costs, (b) outcomes, (c) perceptions by patients and physicians, and (d) the care provided cooperatively by pharmacists, physicians, and patients.

Process of QI: FOCUS

FOCUS is half of the FOCUS-PDCA formula, a common and well-accepted approach to QI. The names of the steps and the acronym are well known and may help to keep the sequence mentally organized.** FOCUS stands for *find*, *organize*, *clarify*, *understand*, and *select*.

Find a Process to Improve

Choosing the process to improve is an important decision. Because most quality managers can identify more possible improvement opportunities than they can act on, priorities have to be set. Criteria are helpful in setting priorities and can include:

---

* From Comprehensive Accreditation Manual for Long Term Care Pharmacies © 1998 by the Joint Commission on Accreditation of Healthcare Organizations. See Chapter 5.

** http://www.rootcauseanalyst.com

- The quality of the data suggesting and describing the problem
- The expected impact on performance, especially concerning high-risk, high-volume, or problem-prone processes
- The relationship of the potential improvement to the dimensions of performance and functions
- The organization's resources (that is, the feasibilty of an alternative project)

In this instance, Dr. Theriz has, in effect, already chosen to improve the quality of medications use among AZHP members, especially among the patients in the Medicare managed care program. However, within that scope, she may need to choose specific patients or problems to address, and will use these criteria to justify her recommendations to corporate management.

The indicator data showed that 75% of patients with congestive heart failure (CHF) who did not receive an angiotensin converting enzyme (ACE) inhibitor had a cardiac decompensation (heart attack) requiring emergency measures. This event occurred in 89% of emergency department visits or hospitalizations for cardiac decompensation by a patient with CHF. Another indicator showed that all patients with asthma who were receiving inhaled bronchodialators but not inhaled steroids had at least one asthma crisis requiring emergency intervention. These accounted for more than half of all asthma emergencies. This treatment violates most consensus guidelines. These guidelines are based on good epidemiology.[2,3]

Other indicators, however, may require more careful interpretation. A performance indicator should have a clear rationale based on evidence and should be valid on its face. Sometimes, however, criterion validity may be desired. In particular, an indicator may be suspected of yielding so many false positives or false negatives that its usefulness in the FOCUS process is actually impaired. The topic of criterion validity was introduced on a conceptual level in Chapter 7.

Validity Example

For example, Dr. Theriz and the QI department at AZHP used medical record review to estimate sensitivity and specificity for some of the indicators in their study. They validated them against the gold standard of professional judgment based on narrative medical records.

They chose indicators that occurred frequently in their database and then identified specific patient cases for which medical records were available, and which represented indicator positives or which represented only the outcome (without the process).

Then a member of the QI department prepared medical record abstracts. The abstractor was not informed whether those patients had been identified as positives or negatives. All chart abstracts were prepared in the same format.

TABLE 11.2

Validity Example (Hypothetical)

MI2PM Indicator	Medical Record Review: Review Positive (S+)	Medical Record Review: Review Negative (S–)	Total
Indicator Positive (I+)	a 14	b 6	a + b 20
Indicator Negative (I–)	c 3	d 12	c + d 15
Total	a + c 17	b + d 18	n 35

Next, the chart abstracts were reviewed by a panel of two clinically trained pharmacists and a gerontologist. Dr. Theriz and the abstractor met with the panel members to explain the instructions for use and to answer any questions. They asked the panel members to decide whether the indicators had been met and whether the patients in the chart abstracts actually experienced a PDRM. Each case was reviewed by the two clinical pharmacists. If they disagreed, the gerontologist was used to break the tie. A case was classified as a true PDRM if and only if two of the three panel members judged it to be a PDRM involving the process and outcome included in the indicator.

For the MI2PM indicator (patient experienced a second myocardial infarction while not taking prophylactic medications), 35 chart abstracts and reviews were performed. They are summarized in Table 11.2. (See also Table 7.2.)

Based on chart review, the sensitivity of the MI2PM indicator was 0.82 (14/17). The 95% confidence interval ranged from 0.57 to 0.96. In words, the indicator identifies about 80% of the cases that would be identified by chart review.

The positive predictive value of the indicator is 0.7 (14/20). In words, about 70% of indicator positives will be true positives.

The specificity was 12 of 18 (0.67). (The 95% confidence interval ranged from 0.41 to 0.87.) In other words, the indicator may correctly classify about two thirds of the true negatives (from chart review). The most important use of the confidence intervals for specificity and sensitivity is to show whether the likely range of values includes zero (invalidity).

Organize a Team to Study the Problem

A FOCUS team is sometimes called a quality circle, especially when its membership is predominately grassroots people, directly involved in production. Dr. Theriz recognized that she would need team members who understood the medications use process well "on the ground," such as physicians, pharmacists, and patients. She also invited others from AZHP, such as the assistant medical director and the QI manager. She invited outside experts, depending on the specific diseases, therapies, or processes chosen for discussion. She was the moderator.

Clarify the Team's Understanding of the Process

The people involved in medications use may actually carry out their roles more or less systematically than team members may suppose. Even something seemingly as straightforward as a patient visit to a physician or pharmacist may take a number of twists and turns as the result of interruptions, delays, etc. More importantly, medications use often is a complicated process involving initiators, co-therapists, and facilitators who have many activities in their lives, of which drug therapy may be only one.

Despite the common (politically correct) assumption that the workers and customers may be the best source of ideas for process improvements, there is no objective reason to believe that. A typical member of a FOCUS team or quality circle may not have reflected carefully on the complexities of medications use beyond his daily experience.

The respective roles of expert leaders and experienced stakeholders in medications use QI are an open question. A number of decision support methods might be necessary in addition to performance data. For example, it may be necessary to discuss the theory of medications use, e.g., the five principles presented in Chapter 8; to discuss typical anecdotes, to clarify mundane issues; to draw a flow diagram of the main ways that tasks get done; and to make lists of contingencies that change the process, e.g., lack of money, transportation problems.

In the AZHP example, Dr. Theriz spent about an hour discussing the theory of medications use with the FOCUS team, in particular the five principles of pharmaceutical care; the functions of initiation, co-therapy and facilitation; and the idea of feedback.

Understand the Root Causes of Variation in the Output

Sometimes a process will run well and achieve the desired results — sometimes not. It is necessary to understand the causes of this variation. Variations can occur in three kinds of quality, roughly equivalent to structure, process, and outcome:

- **Design** — how well a structure (including the processes as designed) has the potential to meet customer needs. Initially, Dr. Theriz will recognize that the medications use process used by AZHP members was not actually designed and is not at all systematic.
- **Conformance** — how well the actual processes being carried out conform to the design.
- **Performance** — how well the processes are actually meeting objectives, e.g., therapeutic objectives and customer needs. The indicators have shown that medications use is frequently not meeting objectives.

This process, called root cause analysis (RCA), is often critically important, because the understanding of variation in quality can powerfully influence the choice of solutions to be implemented in the following PDCA process. Therefore, some specialized techniques have been developed.

In responding to the indicator data in Table 11.1, the team went through two exercises, *search* (nominal group technique) and *organization* (Ishikawa diagram). These procedures should be carried out for each indicator and for all of them collectively. The following example describes a discussion of the fifth indicator in Table 11.1: asthma crisis with albuterol use and without steroid use — rescue without preventer (RWP).

Nominal Group Technique

The nominal group technique (also known as brainstorming) is a well-known technique. It comprises five steps. The following description, while fictional, is based on three actual nominal group exercises using indicator data:

1. *Clarify and agree on objectives.* The moderator stated the objective of the meeting, e.g., "to define the root cause of the asthma rescue overuse without steroid (RWP) indicator performance."
2. *Present the question.* The quality circle members accepted the validity of the indicator, and the question was put to them as "How could it happen that many patients of the AZHP Medicare program experience poor asthma control involving steroid underuse?"
3. *Poll for ideas.* Before polling began, the moderator gave the group a few minutes to think silently about the question. Then the moderator polled the group. Each person in turn offered one idea. The recorder listed the ideas where everyone could see them. Ideas were briefly clarified if necessary, but were not discussed at that time. The moderator discouraged disagreement or criticism of any kind. If a member did not have a new idea to add to the list, he passed his turn. The process continued until everyone passed.
4. *Discussion, clarification, classification.* After everyone passed in the same turn, the group discussed the ideas, mainly to clarify the meaning of each proposed cause and to group similar ideas together.
5. *Voting.* Then each member voted for the ideas that were most important, in his opinion. In this example, the team members each voted for the five most important causes, giving 5 to the most important through a 1 for the fifth most important. The votes were tallied and the leading causes were highlighted.

Table 11.3 shows the condensed results from the nominal group discussion of the RWP indicator.

Organization of Causes: Ishikawa (Affinity) Diagram

The next step is to construct an affinity diagram, also called an Ishikawa, cause-and-effect, or fishbone diagram (Figure 11.2). This exercise is intended to help

TABLE 11.3

Result of Root Cause Analysis

Proposed Cause of Asthma Indicator	Points
Patients need rescue MDI to breathe; they demand prescriptions and refills for rescue medicines like albuterol	40
Some physicians and some patients tend to avoid prescribing or using steroids	27
Lack of patient understanding about disease or correct use of asthma medicines; steroid MDI does not seem to have any effect	25
Pharmacist judgment or practice; some do not ask patients about asthma control, monitor symptoms, or question medications use patterns	18
Physician workload, lack of time/relationship with some patients	14
Pharmacy workload, lack of time/relationship with some patients; workflow, physical arrangements (e.g., lack of a private place to converse)	12
Nonclinical reasons: patients tend to stockpile rescue medicines for home, office, automobile; replace lost medicine	10
MD–patient communication without pharmacist involvement, samples	2
Patient apathy toward health	1
Sharing of medication, e.g., because of insurance	1
Indicator was rising because of pollen season	0

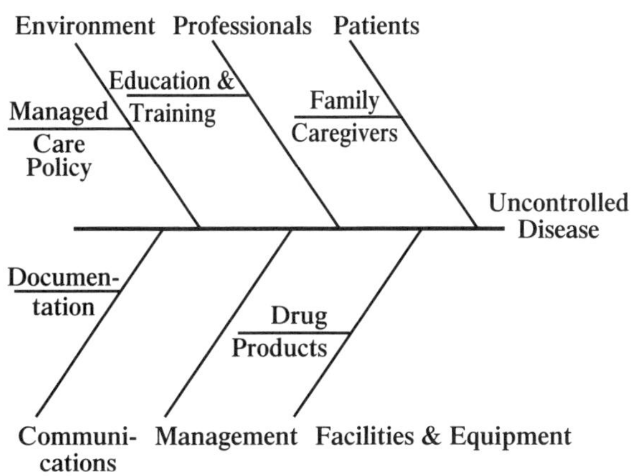

FIGURE 11.2
Structure affinity (Ishikawa) diagram.

the quality circle organize the causes proposed in the nominal group session (Table 11.3). Then they may be more able to develop corrective interventions.

The moderator usually provides a blank fishbone diagram and names the branches according to his or the group's theory of the causes of quality variation. The four M categories are typically used as a starting point: materials, machines, manpower, and methods. Other names and categories can be chosen to suit the problem. Perrow uses seven categories: *design, equipment, procedures, operators, supplies and materials, environment,* and *production pressure* (DEPOSE-P).[4] The example of Figure 11.2 is a hybrid: design is omitted; equipment and supplies and materials are combined; operators was split into professionals and patients; and procedures was split into communications and management. Production pressure was included under management. The objective should be to provide three to six main categories that can encompass all possible influences. Additions can be made to main branches as long as the problem areas can be further subdivided.

The objective of the exercise is not only to sort the results of brainstorming into categories. A more important objective is to stimulate thinking about how individual root causes interact to produce undesired results. These sequences of causes and effects may represent insight into system failure. They may also influence how improvements are described.

Select the Improvement

This is the final step in the FOCUS sequence. The objective is to select the parts of structure or process to change. Changing actual process often requires changing structures (e.g., physical layout, qualifications and number of staff, written procedures, etc.). This step is a description and definition of the selected improvement, which will then be implemented through the PDCA cycle.

For example, the FOCUS team in the fictional AZHP example recommended that AZHP identify patients with a diagnosis of (or a marker for) asthma who had a valid prescription in effect for a steroid inhaler but who were not using it (more precisely, perhaps, not billing AZHP for it). Those patients would then receive education about asthma, e.g., a brochure or a short conversation with a health educator, their pharmacist, or their physician.

Physicians and pharmacists of patients with a diagnosis of (or a marker for) asthma who did not have a valid prescription in effect for a steroid inhaler would receive "Dear Doctor" letters, over the signature of the AZHP medical director, describing asthma treatment guidelines and requesting that they review the patient's asthma management. There were two problems, however.

First, some members were concerned that some "Dear Doctor" letters might lead to unnecessary steroid therapy through overcompliance, in which some physicians accepted the advice at face value without sufficiently reviewing their patients' therapy. Other physicians might find the recommendations to be inappropriate for a few patients and then ignore subsequent letters.

Second, as the FOCUS team worked its way through the top five indicators (Table 11.1), the members began to realize that indicator-specific interventions were becoming quite numerous. The practitioner members, especially, spoke of practitioner burnout and objected that a large number of letters, telephone calls, etc., might be counterproductive.

Therefore, the last few meetings of the FOCUS team were devoted to streamlining the interventions and defining what Dr. Theriz called "fundamental system change" in the way that AZHP provided the prescription benefit to its members. Discussion returned to the theory of medications use, in particular the five principles of pharmaceutical care; the functions of initiation, co-therapy, and facilitation; and the idea of feedback.

These meetings produced the following recommendations to AZHP management:

1. AZHP should continue to use PDRM indicators and should extend their use to other patient groups (a) to assess the quality of medications use among its members, and (b) to provide feedback on performance to its providers.
2. AZHP should identify recurrent and significant problems in medications use among its members and should act directly to improve performance. However, direct action by AZHP should be considered a short-term solution that may be partially replaced by pharmaceutical care systems and practice-level MMSs as described in recommendations 3 and 4.
3. AZHP should strongly encourage its physician network to implement medications management systems for their practices. For example, it should offer financial incentives. To qualify for incentive bonuses, a practice would demonstrate a program based on process indicators derived from the AZHP performance indicator set (a) to systematically identify systemic problems in patient management, and (b) to implement changes to improve them. AZHP should agree to provide data in support of these MMSs.
4. Physician providers should, when possible and appropriate, increase cooperation with selected pharmacies for the purpose of improving medications use through MMSs and should develop PCSs to improve drug therapy outcomes for AZHP members.
5. AZHP should strongly encourage pharmacy providers to cooperate with AZHP physician providers. To qualify for incentive bonuses, a pharmacy would demonstrate cooperation with selected medical practices for direct patient care and demonstrate a program that uses process indicators derived from the AZHP performance indicator set (a) to systematically identify systemic problems in patient management, and (b) to implement changes to improve them. AZHP should agree to provide data in support of cooperating physician–pharmacy MMSs.

Plan, Do, Check, Act

PDCA stands for plan, do, check, act. It is also known as a Shewhart cycle or a Deming cycle. The four steps are as follows.

Plan

First, Dr. Theriz planned the specific implementation and the means for monitoring the implementation, e.g., indicators and a data collection and processing procedure. This was the largest project she had undertaken since joining AZHP. She was convinced that it would succeed if carried out correctly, and was determined to carry it out correctly. She decided that a limited pilot plan would provide her department with valuable experience while limiting the impact of any implementation problems. Success with a pilot program might also justify additional resources that would be needed to implement the program widely.

She further subdivided the planning of the pilot program into two stages. In the first stage, she developed a presentation to senior AZHP management, requesting preliminary approval and an assignment to develop a detailed plan. In the second stage, she developed presentations to provider groups, budgeted bonus payments, developed preferred provider contracts and payment details, and established indicator targets.

As it happened, her proposal was well timed. AZHP's management had foreseen the eventual end of price competition in their market and was looking for opportunities to improve the efficiency of care to its members. Her proposals were accepted.

Do: Implementation of Plan

Family Physician Associates (FPA) is a large group practice, mainly of internists, pediatricians, and family practitioners. FPA is one of the largest independent provider associations in the Acme Zenith Health Plan network. Patients receiving care from FPA physicians were included among the members receiving indicator positives from the screen, with a prevalence near the overall median of AZHP patients.

Dr. Theriz met with the management committee of FPA. She described the FOCUS process and the recommendations that resulted. She described the new AZHP policies. She invited FPA to participate in the pilot program as AZHP's first preferred provider. It would commit (a) to develop a cooperative relationship with selected pharmacies used by FPA and AZHP patients, and (b) to establish an MMS. The management committee estimated that as a preferred provider, it could increase its annual revenue from AZHP by approximately $300 per patient.

The PCS could include a wide variety of specific arrangements. For example, the pharmaceutical care services could be integrated with or separate from prescription services (drug distribution). FPA could choose to provide co-therapy services from physicians, medical residents, clinical pharmacists, clinical nurses, or specially trained physician's assistants. If FPA used pharmacists as co-therapists, they may be full or limited partners in the practice, employees or contractors; and may be located on the practice premises, in clinic facilities, or in community pharmacies. (Each arrangement would have significant advantages and disadvantages that are outside the scope of this discussion.)

Data for the MMS could come from a variety of sources. Dr. Theriz agreed that AZHP would provide what it had available, and even would provide certain reports. FPA's patient records were partially computerized. Most of the pharmacies that FPA would cooperate with in the PCS had computerized prescription records. Developing an MMS might have some long-term benefits to FPA. In addition to the increased revenue from being a preferred provider, an MMS might allow FPA to evaluate its own quality, thus allowing it to justify and sustain the necessary expenditures for the PCS.

The FPA management committee voted to pursue the AZHP proposal further and to invite Hugh DeMann, pharmacist and owner of a local group of pharmacies, to cooperate.

FOCUS within a Pharmacy Practice: Establishment of a PCS

The response of DeMann's Pharmacies illustrates the "wheels within wheels" response of a subsystem to a change in its environment. DeMann's Pharmacies owns four neighborhood community pharmacies, all located within 10 miles of the offices of FPA. DeMann's had been traditional dispensing pharmacies, until FPA's suggestion that DeMann's Pharmacies might cooperate in the AZHP pilot program. This conversation set off a chain of events. The owner, Hugh DeMann, initiated his own FOCUS analysis, summarized as shown in Table 11.4.

PDCA in DeMann's Pharmacies

Following their medications management contract with FPA, DeMann formalized the pharmacies' care process as follows:

- Identify whether a new patient was eligible for the program.
- Describe the pharmaceutical care program to new patients using face-to-face and written communications.
- Ask new patients or their caregivers for some basic information about their disease, or update information on patients already enrolled.
- Review medication profiles, medications use (including recent refill history), symptom status, and quality of life (activities of daily living, etc.).
- Document information and recommendations.
- Communicate essential information to FPA.

DeMann knew that he would have to be able to manage the new program within his pharmacies. He could not directly supervise pharmacists in four locations over all hours of operations, but he could use performance indicators. Many of the process elements in the AZHP performance indicators were easily accessible from the pharmacy dispensing support database, for example, drug use (refill) patterns, duplicate therapies, durations of therapy. Supervising his pharmacists' ability to detect untreated

TABLE 11.4

Example of a FOCUS Process in a Community Pharmacy

Step	Decisions
Find a process to improve	1. DeMann wishes to increase his pharmacies' involvement in patient care: to maintain their relationship with FPA, qualify as a AZHP preferred provider, and if possible develop an MMS service capability that they can use with other group practices. 2. To do this, DeMann recognizes that they must demonstrate increased value, especially to managed care. 3. Their dispensing practice has a low margin, and pharmacists have little discretionary time. The additional reimbursement from preferred provider status is attractive, but they must find feasible improvements within their limited resources. They plan to develop the new programs gradually on the experience, resources, etc., gained from the previously developed programs. 4. They have considered the potential number of patients with *frequent problems* that (a) caused *severe and expensive consequences*, and (b) that they could readily *improve in cooperation with FPA.* 5. *They concluded that their patient advising and monitoring procedures, if redesigned, could contribute to improved outcomes for many patients.*
Organize a team that knows the process	DeMann and his assistant, Utta Lee Wright, will lead the project. DeMann is the business manager, and Wright is the lead pharmacist. In addition, they recruited a professor from a nearby college of pharmacy to meet with them as needed. Each pharmacy would have a lead technician and lead pharmacist for the project.
Clarify your knowledge of the process Understand the causes of variations	They discussed drug therapy problems (DTPs), how pharmacists and pharmacy technicians can recognize DTPs, and how DTPs can be resolved in a busy pharmacy practice. They recognized the need to prioritize some patients, especially in the early days of the program. The key issues would be: 1. Access — patient receiving necessary therapy 2. Effectiveness — patient receiving expected effect, symptom resolution, etc. 3. Safety — patient not experiencing new problems attributable to drug therapy They decided that the main determinants of variation in outcomes are breakdowns in one of the five principles of pharmaceutical care.
Select the process improvement	They decided that pharmacists would interview selected patients to determine the presence of DTPs. They would provide planned and focused monitoring of medication profiles, medications use, health-related quality of life, and physical signs of disease control.

indications would be more difficult within the existing system, but would be possible with the new patient-oriented pharmacy record system that he was instituting.

Check

The objective of the check step is to decide whether the plan is working as intended. If not, in effect another, abbreviated FOCUS procedure may be carried out to correct it. The checking refers to observing the operation and results of the program and comparing them to objectives. At first, checking would concern the start-up of the pilot program. After the program had been operating long enough to stabilize, AZHP evaluated performance indicators and compared them to the goals of the program.

The check step should be, perhaps, the most technical (theoretically based) step in the PDCA cycle. It is potentially the most statistical, because it requires the manager or quality circle to interpret changes in rate-based indicators. This requires an understanding of indicator reliability and control charts.

Reliability Coding Errors

Some understanding of reliability is important, because reliability affects the apparent variability of an indicator, which in turn affects its interpretation in a control chart. Reliability of an implicit indicator refers mainly to the measurement process itself. However, reliability of a highly explicit indicator is not straightforward.

The indicators in this scenario were explicit and were applied automatically to an electronic database. Presumably, no matter how many times an indicator was applied to the database, the same cases would appear as positives and negatives. Therefore, their reliability is perfect.

This does not make the indicator measurements perfect, however. The source of potential unreliability is hidden in the coding of the database itself. For example, an explicit indicator can appear as unreliable if incorrect codes were recorded in the database for disease, drug, or procedure codes and through coding omissions. For example, if the wrong drug code were entered, a patient would appear not to have received a drug he actually did receive. This might result in an indicator false positive. If the coding error happened systematically, it would create a validity problem. It would increase the false positive rate and lower the specificity and positive predictive value of the indicator.

If the coding error happened at random, however, it would have the same effect as measurement error — it would lower reliability. For example, consider that some patients may receive prescriptions but not take them, while others may take medicines for which they do not have prescriptions. The MI2PM (second myocardial infarction, without preventive medications) indicator was used in the validity example earlier in this chapter. A positive indicator shows that a patient who had already suffered one myocardial infarction had another one while he was not receiving aspirin and a beta-blocker. The reliability of this indicator could be lowered if some patients had received beta-blocker prescriptions but had not taken them regularly, and if others took aspirin that was not reflected in a prescription database.

Reliability Example

In the validity example above, two clinical pharmacists reviewed 35 narrative medical records in order to validate the MI2PM indicator. If they disagreed, a gerontologist reviewed the record and broke the tie. The agreement level of the two pharmacist reviewers can provide a measure of reliability. The results are given in Table 11.5.

One index of reliability in this example is given by the total agreement between the two judges, divided by the total sample. (See Table 7.1.)

$$(a + d)/n$$

The two judges agreed in 31 cases (16 positives and 15 negatives):

$$r_{xx} = 31/35 = 0.89$$

A somewhat more sophisticated expression of reliability is the correlation between A's and B's judgments. For data like this, a phi coefficient is a convenient statistic:

$$\phi = [ad - bc]//[(a + b)^*(c + d)^*(a + c)^*(b + d)]$$

In this example,

$$\begin{aligned}\phi &= [(240 - 4)]//88434 \\ &= 236/297.3 \\ &= 0.79\end{aligned}$$

Possible values of phi range from 0, meaning that there is no association between the two sets of measures, to 1, perfect association. Phi can be interpreted approximately as a correlation coefficient. The two observers certainly confirm each other's observations. We conclude that different readings of the same patients with the MI2PM indicator would agree about 79% of the time.

TABLE 11.5

Indicator Reliability Example

	Observer A		
Observer B	**(+)**	**(–)**	**Total**
(+)	a 16	b 2	*a* + *b* 18
(–)	c 2	d 15	*c* + *d* 17
Total	*a* + *c* 17	*b* + *d* 17	n 35

Control Chart

A less than perfectly valid rate-based indicator may still be very valuable in managing a system. This is done with a control chart.

First, baseline statistical data should be collected for the indicator and plotted against time. To construct their control chart, Dr. Theriz and the QI staff at AZHP plotted the prevalence (among the patients of FPA) of the top five performance indicators by month for 15 months. The 15 months constituted the baseline data for the overall prevalence (rate) indicator (Figure 11.3).

In statistical process control, two kinds of variation are recognized: *random* (common) and *special*. Random variation is caused by myriad small events that are usually present in a process. In a stable and high-quality system, random events are not considered to be related to quality.

Special variation is caused by identifiable events that are probably related to quality (at least we hope to identify them). Obviously, Dr. Theriz and her team would waste time and money trying to fix apparent problems that were really only random blips on a control chart. On the other hand, if the system really is out of control, they would like to identify and correct problems.

The problem is that they cannot directly observe special variation. She and her team have to infer its presence. They can directly observe *total variation*, which is usually expressed as the standard deviation of the variable. For example, the standard deviation s of the composite indicator in Figure 11.3 equals 0.31.

Here is how to recognize special variation when it happens. For a normal distribution, the familiar bell-shaped curve, the probabilities related to variation are mathematically known. It happens that 90% of all values in a distribution will be more than the mean m minus 1.65s and less than the m + 1.65s. This distance, from (m – 1.65s) to (m + 1.65s) is called the 90% *confidence interval*. Likewise, 95% of all values will fall within $m \pm 2s$, and 99.99% will fall between $m \pm 2.6s$.* In a control chart, the upper and lower

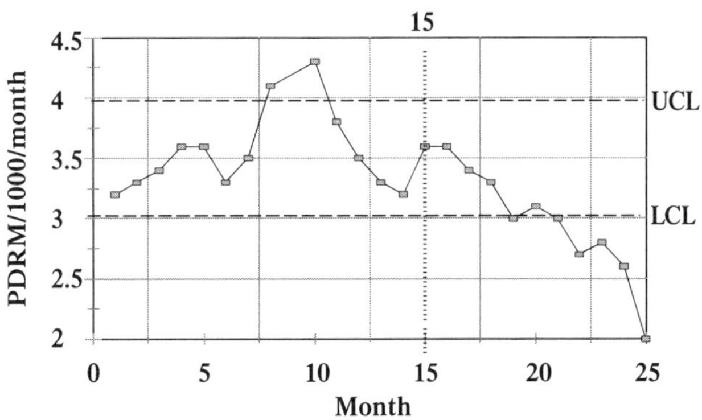

FIGURE 11.3
Control chart for a composite PDRM indicator, with 90% control limits around mean = 3.6.

ends of the confidence interval are called upper and lower control limits (UCL and LCL). In this example, the mean *m* is 3.6. Therefore, the 90% control limits for the composite indicator in Figure 11.3 are:

$$\begin{aligned} UCL &= 3.6 + 1.65*0.31 \\ &= 4.1 \end{aligned}$$

$$\begin{aligned} LCL &= 3.6 - 1.65*0.31 \\ &= 3.04 \end{aligned}$$

Figure 11.3 shows these 90% control limits, based on the mean of 3.6 and the standard deviation of 0.31.

A process should be investigated when special variation or a clear trend is observed, or when a preset threshold is crossed. According to the composite indicator in this fictional example, medications use among AZHP and FPA members appears to have been significantly high (out of control) in months 8 and 9. Except for those months, the remaining variation from months 1 to 15 appears to have been random (in control).

Outliers often help to identify problems and root causes. For example, it would be useful to ask what was different about months 8 and 9 that might (a) have explained the rise in the value of the indicator, and (b) have been under the control of AZHP or FPA. In this example, however, the whole series of indicator values is unacceptable, even if it is in control. AZHP is not willing to accept this rate of PDRM, and it has constructed a control chart to decide when a change is significant rather than to maintain an acceptable status quo. (This may be a common situation when indicators are first used in some drug therapy systems.)

The AZHP preferred provider program, which started in month 17, appears to have been associated with a significant improvement trend in the indicator. If the trend continues, new control limits will be needed, because both the mean and standard deviation for the process will have changed.

Act

Act is the final step in the PDCA cycle. No action is needed at this stage of the example, because the effect of the initial action is evidently still taking place. In the future, however, the indicator may level off at still-unacceptable levels. Dr. Theriz may then choose to implement changes in the way the program is being carried out by FPA. This merges into the *plan* step, and the cycle repeats indefinitely.

Kaizen

Theriz and AZHP are planning significant changes that will take some time to implement. They will have to take care not to move too much faster than their customers (employers and patients) and providers (physicians and pharmacists) can understand. Kaizen is the philosophy of making many small, frequent changes in a process. The changes that work, according to the performance indicators and the quality circle, are made permanent and are made to spread throughout the organization. The ones that do not work may be dropped, while others are tried.

Major quality improvements reportedly have been accomplished gradually by use of kaizen, without the large investment and awkwardness of a major change that takes a long time to implement and sell to customers. However, there still must be a clear goal and consistent commitment; otherwise, kaizen would become mere tinkering. Also, it may seem impossible to apply kaizen to a system that has as many defects as most medications use systems. In other words, drug use outcomes may depend on many factors, and changing just a few at a time may produce small and inefficient results.

Connective Summary

Chapter 10 and this chapter described two interrelated systems, one on a patient level and the other on a group or population level. These systems complement and support each other.

The idea of pharmaceutical care has been advocated for over 10 years, and accepted by many professional organizations, including the World Health Organization, the International Pharmaceutical Federation, and pharmacy societies of many nations, such as the Royal Pharmaceutical Society of Great Britain and the American Pharmaceutical Association.

Still, few patients receive pharmaceutical care. There is little evidence that PDRMs are any less prevalent now than they were 10 years ago. Few managed care organizations or professionals consistently provide pharmaceutical care, perhaps because they cannot recognize the prevalence of PDRMs in their own patients. Pharmaceutical care systems are being adopted, but the rate of adoption is inappropriately slow, given the magnitude of the problem described in Chapter 2. Their rate of adoption is too slow to keep pace with other changes in health care.

This chapter described a way for managed care organizations and professional group practices to manage (evaluate and improve) the quality of medications use among their own patients. The example emphasized medications management with performance indicators in a managed care organization. A pharmacy or medical practice manager could also use medications management with process indicators on the practice level.

It would be difficult to overstate the importance of medications management systems as a means of improving the safety, effectiveness, and efficiency of drug therapy. It seems essential that managed care organizations adopt them. However, if they did and if they found severe problems, many of those problems could not be resolved without instituting pharmaceutical care systems on the practice level.

Chapters 12 and 13 return us to present-day reality. They provide an introduction to managed care, a very influential aspect of the environment within which pharmaceutical care and medications management would take place. That discussion then leads to the concluding chapter (Chapter 15), which addresses broad issues and ideas concerning how medications management can become a normal part of health care delivery.

References

1. Angaran, D.M. and Hepler, C.D., Outcomes of drug therapy, in *Pharmaceutical Care*, Knowlton, C.H. and Penna, R.P., Eds., Chapman & Hall, New York, 1996, p. 176.
2. Ernst, P. et al., Risk of fatal and near-fatal asthma in relation to inhaled corticosteroid use, *JAMA*, 268, 3462, 1992.
3. Spitzer, W.O. et al., The use of beta-agonists and the risk of death and near death from asthma, *N. Engl. J. Med.*, 326, 501, 1992.
4. Perrow, C., *Normal Accidents: Living with High-Risk Technologies*, Princeton University Press, Princeton, NJ, 1999.
5. Institute of Medicine, *Crossing the Quality Chasm: A New Health System for the 21st Century*, National Academy Press, Washington, D.C., 2001.

12

Managed Care

Finding solutions to reduce preventable drug-related morbidity (PDRM) requires an understanding of the health care environment. There are a number of entities found in health care today such as insurance companies, managed care organizations, medical groups and practitioner associations, pharmacy benefit managers, patients, and providers. Each of these shapes the complex health care system we have today. Understanding the structures, rules, and customs of these organizations can be helpful in explaining why medication problems occur and why many interventions fail to fix the problems. Considering all of the players in health care today, managed health care organizations along with insurance companies are having a profound impact on how health care providers and patients behave in the context of the medicines use process. Consequently, Chapters 12 and 13 will examine the role of managed care in today's health care environment and its influence on the medicines use process.

Managed health care, in a variety of forms, has been in place in the United States for most of the 20th century. In the United Kingdom, the National Health Service (NHS) has been in effect since 1948. While the details of the structure of health plans differ among nations and will undoubtedly change in response to social, political, and economic forces, some form of managed care probably will provide the underlying framework for health care delivery in the United States and U.K. for the foreseeable future.

The objectives of this chapter are to outline:

- The types, terminology, and basic concepts of managed care
- The structures, standards, principles, and methods of managed care

This introduction is a prerequisite to understanding how managed care influences health care delivery, including medicines use.

Introduction: Scope of Managed Care

The term *managed care* is used broadly in this book to denote a method of providing and paying for health care services that organizes physicians, hospitals, and other health care providers into health care delivery groups ostensibly for the purpose of improving the quality and cost-effectiveness of health care. Managed care usually reduces or replaces the traditional fee-for-service (FFS) professional payment basis with other methods, as described below.

Managed care organizations (MCOs) contract with *purchasers* (e.g., employers; labor unions; business coalitions; federal, state, and provincial governments; and individuals) to provide health care to people (members) in *defined populations*. Organizational structures include health maintenance organizations (HMOs), preferred provider organizations (PPOs), and others.

In the United States, private organizations have traditionally provided the vast majority of health care coverage. The U.S. government operates some publicly funded health finance programs, but access is limited to specific groups. Most Americans obtain private health insurance through their places of employment. Although many American managed care organizations are private, governmental programs like the Veterans Administration and U.S. Public Health Service operate programs that are, in essence, managed care programs. *Managed care* is an American term. Although Canadians and Europeans may think of it as an American idea, highly regulated single-payer systems like the British National Health Service and government health insurance programs like Canadian provincial health care programs have many similarities to American managed care.

Since the 1980s, the percentage of Americans cared for by MCOs has increased rapidly. Today, managed care dominates the health care financing and delivery system in the United States. In 2000, for example, more than 90% of insured Americans were enrolled in some form of a managed care plan, representing an increase of more than 30% over 1988.[1] Likewise, most of the few remaining commercial traditional health insurance plans have adopted techniques used by managed care organizations such as case management and preauthorization programs. Additionally, public sector programs such as Medicare and Medicaid have increased their reliance on managed care as a method for delivering care to its enrollees.

History of Managed Care

The Western Clinic in Tacoma, Washington, may be the first example of an HMO or prepaid practice group (as HMOs were commonly referred to before the 1970s). Starting in 1910, the Western Clinic offered a broad range of medical services to an employer's workers in return for a premium payment of $0.50 per member per month.[2] A decade later, Baylor Hospital in Houston, Texas, agreed to provide approximately 1500 teachers prepaid care at its hospital, an arrangement that represented the origins of Blue Cross, and in 1939, state medical societies in California and elsewhere created Blue Shield plans, which reimbursed for physician services.[3] Because physicians wanted to protect and enhance patient revenues in the midst of the Great Depression, the number of Blue Cross and Blue Shield plans increased. However, many of these plans, and especially prepaid plans, were considered by organized medicine as a threat. In 1932, the American Medical Association (AMA) stated its opposition to prepaid group practices and favored, instead, indemnity-type insurance.[4]

The period immediately following World War II saw the formation of several HMOs that remain prominent today. Examples of HMOs that had their origins during that period include the Kaiser Foundation Health Plans, the Group Health Association (later acquired by Humana Health Plans and then sold to the Kaiser Foundation Health Plans), Health Insurance Plan (HIP), and Group Health Cooperative of Puget Sound. In reaction to prepaid group practice HMOs such as the Kaiser Foundation Health Plans, an alternative type of managed care called independent practice association (IPA) HMOs began to emerge during the 1950s.[4]

Through the early 1970s, HMOs played a relatively small role in the financing and delivery of health care in the United States, although they had been large players for a period of time in some geographic markets such as Seattle and regions within California. In 1970, the total number of HMOs was fewer than 40. However, the HMO industry received significant support with the enactment of the 1973 Federal HMO Act. This act provided start-up funding for new HMOs and required most employers that offered traditional indemnity coverage to also offer two federally qualified HMOs, when HMO plans had formally requested it.* Discussions about health care in the U.S. government leading up to this act raised concerns about the fee-for-service model used by traditional indemnity insurance in public sector programs such as Medicare as well as private sector programs. Fee-for-service rewards physicians based on their volume of services, arguably incorporating financial incentives to provide unnecessary services to their patients.[5] Spurred by this act, the number of HMOs increased dramatically until the rate of growth started a small decline beginning in the early 2000s.[2,6]

Other managed care developments that occurred during the 1970s and the early 1980s included the rise of modern preferred provider organizations. PPOs are believed to have been started in Denver during the early 1970s when a benefits consulting firm negotiated fee-for-service discounts with physicians.[4]

Types of Managed Care Organizations

So many changes have been occurring in the structure and financing of health care that it is difficult to describe the many forms of managed care in today's

* This provision was eliminated in 1995.

market. Even more difficult is predicting the specific characteristics of managed care 10 years from today. Previously, the various types of MCOs were reasonably distinct; however, today the differences have become blurred. For example, many HMOs traditionally limited their members to care received from an exclusive provider group. Today, many allow members to use nonparticipating providers at a reduced coverage level, mimicking PPOs or even traditional indemnity insurance to some extent.[7] While there are many variations of managed care organizations, three major types are described below: preferred provider organizations, health maintenance organizations, and point-of-service plans (POSs).

Preferred Provider Organizations

PPOs include the following characteristics. First, PPOs typically establish a network by contracting with selected providers to offer health services for covered members. Participating providers included in the network often consist of hospitals, physicians, diagnostic facilities, and pharmacies. Second, most PPO participation agreements involve a negotiated payment rate with providers in which providers accept the PPO's payments as payment in full for covered services (excluding co-insurance or deductibles paid by patient members). Negotiated rates often take the form of fixed-fee schedules or discounts from charges or payments based on diagnosis-related groups. These are sometimes called negotiated FFS rates. PPOs are generally different from HMOs in that they do not accept capitation risk; rather, financial risk remains with the insurance company or self-insured employment-based entity. Third, most PPOs use utilization management programs to control the utilization and cost of health services provided to their patient members. The last characteristic involves consumer choice. Unlike the more traditional HMOs found during the 1990s, PPOs generally allow members to use non-PPO providers instead of PPO providers, although these health plans will generally ask the member to share more of the costs. Another aspect of consumer choice found in PPOs is that patient members may choose to receive a service from any provider in the PPO network. In other words, patient members may switch their providers as frequently as they wish based on provider availability.[7]

Health Maintenance Organizations (HMOs)

HMOs are organized health care systems that are responsible for both the financing and delivery of a broad range of comprehensive health services to an enrolled population. The earlier HMOs all shared a common financial arrangement referred to as prepaid fixed fees. While prepaid fixed fees are still common, every HMO no longer uses them. In many ways, an HMO may be considered as a combination of a health insurer and a health care delivery system in contrast to traditional health insurance companies, who are responsible for only reimbursing providers for the cost of health care delivered to the insurance company's members.

Because HMOs are responsible for providing or coordinating covered health services, they create systems that allow their patient members to have access to covered health services. Additionally, HMOs generally are responsible for ensuring the quality and appropriateness of the health services they provide to their members. There are four commonly recognized models of HMOs, including staff, group, network, and IPA. The major differences between these models generally pertain to the relationship between the HMO and its participating providers.

Most HMO models share some similar characteristics, including a requirement that a member (patient) go through many cost containment procedures before getting care, the most prominent of which is referred to as the gatekeeper provision. A primary care provider (PCP) is assigned to each member, and that physician controls all care for that member. In order to see a specialist or consult with a dietician, for example, an HMO member must first get permission from their gatekeeper provider. Another feature found in each of the HMO models is the use of some form of performance or risk-based reimbursement to pay a group practice of physicians or even individual physicians, especially primary care providers.[8] At a simple level, there are two basic ways to compensate providers for services: capitation or negotiated fee-for-service. Capitation is prepayment for services on a per member per month (PMPM) basis. In other words, a PCP is paid a fixed amount of money every month for an HMO member enrolled in his or her practice regardless of whether that member receives services and regardless of how expensive those services are.

There are many different forms of capitation that are beyond the scope of this chapter; however, one example is offered to provide the reader with an understanding of generally how this reimbursement method works. In setting a capitation rate for a PCP, an HMO may begin by calculating what a physician would receive from FFS for a particular membership base, assuming appropriate utilization. If a physician receives approximately $55 per visit in collected fees under FFS, and a reasonable estimated visit rate is three primary care visits per member per year (PMPY), then multiplying 3 by $55 and dividing the result by 12 yields $13.75 PMPM. An HMO may then specify that as the capitation rate. This example is simplistic and does not accurately describe precisely how HMOs calculate capitation rates because it does not account for other variables that are often considered, such as varying scope of services, actual visitation rates for a particular area by age and gender, effects of copayments, and so on. Furthermore, many HMOs will withhold some percentage of the capitation rate to cover cost overruns, such as those caused by larger numbers of referrals to specialists than originally budgeted, or increased use of institutional services or pharmacy expenses. The withheld payments are used at the end of some period for reconciliation of cost overruns, and the remainder is returned to the PCP. In other words, money from the "withhold account" may or may not be given back to physicians based on whether or not utilization is well managed.[8] The following section provides brief descriptions of these major HMO types.

Staff Model

Physicians and most of the other providers who offer care to patient members of staff HMOs are employees of the HMO. These providers are typically paid on a salary basis and may also receive bonuses or other types of incentive payments based on their performance. A staff HMO employs physicians representing most of the common specialties needed to provide care to its members (patients). In some cases, staff HMOs will enter into contracts with select community subspecialists to provide care for infrequently needed health services.

Staff model HMOs are sometimes referred to as *closed-panel* HMOs because most participating providers are employees of the HMO and community physicians generally cannot participate. Physicians in staff model HMOs usually practice in one or more centralized ambulatory care facilities that may often resemble outpatient clinics, with physician offices and ancillary support services to support the health care needs of the HMO's members. Many staff HMOs contract with hospitals and other inpatient facilities in the community to provide nonphysician services for its members.[7,8] Some staff model HMOs, such as Kaiser Permanente, thrived during the early 1990s, while others did not. Many that do exist today are incorporating other types of physician relationships into their delivery system.

One theoretical advantage of staff HMOs over other types of HMOs is their greater degree of control over the practice patterns of employed physicians. As a result, it can be easier for a staff model HMO to manage and control utilization of health services. They also offer the advantage of one-stop medical care for their members because of the centralized HMO facilities. Staff HMOs, however, also suffer from several weaknesses that may threaten their financial solvency. These include the costly financial requirements associated with developing and maintaining a complete (or nearly complete) health care delivery system with large fixed-salary expenses, and costly buildings for what often is a relatively small membership of patients. Second, staff HMOs control access to care by providing a limited number of providers from which patients may choose to receive care.[7]

Group Model HMOs

In a pure group model HMO, the HMO contracts with a multispecialty physician group practice to provide all physician services to its HMO members. Physicians and other PCPs are employed by the group practice and not by the HMO. In some cases, these physicians may be allowed to see both HMO patients and non-HMO patients, but often the HMO enters into a contract that limits the physician members of the group practice from seeing non-HMO patients.

Physicians in the group practice share facilities, equipment, medical records, and support staff. The physician group practice may contract with the HMO on an all-inclusive capitation basis to provide physician services to HMO members. *Capitation* means that the group practice is paid a certain sum per enrolled HMO member per month. This payment is made to the practice group whether they see the member or not. With the capitation contract comes some risk for the physician group practice, because if they see every member that is enrolled each month, they will not have enough money to pay their expenses. If their patients are healthy or if they limit care, however, and see only a percentage of the members, then they can make a profit on a capitated contract.[7,8] For many contracts, the group is responsible for providing all physician services to HMO patient members assigned to the group and may refer to other physician specialists when necessary. The group is typically financially responsible for reimbursing specialists for any referrals it makes.

Like staff model HMOs, group model HMOs are sometimes referred to as closed-panel HMOs because physicians must be members of the group practice to participate in the HMO. Similar to staff model HMOs, it is easier to conduct utilization management because of the centralized nature within which care is delivered and because physicians are part of one medical practice group. Group practice HMOs frequently have lower capital needs than do staff model HMOs because the HMO itself does not support the large fixed-salary costs such as the case in a staff model HMO. Like staff model HMOs, group model HMOs share some common disadvantages. For example, both HMO models provide a limited choice of participating providers from which HMO members can select. Because providers provide care in a limited number of sites, there is generally a limitation in the geographic accessibility of physicians for HMO members.[7]

Network Model HMOs

A network HMO contracts with more than one group practice to provide physician services to its HMO patient members. These group practices may be broad-based multispecialty groups, in which case the HMO resembles a group model HMO. Alternatively, the HMO may contract with several small groups of primary care providers, in which case the HMO is classified as a primary care network model. In the primary care network model, the HMO contracts with several groups typically consisting of 7 to 15 PCPs each, representing the specialties of family practice, internal medicine, pediatrics, and obstetrics/gynecology to provide physician services to its patient members. Most frequently, the HMO compensates these groups on an all-inclusive physician capitation basis with similar arrangements found for group model HMOs.[7]

In contrast to staff and group model HMOs, network HMOs may be either closed or open panel. If the network model is a closed panel, it will contract with only a limited number of existing group practices. If it is an open-panel plan, participation in the group practices will be open to any physician who meets the HMO's and the group's credentialing criteria. Unlike staff and group model HMOs, network model HMOs typically offer much broader physician participation, overcoming the geographic restrictions associated with providing care in only several locations, as found with staff and group HMOs.[7,8]

IPA Model HMOs

IPA model HMOs contract with an association of physicians, called an independent practice association, to provide physician services to the HMO members. The physicians are members of the IPA, which is a legal entity, but they remain individual practitioners and retain their separate offices and identities. IPA physicians will often see patients from many HMOs as well as PPO members or even patients that are covered by traditional indemnity-type insurance.

Generally, IPAs recruit physicians from all specialties to participate in their plan. Broad participation of physicians allows the IPA to provide all necessary physician services through participating physicians. It minimizes the need for participating providers to refer patients to nonparticipating providers to obtain services.

Most HMOs compensate their IPAs on an all-inclusive physician capitation basis. The IPA then compensates its participating providers on either a fee-for-service basis or a combination of fee-for-service and primary care capitation. In the fee-for-service variation, IPAs pay all of their participating physicians on the basis of a fee schedule and usually withhold a portion of each payment for incentive and risk-pooling purposes. Under the primary care capitation approach, IPAs pay their participating PCPs on a capitation basis and pay their specialist physicians on the basis of a fee schedule. The primary care capitation payments are based on fixed amounts per member per month and may vary depending on the HMO member's age and gender.[8]

IPA model HMOs overcome some disadvantages associated with staff, group, and network HMOs. They require less capital to establish and operate. In addition, they offer a broad choice of participating physicians who practice in their private offices. From the HMO's perspective, there are several disadvantages associated with IPAs. One is that the process of utilization management can be more difficult in an IPA model HMO because physicians remain individual practitioners with little sense of being part of the HMO. As a result, IPA model HMOs may devote more resources to managing inpatient and outpatient utilization than would be the case for staff and group model HMOs.[7,8]

Point-of-Service (POS) Plans

Some people believe that they may need the services of a nonparticipating provider occasionally and may wish to have those services financially covered to some degree by their health plan. In response to patient demand, many HMOs have therefore developed some level of indemnity-type coverage for their members (patients), allowing the member to choose either HMO coverage or indemnity coverage at the point of service when medical care is needed. The indemnity coverage available under POS options from HMOs typically requires high deductibles and co-insurance to encourage patient members to use HMO services within the network instead of out-of-plan services.[7]

Recent Managed Care Trends

Shifting Enrollments

Managed care constitutes one of the most complicated industries in the United States. Enrollment in traditional indemnity plans dropped from 23% of all active employees covered in employer-sponsored health plans in 1996 to only 8% in 2000. As of 2000, more than 90% of insured Americans were enrolled in some form of a managed care plan, representing an increase of more than 30% over 1988. The following is a breakdown of plans that MCO members are in:

- 44% in a preferred provider organization, up from 31% in 1996
- 32% in an HMO, up from 27%
- 16% in a point-of-service plan, down from 19%
- 8% in other plan types[1]

HMO enrollment growth is slowing, from a peak rate of 16% in 1996 to an average annual rate of less than 5%. Total HMO enrollment was 80.8 million at its peak during 1999 and dropped to approximately 78 million during 2001.[6,9] The relatively flat rate of growth appears to be caused by increases in HMO premiums and the saturation of certain geographical markets in the country. Double-digit commercial premium increases in 1998 and 1999 have hurt HMO profitability, with about 60% of HMOs experiencing negative profit margins in 1998.[9] Currently, California and Massachusetts are the only states with an HMO penetration rate around 50%. It is forecast that by the year 2005, penetration will exceed 50% in those two states as well as in Colorado, Delaware, Kentucky, Maryland, New Mexico, Pennsylvania, Rhode Island, and Tennessee.[9]

More than 40% of total HMO enrollment is in IPA model HMOs. Enrollment in staff model HMOs continues to decline and now contributes less than 1% of total enrollment. HMO enrollment continues to be concentrated in the largest and oldest plans — more than 80% of enrollment is in plans that are at least 10 years old and have at least 100,000 members.[10]

Currently, the strongest competition for HMOs is PPOs. During the past few years, consolidation in the PPO industry has escalated, and diversified national firms appear to have selected a strategy, which includes increasing their market strength through high provider penetration in specific key metropolitan markets.[9,10]

Medicare Managed Care

The HMO Medicare annual growth rate also showed a sharp decline recently, dropping from 18.6% in July 1998 to just 4% in July 1999. HMOs added slightly fewer than 250,000 Medicare enrollees for the 12-month period starting July 1998, bringing Medicare HMO enrollment, as of July 1, 1999, to its peak at 6.4 million. Since 1999, the number of Medicare

HMO enrollees has dropped.[6] Recent slow growth can partially be attributed to numerous HMOs across the country dropping out of Medicare service areas. Citing high costs and low reimbursement rates, many HMOs are condensing their service areas or withdrawing from the program entirely.[9]

Medicaid Managed Care

Medicaid enrollment added only slightly more than 475,000 enrollees during the 12 months ending on July 1, 1999, with total enrollment of 10.8 million. Unlike the growth rates for total and Medicare HMO enrollment, the annual growth rate for Medicaid increased slightly, rising 4.6% since January 1999. One reason for this growth is that many states still require Medicaid enrollment in a managed care program. The bulk of new Medicaid enrollees are in the Pacific and Mountain regions, which added 208,675 and 143,947 enrollees, respectively, since January 1, 1999.[9]

Medical Groups

The percentage of medical practice groups with managed care contracts that had contracts with preferred provider organizations during 1998 was 81%. By comparison, 49% of medical groups with managed care contracts had contracts with network HMOs, and 48% had contracts with IPA model HMOs.[11]

Costs

During 1998, slightly more than half of all HMOs reimbursed more than 60% of primary care services through capitation contracts.[10] In many areas, PCP capitation rates have been dropping, for example, in California from an average of $45 PMPM in 1993 to $29 PMPM in 1999.[12]

In 2000, employer-sponsored health benefit costs rose 8.1%, the third straight year in which increases were more than double the rate of general inflation. The average cost per employee rose from $4097 in 1999 to $4430 in 2000 (see Figure 12.1). The slowing of the rate of increase in health care costs noted during the early years of managed care now seems to have ended. Current projections suggest that the average health benefit cost will increase annually by a double-digit value during the first decade of 2000, with HMO costs rising more sharply than PPO costs.[1]

Prescription drug costs played a major role in the overall cost increase in 2000, with employers reporting an average drug cost increase of 17.5%. (Drug cost rose 11.5% in 1998 and 15.2% in 1999.) Between 1991 and 1998, the average retail price of a prescription increased almost 60%, from $23.68 to $37.38. Since 1998, the average retail price of a prescription has continued to rise, reaching almost $45 in 2002. During this period, the average price of a prescription for a brand-name drug increased 80%, which is much larger than the 55% increase for generic drugs.[13–16]

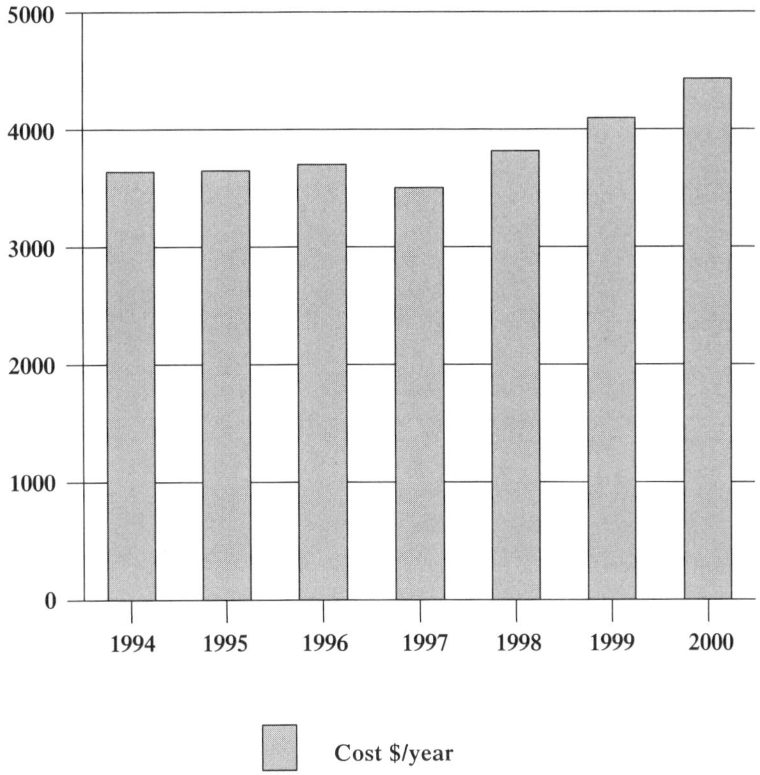

FIGURE 12.1
Average annual health care cost per employee.

The average reimbursement rate for retail pharmacies, based on average wholesale price (AWP) and dispensing fee, is stable. The average AWP discount is 13.1%, and the average dispensing fee is $2.30.[15] When a pharmacy sells a prescription to a consumer, on average, about $0.74 of each dollar in sales goes to the pharmaceutical manufacturer, $0.03 to the wholesaler, and $0.23 to the pharmacy.[15]

Price changes for existing drugs have contributed less (18%) to the increase in prescription drug expenditures since 1993 than have increased utilization rates (43%) or changes in the types of drugs used (39%), with new and more expensive drugs typically replacing older drugs in the same therapeutic category.[13] Overall, utilization of drugs grew from an average of 8.3 prescriptions PMPY in 1999 to 8.6 prescriptions PMPY in 2000 — a 3.6% increase. Widely used gastrointestinal, antidepressant, antirheumatic, and cardiovascular drugs showed the most significant utilization increases.[14]

Persons older than 65 account for approximately 13% of the U.S. population, with the average patient older than 65 filling approximately 20 prescriptions per year, compared with the average patient in his or her 20s filling approximately 3 prescriptions per year. In addition, the average PMPY cost for a person between the ages of 66 and 70 years ($704.52) is nearly nine times higher than for a person younger than 20 years ($81.06). Remarkably, 5% of the people receiving drug benefits account for more than 50% of the spending, with most of the high-cost prescription drug users receiving treatment for conditions such as cancer, diabetes, and cardiovascular disease. In addition, the likelihood is very high that a high-cost prescription drug user in 1 year will be a high-cost user in a subsequent year. Rates of use for certain drug classes are very high among the highest cost adult patients. Specifically, 48% use antidepressants or antianxiety medications, 46% use pain medications, 40% use antiulcer medications, and 59% use antihypertensives.[17]

With pharmaceuticals now accounting for approximately 14% of the total medical plan cost, nearly all managed care organizations and contracted pharmacy benefit management companies have instituted a number of intended cost-saving strategies to lower the cost of pharmaceuticals (see Chapter 13).[1]

Performance Measurement in Managed Care

Accreditation and performance measurement have been dominant features within hospitals for many decades. Spurred by concerns raised by employers, a performance measurement system was introduced to help gauge whether employers were receiving value from their health care compensation program. More than half of HMO and POS plans now participate in some type of accreditation offered by either the National Committee for Quality Assurance (NCQA), the Utilization Review Accreditation Commission (URAC), or the Joint Commission on Accreditation of Healthcare Organizations (JCAHO). Over a number of years, NCQA has refined a set of performance measures for managed care plans through its Health Plan Employer Data and Information Set (HEDIS).

HEDIS, designed to ensure that purchasers and consumers have the information they need to reliably compare the performance of MCOs, is a performance measurement tool used by more than 90% of health plans. The measures in HEDIS are related to many significant public health issues such as cancer, heart disease, smoking, asthma, diabetes, mental health, controlling high blood pressure, and menopause. HEDIS consists of approximately 60 measures that fall into eight broad areas, including:

- Effectiveness of care
- Access and availability of care
- Member satisfaction
- Use of services
- Cost of care

- Informed health care choices
- Health plan descriptive information
- Stability of the health plan

The standards for including a measure in HEDIS include evaluations of each measure's reliability and validity.[18,19] For a health plan to earn NCQA accreditation, it must report on a number of performance measures, including, but not limited to, the following HEDIS *effectiveness of care* measures: beta-blocker treatment after a heart attack, childhood and adolescent immunizations, breast cancer and cervical cancer screening, prenatal care in the first trimester, advising smokers to quit, and eye exams for people with diabetes.[18]

Each HEDIS measure specifies not only what to measure but also how to measure it to allow all MCOs to be measured similarly. The development of valid and reliable measures presumably help managed care organizations to measure data consistently, permitting direct comparisons between health plans. An example of a HEDIS indicator concerning drug therapy is appropriate medications for people with asthma. This indicator measures the percentage of members with chronic asthma who receive medications recommended as primary therapy for long-term control, such as inhaled corticosteroids. Another example related to drug therapy concerns beta-blocker treatment after a heart attack in members age 35 and older who were hospitalized and discharged with the diagnosis of acute myocardial infarction.

Efforts to measure performance in managed care organizations have seemingly resulted in improvements in the way care is delivered. Nonetheless, the literature suggests that there are far too many instances in which providers, most of whom practice within a managed care environment, do not provide care consistent with evidence-based best practices. For example, while the benefits of aggressive, intensive treatment of diabetes are well established and are reflected in consensus recommendations for prevention of diabetic complications, primary care physician adherence to certain guideline recommendations has been found to be low.[20] This was found to be particularly true for recommendations regarding examination of teeth and gums, examination of the feet, and laboratory tests involving urine; while compliance with recommendations for eye exams, neurological and circulatory exams, and laboratory procedures using blood were relatively high.

Conclusion

Managed care organizations, in their many manifestations from an American IPA to a government program like the U.S. Veterans Administration or the British NHS, are a fact of life in health care delivery throughout the industrialized world. American managed care offers an alphabet soup of organizational variation and appears nearly unique in its use of business models.

The structure of managed care obviously offers many opportunities to control expenditures for health care, either through market power and prudent buying in an open market model or through negotiated price controls in governmental and single-payer approaches. It also offers enormous potential to improve quality.

The next chapter will describe some familiar (and some not-so-familiar) managed care strategies to improve medicines use. Then Chapters 14 and 15 will explore ways to close the gap between the reality and the promise of managed care in improving the quality of medicines use in populations.

References

1. Thirteenth Annual Mercer/Foster Higgins National Survey of Employer-Sponsored Health Plans, 2000, William Mercer, Inc., Chicago, IL.
2. Mayer, T.R. and Mayer, G.G., HMOs: origins and development, *N. Engl. J. Med.*, 312, 590, 1985.
3. Starr, P., *The Social Transformation of American Medicine*, Basic Books, New York, 1982, p. 295.
4. Fox, P.D., An overview of managed care, in *Essentials of Managed Health Care*, 4th ed., Kongstvedt, P.R, Ed., Aspen Publishers, Gaithersburg, MD, 2001, chap. 1.
5. Stumpf, G.B., Historical evolution and political process, in *Group and IPA HMOs*, Mackie D.L. and Decker, Eds., Aspen Publishers, Gaithersburg, MD, 1981, p. 17.
6. HMO enrollment in big U.S. cities drops slightly, in *Reuters Health*, June 26, 2002, http://www.lifeclinic.com/healthnews/article_view.asp?story=19980.
7. Wagner, E.R., Types of managed care organizations, in *Essentials of Managed Health Care*, 4th ed., Kongstvedt, P.R, Ed., Aspen Publishers, Gaithersburg, MD, 2001, chap. 2.
8. Kongstvedt, P.R., Compensation of primary care physicians in managed health care, in *Essentials of Managed Health Care*, 4th ed., Kongstvedt, P.R, Ed., Aspen Publishers, Gaithersburg, MD, 2001, chap. 7.
9. The InterStudy HMO Industry Report 10.1, InterStudy Publications, Minneapolis, MN, 2000.
10. The InterStudy Competitive Edge, InterStudy Publications, Minneapolis, MN, 1999.
11. The Hoechst Marion Roussel, Managed Care Digest Series™, 1999 Medical Group Practice Digest, 1999, Kansas City, MO.
12. Low fees cited in doctors' demise, in *The Press Democrat*, Santa Rosa, CA, September 4, 1999, http://healthcare.newsreal.com/story/19990904/08/54/5695396_st.html.
13. *Prescription Drug Trends: A Chartbook*, Henry J. Kaiser Family Foundation, Menlo Park, CA, 2001.
14. Prescription drug use patterns complicated by wide regional variation, in *Express Scripts Drug Trend Report*, St. Louis, MO, 2001.

15. Wyeth-Ayerst Prescription Drug Benefit Cost and Plan Design Survey Report, Phamacy Benefit Management Institute, Inc., Tempe, AZ, 1999.
16. Lee, K., Analysts Promote OTC Drugs as Defensive Medicine, *Employee Benefit News*, May 1, 2001.
17. Prescription drug trends in *U.S. 2000: Utilization and Cost Implications for Pharmacy Benefit Plans*, PCS HealthSystems, Irving, TX, 2000.
18. O'Kane, M.E., Accreditation and performance measurement programs for managed care organizations, in *Essentials of Managed Health Care*, 4th ed., Kongstvedt, P.R, Ed., Aspen Publishers, Gaithersburg, MD, 2001, chap. 26.
19. NCQA releases final HEDIS 2000 measures: focus is on heart disease, asthma, women's health, June 29, 1999, http:///www.ncqa.org.
20. Kenny, S.J., Smith, P.J., Goldschmid, M.G., et al., Survey of physician practice behaviors related to diabetes mellitus in the U.S., *Diabetes Care*, 16, 1507, 1993.

13

Managed Care Strategies to Influence the Cost, Access, and Quality of Medicines Use

This chapter describes strategies used by managed care organizations (MCOs) to manage medicines use and offers a critical assessment of its impact on outcomes. Managed care organizations can use four major strategies to influence medicines use (see Table 13.1):

- Creating an efficient drug distribution network
- Controlling patient behavior
- Controlling physician behavior
- Promoting best practices

These strategies are intended, presumably, to improve the quality of medicines use and to reduce preventable drug-related morbidity (PDRM). They can affect outcomes very significantly, as discussed in Chapter 6. The effect on quality, however, may depend in large part on how each type of strategy is implemented and on the mix of programs.

Medication Carve-Outs and Pharmacy Benefit Managers

Approximately 90% of MCO health plans separate (carve out) medicines from other medical services and contract directly with a pharmacy benefit management company (PBM) to administer drug consumption (the pharmacy benefit) under their health plans.[1] Carve-outs are not unique to pharmacy as it is common for MCOs to carve out certain clinical services such as mental health and dental services. According to Gondek,[2] PBMs are organizations that apply managed care principles to prescription drug programs to promote optimal, cost-effective drug use for a positive impact on the total cost of care. Among their functions, they manage drug and dispensing costs and provide a broad array of administrative functions

TABLE 13.1

Managed Care Strategies

Efficient Drug Distribution
Pharmacy network
Claims adjudication
Contracts with pharmaceutical manufacturers that provide discounts and rebates
Formulary
Utilization Controls (Patient)
Copayments, tiered pricing programs
Drug cap programs
Education
Utilization Controls (Physicians)
Prior authorization, drug formulary, therapeutic interchange, drug utilization review
Education
Provider profiling and penalties for violation of prescribing policies
Promotion of Best Practices
Pharmaceutical care
Disease management

(claims processing, adjudication, development and management of pharmacy networks, and data reporting) and clinical functions (formulary management, utilization management, and disease state management).[3] Due to the complexity of the medicines use process, PBMs work with patients, managed care organizations, employers, pharmaceutical manufacturers, physicians, and pharmacy providers.

HMOs represent about 40% of the total PBM market, and preferred provider organizations (PPOs) represent about an additional 25% of the market. A 1998 survey of 604 HMOs conducted by the Pharmacy Benefit Management Institute found that fewer than 1% did not offer a pharmacy benefit to their members, 10% did not use a PBM (primarily staff and group model HMOs that dispensed prescriptions through their own pharmacies), and 90% offered a drug benefit in which a PBM played some role.[4]

Corporate acquisitions have frequently occurred in the PBM industry during the past decade, with the three largest PBMs (Advance Paradigm/PCS, MedcoHealth, and Express Scripts) leading the rest of the industry in terms of sales and volume of prescriptions processed. The total number of patient lives managed by PBMs increased to more than 230 million in 2000, compared to 176 million in 1998. According to data collected in 1999, PCS (merged with Advance Paradigm in October 2000) reported the largest number of lives (56.1 million), compared with MedcoHealth's 53.5 million.[4]

PBMs generally contract with community pharmacy providers, mail service pharmacies, and Internet pharmacies to control both the ingredient cost and administrative costs associated with the processing of prescriptions. Most PBMs contract with a broad network of community-based retail pharmacies, which often include both independent and chain community pharmacies to provide more distribution points for their MCO patient members. PBMs negotiate payment for services with these pharmacies. The negotiated price may vary based on market penetration of managed care organizations in specific geographic regions and other factors. As part of their distribution network, most PBMs also make mail service pharmacies available to their MCO members.[5] In 1999, approximately 87% of 446 employers, representing more than 15 million beneficiaries, reported that they offered a mail-order pharmacy benefit in their health plans. Mail service pharmacy sales are growing, accounting for $11.2 billion outpatient prescription sales in 1998, up 19% from 1997.[6] One reason for the increased sales is due to PBMs' encouragement of the use of mail service pharmacies to fill prescriptions for chronic conditions. In 1997, mail service accounted for approximately 10% of all prescriptions for HMO members, with almost 20% of all prescriptions for members of network model HMOs filled by mail service pharmacies.[7]

PBMs commonly negotiate discount contracts with pharmaceutical manufacturers. Contracts are usually performance based and provide financial rewards to the health plans or to the PBM if the market share or volume of products under contract increases. Based on the contract between an MCO and its PBM, these discounts may be kept by the PBM, or they may be passed on to the managed care organization, to patient members, or to physicians and pharmacists as incentives for prescribing and dispensing preferred (or formulary) medications.[5]

Drug Formulary

A drug formulary is a listing of preferred medications, developed by the MCO's health plan or PBM, to guide physician prescribing and pharmacy dispensing. By the end of the 1960s, formulary systems had been introduced into almost every hospital in the United States. The Joint Commission on Accreditation of Hospitals — now the Joint Commission on Accreditation of Healthcare Organizations (JCAHO) — had encouraged hospitals to form pharmacy and therapeutics committees (PTCs) and to establish formularies as early as the 1950s.[9]

The American Society of Health-System Pharmacists (ASHP) describes a formulary as a list of drugs approved for use within a health care setting and describes formulary systems as "a uniquely dynamic system that represents the current body of pharmaceutical knowledge and medical community standards resident in the health care setting it serves."[10] Formularies are almost always developed and evaluated by multidisciplinary groups or PTCs including physicians, pharmacists, and nurses. According to ASHP, the primary purposes of the PTC is to determine drug coverage policy development, policy enforcement, and education to promote safe, effective, and cost-effective pharmaceuticals.[10]

In the 1970s, formularies began to be applied beyond the confines of the hospital. Initially, these formularies, in staff or group model HMOs, were similar to hospital formularies in control and standardization of drugs. They reflected staff and PTC views on drug use. Many states also operated formularies for outpatient medications in managing their Medicaid programs, with varying degrees of success or even outright failure, depending on the outcome of interest.[11,12]

Later, independent practice association (IPA) and network model HMOs also began to use formularies to control their outpatient pharmacy benefits,[13] and use of formularies by HMOs to help manage drug benefits grew from 39% in 1989 to 93% in 1997. Today, formularies and formulary systems affect most HMO patient members and the more than 230 million covered lives managed by PBMs.[14–16]

Some advantages and disadvantages of formularies are described in Table 13.2. Formularies can be separated into two groups: open or closed. Open formularies allow many drug products, and those that are not listed are generally available and reimbursed. Closed formularies contain fewer drug products. Those that are not listed are generally not available or reimbursed. Some formularies are described as partially closed, meaning that they are restricted in one or more ways for some drug products and open for others.[14–16,19] Other terminology used for describing formularies is positive (drug products are explicitly listed for coverage or reimbursement) or negative (drugs are specifically identified for exclusion), which is often a method used for Medicaid formularies.[18,19]

Restrictions of reimbursement and access to drugs tend to be stricter in closed formulary systems. These controls may consist of required generic substitution; therapeutic interchange; tiered copayments; prior authorization, preferred, and excluded drug products; and limits on the number of prescriptions, quantity of drug, or day's supply per prescription.

TABLE 13.2

Advantages and Disadvantages of Formulary Systems[17]

Advantages	Disadvantages
Educates physicians and patients about drugs	Administrative burden and inconvenience to participants
Can reduce adverse drug events	May not be an effective drug list for 100% of the population served
Can enhance cost-effective prescribing	Can decrease quality of care by denying access to needed medications
Can increase quality of care through evidence-based management of disease	May cause unwanted or unexpected outcomes due to discontinuation of drug therapy
Can assure use of quality drug products	

With open formulary systems, prescribing tends to have fewer controls. Open formularies generally do not require generic substitution or therapeutic interchange, although some do encourage generic drug utilization. Of managed care plans surveyed in 1997, 93% used formularies,[15] with 27% reporting closed formularies in 1999 and 45% reporting partially closed formularies.[16]

Critique

Although formularies have been around for a long time, there is little evidence to support their effectiveness in improving the quality of care and reducing overall health care costs, particularly in managed care settings. The National Pharmaceutical Council (NPC) in its 1999 report concerning formularies[20] concluded:

> This body of literature indicates that such formularies often have a negative impact on overall costs and quality of care, that they often fail to achieve their fundamental goals, and may paradoxically exert adverse effects on budgets, patients, doctors, and pharmacists ... none of the studies clearly showed an association between drug restriction and reduced costs in other health service categories.

Many of the studies considered by NPC in reaching its conclusions focused exclusively on hospital formularies and state Medicaid program formularies. Only a few of the studies considered formularies in the managed care environment, although one study that examined formulary use in six HMOs did find an association between restrictive formularies (i.e., formulary limitations in drug class) and higher utilization of medical services.[21] Chapter 6 reviews additional literature suggesting that restrictive formularies may sometimes reduce quality and increase total costs of care.

Utilization Controls on Patient Behavior

Although almost 45% of all prescriptions dispensed are for generic drugs, they account for less than 20% of prescription sales in dollar terms because they are less expensive than brand-name drugs.[22] Because of the cost savings when generic drugs are prescribed, many health plans encourage the use of generics by offering financial incentives, usually through a strategy of varying copayment levels.

Deductibles and Copayments

One reaction by managed care organizations and employers to rising prescription costs has been to increase the level of its cost sharing with MCO members. Cost sharing often takes the form of patients being required to pay a deductible before the MCO will reimburse for pharmaceuticals and also a copayment for each prescription dispensed. Overall, 12.6% of HMO members paid an annual deductible before receiving pharmacy reimbursement during 1999, and the average annual deductible across all types of HMO plans, including commercial, Medicaid, and Medicare, was $84.[23]

Managed care members are often also required to pay a copayment for each prescription medication. Several reasons have been offered in support of this practice. First, sharing the cost of the prescription with the patient directly reduces the cost of drug products to the health plan. Second, copayments provide financial incentives to patients to use the MCO's preferred drugs. Third, copayments have been shown to reduce the number of prescriptions dispensed, perhaps because patients may elect to not spend their own money to have certain prescriptions dispensed when the patient perceives that the medication may be unnecessary.

Managed care organizations and PBMs generally attempt to structure copayment levels high enough to achieve their financial aims but not too high as to discourage the use of needed medications. One of the more recent changes introduced to drug benefit design is the introduction of *tiered copayments*, essentially providing MCO members with financial incentives to choose lower-cost drugs.

Tiered Copayments

Most MCO members now participate in a plan with either a two-tier or three-tier cost-sharing (copayment) formula for prescription drugs. In a two-tier plan there is one copayment for generic drugs and one for brand names. In most three-tier plans, there is one copayment for generic drugs, another for name brand drugs with no generic substitute or a preferred brand product, and a third for name brands with generic substitutes or a nonpreferred brand product. The amount that MCO members pay per prescription varies and has been rising in more recent years. In 2000, copayments for prescription drugs averaged $10 for generics, $25 for brand-name drugs without generic substitutes, and $40 for brand-name drugs with substitutes, although copayments for some tiers may be as high as $50 or more for some plans.[22,24]

Three-tier copays are realizing rapid, widespread adoption, and in 2000, they were required in health plans for about 35% of IPA HMO enrollees. This percentage is expected to rise considerably. MCOs, PBMs, and employers are also experimenting with three-tier percentage copay (or co-insurance) that requires consumers to pay a fixed percentage of drug costs. This may represent the next leap in pharmacy benefit redesign. Percentage copays presumably would serve to sensitize patients to the actual product costs of drug therapy, providing a stronger financial incentive for using lower-cost drugs.[22,24]

The level of copayment is often tied to contractual relationships between PBMs and pharmaceutical manufacturers. These contracts determine the cost of the drug to the PBM and each drug product's positioning in the formulary. For example, a contract may limit the number of drug products (e.g., to only Prilosec®) within a particular therapeutic category (e.g., proton pump inhibitors) to preferred status in the formulary, thereby driving up market share for those preferred agents in exchange for a lower cost for a drug product to the PBM. The implication is that unless a preferred drug product is prescribed, the patient will be faced with paying a larger copayment for a nonpreferred medication.

Rx to OTC Switch

Another strategy used by managed care organizations to share health plan costs with patients involves the growing phenomenon of switching from prescription to over-the-counter (OTC) drugs.[25] Based on recommendations from managed care organizations and PBMs, many employers have opted to not pay for most OTC products, relieving the health plan of paying the cost of a prescription when an OTC form of a prescription product is available. To save money, some MCOs have aggressively pursued this form of cost shifting by petitioning the Food and Drug Administration (FDA) to sell some prescription products directly to consumers.

The potential savings to the health plan from using over-the-counter medications rather than prescription products can be very large; the average nonprescription drug cost, at $4.75, is only about a tenth of the average prescription drug cost, $44.42. Additionally, using OTCs may help some patients avoid scheduling a visit to see their physician, saving the health plan even more money.[26]

Drug Caps

Limits on the number of prescriptions, quantity of drug, or day's supply per prescription are collectively known as drug cap programs. Drug caps are used by some MCOs to control patient behavior. These types of caps are not common in employer-provided or commercial health benefit programs yet. Just 4% of workers in small firms (3 to 199 employees) and 2% in all large firms (200 or more employees) face a cap on drug benefits.[22]

However, several state Medicaid programs have used drug cap programs that limit the number of prescriptions that can be dispensed during a specific period of time, for example, five prescriptions per month or three brand-name prescriptions and an unlimited number of generic prescriptions per month. While these programs are sometimes successful in reducing prescription costs, their impact in terms of human costs and total health care costs is often far outweighed by any savings in prescription expenses. For example, when the Medicaid agency in Mississippi introduced a cost-containment strategy that limited the number of prescriptions that would be paid for by Medicaid each month to five prescriptions, some of the state's most vulnerable patients were faced with making decisions about whether to have a prescription filled or pay for food or housing. The implications of not having some prescription medications dispensed can be significant, as seen in the case of Donald Ashwell of Harrison County, Mississippi, who died because he did not get the antibiotic he needed as a result of a drug cap policy.[27] Not only do people sometimes die as a result of policies that limit access to necessary health care services, but overall health care costs increase, even when the expenses of drugs decrease, as found in the case of the drug cap policy introduced by the Medicaid agency in New Hampshire (see Chapter 5).[12]

Improving Prescription Information Exchange between Providers

PBMs acknowledge that any formulary-related strategy that is intended to successfully control costs while ensuring continued access to prescription drug therapy ultimately requires more active and earlier participation by physicians with better and more useful information. One example is RxHub (expected launch during the first decade of 2000), a joint venture involving leading pharmacy benefit management companies, to improve the prescribing process for physicians using the latest in information technology.[28] RxHub is essentially an electronic exchange for prescription management that creates a universal standard to connect the data transmission devices in physician offices with the PBMs and pharmacies, allowing for the transmission of prescriptions directly from a physician to the patient's pharmacy of choice. It lets the physician and the pharmacy know exactly what the patient's PBM will cover and what tier each medication belongs to.[29]

Critique

Little literature is available concerning whether physicians understand or use formulary information, such as whether a product is a preferred agent according to an MCO's formulary, in guiding their prescribing choices. What little is known suggests that many physicians, particularly those who are part of PPOs, network model HMOs, and IPA model HMOs, pay little attention to MCO formularies since these physicians see patients that are members of many health plans, each with its own formulary. The challenges associated with a physician being able to keep track of the provisions associated with each MCO's formulary are significant.[5] Furthermore, the extent to which patients initiate conversations with their physicians about the role of an MCO's formulary on copayments paid for specific medications is also unknown, as is their influence on prescribing behavior.

However, some MCOs track each medical group's or each physician's prescribing patterns to identify practitioners who tend to prescribe large numbers of nonpreferred drug products.[25] Information about prescribing patterns has been used by some health plans to design educational interventions about their formulary system, with the aim of influencing physicians to prescribe preferred agents more frequently. In other cases, some health plans have included adherence to preferred prescribing patterns as a performance measure for its panel of providers, presumably for the purpose of influencing prescribing patterns through the use of either financial incentives or disincentives for the physician.

The techniques used by managed care for controlling patient behavior are largely focused on reducing health plan drug costs. While some techniques, such as encouraging the use of generic drugs, seem relatively harmless to patients, others, such as drug caps, have harmed patients by reducing access to necessary medicines. Due to the enormous pressures to reduce health care costs, sometimes managed care organizations and pharmacy benefit managers implement pharmacy benefit plan changes that appear to be helpful in decreasing drug costs in the short run. While many are indeed successful in reducing drug costs in the short run, the consequences can be most severe. Not only are some patients harmed by these policies because they forego medicines they really need, but also overall health plan costs may rise in the long term because patients who become ill from not taking their medicine will be more likely to require expensive health care services, including hospitalization.

Utilization Controls on Physicians

Managed care organizations' efforts to control physician behavior tend to involve the use of formularies, prior authorization, therapeutic interchange policies, drug utilization review, and provider profiling. Prior authorization, sometimes referred to as a medical necessity review, requires physicians to obtain certification of medical necessity prior to drug dispensing. Prior authorization is commonly used by managed care to review the medical necessity of clinical services such as specialist referrals, hospitalization, and certain procedures, as well as certain drug therapies. Most PBMs have established protocols for physicians to receive prior authorization over the telephone. In some programs, physicians are prompted through a series of interactive menus asking for clinical and patient information. At the end of the telephone menus, the physician is either given a prior authorization number or connected to a pharmacist, who asks further questions.[30,31]

Drug utilization reviews (DURs) may be used by PBMs to ensure appropriateness of drug therapy (as a quality assurance activity) or to assure compliance with a formulary.* Approximately 75% of HMOs have their PBMs perform utilization management programs, such as concurrent DURs and retrospective DURs.[30] DURs are frequently implemented on a population basis, although interventions are commonly directed at individual

* To the extent that the formulary was developed to improve prescribing quality, these may be similar objectives; however, prescribing is only a part of medicines use. See Chapters 4 and 6.

patients. DURs have been required for all Medicaid recipients since 1993, based on the requirements set by the Omnibus Budget Reconciliation Act of 1990. DUR activities are varied in managed care, but they all appear to be designed to review physician prescribing, pharmacist dispensing, and patient use of medications in an attempt to reduce costs and purportedly to reduce treatment variations and optimize patient care outcomes.[31]

Physician profiling involves generating data on physician prescribing and comparing physicians to expected prescribing patterns within select therapeutic categories. Profiling focuses on the patterns of an individual prescriber's care rather than that provider's specific clinical decisions for an individual patient. Often the practice pattern of an individual prescriber, or perhaps even of a medical group, is expressed as a rate or a measure of resource use during a defined period of time and for a defined population.[32]

The resulting profile can then be compared against a peer group or a standard that is typically specialty specific and regional. Today, MCOs tend to use profiling to measure provider performance, to guide quality improvement activities, to select providers for managed care networks, to decide how much money may be returned to individual physicians from capitation withhold fees or to reach bonus decisions for its provider panel, and to decide whether providers will be invited to continue in an MCO's provider panel.[33] About three fourths of HMO plans provide feedback to physicians on a plan-wide basis, while about four fifths of HMO plans provide at least some clinical feedback to individual physicians.[34]

Examples of measures used in provider profiling are not limited to drug therapy. In some MCOs, these measures may be driven to a large extent by HEDIS indicators or an MCO's financial performance indicators. Indicators may include percentage compliance with the MCO's preferred drug formulary, monthly drug costs, appropriate medications for people with asthma, beta-blocker treatment after a heart attack, average wait time to schedule a routine physical, number of hospital admissions, number of referrals out of network, member satisfaction, and the percentage of children receiving appropriate immunizations. In the case of drug therapy, PBMs usually target aberrant prescribers for educational intervention and share the results of the profiling with the MCO. During prescriber education, the PBM may review with physicians the appropriateness and cost of their prescribing patterns. These educational sessions typically occur via mailings, telephone calls, or face-to-face visits.

Promotion of Best Practices

Because of growing recognition of large practice pattern variations found in health care (see Chapter 5), managed care organizations have shown interest in implementing programs intended to reduce the gap between evidence-based best practices and actual medical practices. There are now hundreds of studies in the medical literature showing that this gap is a significant cause of preventable morbidity.

For example, regardless of the availability of well-accepted guidelines for diabetes, adoption of American Diabetes Association (ADA) guidelines has been poor. Lawler and Viviani[35] compared self-reported physician advice to patients about glucose testing and patient-reported physician advice among a group of 47 providers at an academic family practice center. The researchers reported that physician beliefs and practices were divergent and that provider performance of the ADA guidelines was low.

Worrall et al.[36] found that only 53% of patients cared for by family physicians in Canada had HbA_{1C} measurements done in the previous year and concluded that compliance with the Canadian Diabetes Association (CDA) guidelines was poor and that physicians were doing about half the recommended checks and procedures.

Programs aimed at the improvement of medical practices are often referred to as disease management programs. Some managed care organizations have created comprehensive programs that address all of the needs of their members rather than focusing on the management of specific medical conditions. Such programs are referred to as *health management*. When focusing on the drug therapy needs of patients, health management programs have sometimes been referred to as *pharmaceutical care*.[37]

Disease management is a concept that is gaining widespread acceptance and creating significant enthusiasm in managed care organizations. Although there are few documented successes, disease management has been embraced by multiple healthcare organizations as a promising approach to improve quality and decrease costs for selected patient populations. Disease management strategies have focused on chronic conditions with significant long-term clinical and economic impact and may be defined as follows: "Disease management is an approach to patient care that coordinates resources across the entire healthcare delivery system and throughout the life-cycle of a disease."[38]

The critical distinction between a disease management approach and traditional attempts to control costs and improve quality is a change of focus from discrete episodes of care to the health care continuum. This is an attractive concept in an era of managed care full-risk contracting due to its emphasis on continuity of care and prevention of health problems. Many "players" or disease management vendors have emerged in this area, including integrated delivery systems, MCOs, pharmaceutical companies, and information technology vendors.

One tool used in many disease management programs is clinical practice guidelines. Practice guidelines, defined as "systematically developed statements to assist practitioners and patient decisions about health care for specific clinical circumstances,"[38] are becoming increasingly common in the practice of medicine. Interest in the use of practice guidelines seems to be based on the inherent difficulty in keeping practitioners up-to-date in terms of which treatments best affect desired patient outcomes. With more than 33,000 medical articles published monthly, practitioners cannot easily incorporate this knowledge into their practices, suggesting the importance of guidelines in helping physicians and other providers keep up-to-date.

Guidelines are intended to synthesize all relevant information into a single document and make it possible for providers to integrate the data being published into their daily routines. Guidelines have been credited with the following objectives:[39–42]

- Reducing unnecessary variations in medical practice
- Reducing inappropriate care
- Eliminating or reducing unnecessary health care costs
- Facilitating care based on scientific knowledge and new technology

The attainment of these objectives may be made possible through the provision of, and effective implementation of, well-developed, up-to-date best practices that are accessible to practitioners in an easy-to-follow, user-friendly format. Guidelines, although recognized as tools for improving the quality of health care and for guiding health care providers in their practices, are not expected to replace clinical judgment. Practice guidelines are intended to assist providers in incorporating best practices from the literature and from expert opinion into the care provided to specific patients.[43]

Worrall et al.[44] reported that there is very little evidence that the use of clinical practice guidelines improves patient outcomes in primary medical care based on a review of 13 randomized clinical experimental or quasi-experimental studies. However, the researchers noted that the guidelines used in these studies were old, and the methods used to study the impact of the guidelines may have been insensitive to small changes in outcomes. Grimshaw and Russell[45] reached somewhat different conclusions about the effectiveness of clinical practice guidelines. Based on an analysis of 59 published evaluations of clinical guidelines, these researchers found that explicit guidelines do improve clinical practice, when introduced in the context of rigorous evaluations, although the size of the improvements in performance varied considerably.

A 1996 survey conducted by the American Association of Health Plans[46] found that 86% of surveyed HMOs promoted clinical practice guidelines, and 90.2% of the HMOs have staff members assigned to develop and implement practice guidelines. This survey also revealed that the two most common guidelines found within HMOs are for diabetes and asthma. The use of guidelines has been growing; in 2000, almost 90% of all HMOs had one or more clinical protocols to guide physician activities, and 40% of all HMOs developed more than eight sets of clinical guidelines for physicians to use.[47]

Much of the responsibility for guideline implementation and assimilation ultimately resides with individual providers and health care organizations at the local level.[48] However, some MCOs ask PBMs to provide clinical functions including disease management. When asked, HMOs indicated that of all functions provided by PBMs, they were least satisfied with the disease management services provided.[49] Interestingly, clinical interventions, sometimes referred to as disease management programs by PBMs, are fundamentally distinct from the model of disease management discussed earlier in the chapter, which is locally based and provider driven.

Clinical interventions or disease management programs provided by PBMs include the following:

1. Direct contacts with physicians made from an outbound call center attached to a mail service pharmacy, providing PBMs with a tool for encouraging drug product switches consistent with formulary objectives
2. Therapeutic interchange programs in which a PBM representative telephones physicians who have prescribed nonpreferred drug products in an attempt to persuade physicians to substitute a preferred agent, often one that is rebated by a pharmaceutical manufacturer
3. Physician counterdetailing performed by field-based pharmacists or physicians who meet with physicians as representatives of a managed care plan or a PBM
4. Promotion of drug-specific clinical protocols specifying the conditions that a patient member must meet for a physician to prescribe a specific drug

Conclusion

It seems clear that managed care organizations have the power and the will to change the manner in which drug therapy is provided, *by* large numbers of providers, *to* large numbers of people. Perhaps managed care organizations have used this power to control total costs of care and to improve people's lives more efficiently. However, as well intentioned as the industry may be, there is little evidence to support this assumption.

Moreover, some activities have been shown to hurt people and to increase total costs. The use of prescription drug caps and prescription limits in poor populations is an obvious example. Some readers by now may be tiring of this example, but we raise it repeatedly because parts of the industry, at least, appear either not to learn from such mistakes or not to care.

Avoiding harmful and pointless policies is not really the point, however. Managed care should have an enormous capacity to influence the environment of medicines use in ways that might greatly improve medicines use in large populations of people.

It is puzzling that managed care organizations have not succeeded more toward this end. A key element was mentioned in Chapter 6. Managed care organizations have apparently exempted themselves from the rules that they have laid down for providers, namely, that practices should conform to the evidence. The evidence, to say the least, does not encourage a continuation of past practices. Managed care organizations — government programs certainly included — should begin to systematically evaluate not only the quality of medicines use in their populations, but also the impact of their own policies and programs.

Chapter 11 described how that might look. Chapters 14 and 15 will explore some of the issues in getting there.

References

1. *1999 HMO-PPO/Medicare-Medicaid Digest,* Hoechst Marion Roussel Managed Care Digest series, 1999.
2. Gondek, K., Assessment of the Impact of Pharmacy Benefit Managers, HCFA-95-023/PK, Health Care Financing Administration, Washington, D.C., September 30, 1996.
3. Health Industries Research Center, National Accounts: Marketing Challenges and Opportunities for the Late 1990s, Health Industries Research Center, Santa Cruz, CA, 1998/1999.
4. Pharmacy Benefit Management Institute, Inc., HMO-PBM Market Share and Formulary Management Report, 1998, www.pbmi.com.
5. Navarro, R.P., Prescription drug benefits in managed care, in *Essentials of Managed Health Care,* 4th ed., Kongstvedt, P.R., Ed., Aspen Publishers, Gaithersburg, MD, 2001, chap. 15.
6. Wyeth-Ayerst Prescription Drug Benefit Cost and Plan Design Survey Report, 2000.
7. The New Pharmacy, May 19, 1999, http://www.bergen.com/biz/mail191999905193.htm.
8. Novartis, Pharmacy Benefit Report: 1998 Facts & Figures, 1998.
9. Rascati, K.L., Survey of formulary system policies and procedures, *Am. J. Hosp. Pharm.,* 49,100, 1992.
10. American Society of Health-System Pharmacists, ASHP statement on the formulary system, in *Practice Standards of ASHP 1997-1998,* ASHP, Bethesda, MD, 1997.
11. Meyer, M.C., Bates, H., Jr., and Swift, R.G., The role of state formularies, *J. Am. Pharm. Assoc.,* NS14, 663, 1974.
12. Soumerai, S.B., Avorn, J., Ross-Degnan, D., and Gortmaker, S., Payment restrictions for prescription drugs under Medicaid: effects on therapy, cost and equity, *N. Engl. J. Med.,* 317, 550, 1987.
13. Dillon, M., Drug formulary management, in *Managed Care Pharmacy Practice,* Navarro, R.P., Ed., Aspen Publishers, Gaithersburg, MD, 1999.
14. Cook, A., Kornfield, T., and Gold, M., *The Role of PBMs in Managing Drug Costs: Implications for a Medicare Drug Benefit,* Mathematica Policy Research, Inc., Washington, D.C., 2000.

15. Novartis, Pharmacy Benefit Report, Novartis Pharmaceutical Corp., East Hanover, NJ, 1998.
16. Novartis, Pharmacy Benefit Report, Novartis Pharmaceutical Corp., East Hanover, NJ, 1999.
17. Blumenthal, D. and Herdman, R., Eds., *Description and Analysis of the VA National Formulary*, National Academy Press, Washington D.C., 2000.
18. Goldberg, R.A., Managing the pharmacy benefit: the formulary system, *J. Manag. Care Pharm.*, 3, 565, 1997.
19. Rucker, T.D., A Public Policy Strategy for Drug Formularies: Preparation or Procrastination Necessity for Implementing an Effective National Formulary, 1999.
20. Component Management Fails to Save Health Care System Costs: The Case of Restrictive Formularies, National Pharmaceutical Council (NPC), 1999.
21. Horn, S.D., Sharkley, P.D., and Phillips-Harris, C., Formulary limitations and the elderly's results from the Managed Care Outcomes Project, *Am. J. Manag. Care*, 4, 1105, 1998.
22. Employer Health Benefits, Kaiser Family Foundation and the Health Research and Educational Trust, 2000.
23. Novartis, Pharmacy Report: Facts & Figures, 2000.
24. HIRC Releases Spring 2001 Data on Pharmaceutical Three-Tier Copays and Percentage Copays across HMOs, PBMs, Employers, and Coalitions, June 18, 2001, http://biz.yahoo.com/bw/010618/0575.html.
25. CDER Report to the Nation: 2000, FDA Center for Drug Evaluation and Research, Washington D.C., 2001, http://www.fda.gov/cder/reports/RTN2000/RTN2000-1.HTM.
26. Lee, K., Analysts Promote OTC Drugs as Defensive Medicine, *Employee Benefit News*, May 1, 2001.
27. Neergaard, L., Mississippi Death Raises Questions about Medicaid Prescription Limits, Associated Press, June 30, 1999.
28. Prescription drug use patterns complicated by wide regional variation, in *Express Scripts Drug Trend Report*, 2001.
29. Script Central: PBMs Create Electronic Hub to Link Pharmacies, Physicians, *Modern Physician*, March 12, 2001, http://web.lexis-nexis.com/universe/document?_ansset=A-WA-A-V-MsSEWY.
30. Wyeth-Ayerst Prescription Drug Benefit Cost and Plan Design Survey Report, 1999.
31. Peterson, A.M. and Wilson, M.D., Drug utilization strategies, in *Managed Care Pharmacy Practice*, Navarro, R.P., Ed., Aspen Publishers, Gaithersburg, MD, 1999, p. 176.
32. Lee, P.R. et al., Managed care: provider profiling, *J. Insurance Med.*, 24, 179, 1992.
33. Walker, L.M., Can a computer tell how good a doctor you are? *Med. Econ.*, 71, 136, 1994.
34. 1999 BD Becton, Dickinson and Company Report on Physicians in Managed Care, 1999.
35. Lawler, F.H. and Viviani, N., Patient and physician perspectives regarding treatment of diabetes: compliance with practice guidelines, *J. Fam. Pract.*, 44, 369, 1997.
36. Worrall, G., Chaulk, P., and Freake, D., The effects of clinical practice guidelines on patient outcomes in primary care: a systematic review, *CMAJ*, 156, 1705, 1997.

37. Hepler, C.D. and Strand, L.M., Opportunities and responsibilities in pharmaceutical care, *Am. J. Hosp. Pharm.*, 47, 533, 1990.
38. Field, M.J. and Lohr, L.N., Eds., *Clinical Practice Guidelines: Directions for a New Program*, Institute of Medicine, National Academy Press, Washington, D.C., 1990, 8, 106.
39. Tunis, S. et al., Internists attitudes about clinical practice guidelines, *Ann. Intern. Med.*, 120, 956, 1994.
40. Durieux, R.N., Clinical practice guidelines: from methodological to practical issues, *Intensive Care Med.*, 20, 593, 1994.
41. Woolf, S.H., Practice guidelines: a new reality in medicine III: impact on patient care, *Arch. Intern. Med.*, 153, 646, 1993.
42. Fang, E. et al., Use of clinical practice guidelines in managed care physician groups, *Arch. Fam. Med.*, 5, 528, 1996.
43. Kernodle, S.J., Improving health care with clinical practice guidelines and critical pathways: implications for pharmacists in ambulatory practice, *Pharm. Pract. Manage. Q.*, 17, 76, 1997.
44. Worrall, G., Chaulk, P., and Freake, D., The effects of clinical practice guidelines on patient outcomes in primary care: a systematic review, *CMAJ*, 156, 1705, 1997.
45. Grimshaw, J.M. and Russell, I.T., Effect of clinical guidelines on medical practice: a systematic review of rigorous evaluations, *Lancet*, 342, 1317, 1993.
46. American Association of Health Plans, By the number, *HealthPlan,* 37, 84, 1996.
47. 1999 Becton, Dickinson and Company Report on Physicians in Managed Care, 2000.
48. Agency for Health Care Policy and Research, AHCPR Clinical Practice Guideline Program: Report to Congress, AHCPR Pub. 95-N012, U.S. Department of Health and Human Services, Public Health Service, Washington, D.C., 1995.
49. Pharmacy Benefit Management Institute Customer Satisfaction Survey Report, Scottsdale AZ, 1996.

14

A Market Perspective

The next decade may bring changes in the delivery of health care in the United States that rival or exceed the changes wrought by the introduction of managed care. The Institute of Medicine (IOM) report *Crossing the Quality Chasm* has called for fundamental redesign of the present health care arrangements toward an adaptive systems model.[1,2] That overlaps, by the way, with part of managed care's original objective. We have been here before. Managed care, in its present incarnation, seems to have developed the *managed* part a bit more than the *care* part. The IOM is asking for more than a rebalancing, however. It has called for a complete overhaul of present-day arrangements and the formation of adaptive systems, perhaps something like the one described in Chapter 11.

Until that bright future comes, a strategy to improve medications use must recognize present-day market influences. Present market forces, as symbolized by managed care organizations (MCOs) and third-party payment, now influence the delivery of health care greatly, rivaling scientific and professional opinion. Pharmacists are filling more prescriptions; physicians are seeing more patients. Most professionals have changed, and will continue to change, their practice to fit the demands of managed care. A permanent change from the status quo to medications use systems (MUSs) requires a change in the market for professional services.

This chapter will describe issues in the marketing and adoption of pharmaceutical care and medications management systems. The discussion is fairly long and detailed, but the conclusion is short. *Managed care organizations should evaluate the quality of medications use among their members.* They should expand present drug use evaluation (DUE) programs with measures that link inappropriate medications use processes to adverse outcomes. Inappropriate medications use should include, but certainly not be limited to, prescribing. Examples of such performance indicators were given in Chapters 3, 7, and 11. These can be computerized, and the process would not be expensive.

An unacceptable prevalence of poor process–poor outcome events might show the MCO whether it should implement a medications management system (FOCUS-PDCA) to follow up serious and recurring problems.

Professions as Marketing Mechanisms

Professions are, fundamentally, a means of marketing certain kinds of services. This idea, while perhaps familiar to sociologists, is unfamiliar to many people. A brief historical and sociological introduction may help to cut through sentimentality and posturing on the one hand, and irrational cynicism on the other. A balanced understanding is necessary to appreciate the monumental significance of organizing the delivery of health care services into MCOs.

According to Larsen's historical analysis, modern professions developed in England and America in response to the Industrial Revolution. Industrialization was creating the mercantile system, intended for industrial output. Factories were producing newly standardized, impersonal products to be distributed through organized channels of distribution. The basic ethical principle of the mercantile system was *caveat emptor* (let the buyer beware). Industrial firms were heteronomous; i.e., they included workers with many status levels and skill sets. Management of industrial firms was hierarchical. At first, industrial firms operated autocratically. Later, management became subject to rules and procedures, especially according to Max Weber's notion of bureaucracy (rule by officials).[3]

Industrialization was highly effective for producing and marketing standardized products, as history attests. It was quite ineffective, however, for producing and marketing nonstandardized, highly individualized, personal services, especially those that (1) involved priceless values (health, legal rights, spiritual or religious support, and advanced education); (2) were difficult or impossible for a consumer to evaluate in advance of using them; and (3) required the provider to possess advanced knowledge and skill (as do medicine, law, the clergy, and the professorate). Larsen referred to such services collectively as services that required *trust between strangers* before buying and selling could occur.

As the middle class expanded, learned professionals (who had served the aristocracy) began to market their services to the newly rich with promises of a special ethic of responsibility for client interest, briefly stated as *caveat vendor* (let the seller beware). Some trades, such as apothecaries, which had not had access to the aristocracy, sought to market their services to the middle class through the same system and began to professionalize. The professional promised to be bound by a code of ethics that placed the interest of the client ahead of his own convenience or immediate financial gain, as illustrated by the Hippocratic oath. (Guarantees of success, however, were considered a sign of a charlatan.)

Professionals also organized themselves into homogenous societies of fraternal, politically equal, largely autonomous members. These societies imposed admission requirements (e.g., educational standards and licensure) that limited entry to their markets and regulated the behavior of members through codes of ethics.

So, we can discern two sets of shared beliefs, assumptions, and values: the mercantile culture, which was heteronomous, hierarchical, and bureaucratic, and the professional culture, which was homogeneous, fraternal-egalitarian, and collegial. As with most cultures, members tend to be more comfortable with others from their own culture. Diplomatic missions to the other culture usually involved emissaries (e.g., change agents), but the two cultures pretty much coexisted independently until the mercantile culture began to pay for services from the professional culture (more about that later).

The two cultures were assumed to be incompatible, although professionals are often employed in bureaucracies, and bureaucrats (in the nonpejorative meaning) are often better practice managers than the professionals themselves. Research suggests that the two systems are, indeed, largely incompatible. The professional and bureaucratic cultures, however, have one important value in common: respect for technical competence as a basis for differentiation by rank, pay, responsibility, and privilege.[4–6] This may be the strongest and most permanent basis for cooperation between MCOs and health professionals.

None of this is intended to suggest that the professional system was superior, to look back with nostalgia on the "good old days" of independent practice, or to denigrate the idea of managing the care provided by professionals. Rising expenditures for health care had to be controlled. The professional notion of quality had often become myopic and self-serving. American business and consumer interests needed to replace it with a consumer-oriented idea. Professions surely suffered from hubris and abused their power in many large and small ways.[7] They have met nemesis.

Replacing independent professional practice with managed care (as a social institution) should mean a merging of these two partly incompatible cultures, each with incompatible approaches to the market. This is especially clear in the implicit decision in the United States to use managed competition as a means of controlling price and value. This discussion leads to four observations about the overall enterprise of managed care:

1. The basic issues of buying and selling professional services have not changed. People still need complex services involving priceless values, great uncertainty, and accommodation of specific human needs. The mercantile system may be no more effective at providing valued, complex, and specific services now than it was in the 19th century.
2. The goal must be a new organization of health care delivery through synthesis and compromise, between business and profession. If there must be winning and losing, it should be according to some realistic notion of the national interest, and fairly distributed across business and profession. Organized purchasers may feel that their time has come, but managed care cannot be permitted irresponsible domination of health professions. If that happens,

neither they nor their members, business customers, or employees will be better served than they were under the professional system. In particular, the economic power of managed care does not justify the substitution of mercantile ethics for professional ethics.

3. If managed care wishes to achieve such a synthesis, it must avoid its own version of professional hubris. Managed care was needed because the health professions (not just medicine) used their virtual monopoly control over information and professional labor to resist needed change. Turnabout may be fair play, but it is not in the public interest. Managed care should, therefore, avoid recourse to raw economic power lest it eventually suffer the same fate.
4. The basis of compromise and synthesis between the health professions and managed care, theoretically if not actually, is respect for technical competence. If managed care cannot provide outcomes that professionals can agree are technically good, and cannot offer at least as much value for money as the "old way," then it will not keep its fundamental promise, and its raison d'etre will vanish. If it is not seen to pursue technical excellence, e.g., by voluntarily embracing quality standards, then public regulation should require it, or the experiment should be allowed to fail.
5. Likewise, professionals must preserve the traditional ethic of beneficence, despite economic or any other inconvenience. If professions will not stand up for the *professional thesis* and fight for their patients' needs when necessary, there will be no synthesis of ideas, no powerful noneconomic mandate to recognize, no higher values to accommodate. Managed care and profession would simply be haggling over price, to coin an old joke.

Stakeholders in the Market for Medications Use Systems

For convenience, we will use the word *market* broadly to mean more and less regulated arrangements for buying and selling. The market of main interest is the market for pharmaceutical care (drug products and professional services concerning their use). The market for medications management is related intimately. This market requires three components: supply, demand, and a way of transacting business, i.e., a bringing together of sellers and buyers, a basis of payment, and a means of payment.

The market for pharmaceutical care is not a typical market. It comprises many providers (pharmacists, nurses, and physicians) on the supply side and many clients (patients, third-party payers, MCOs, and the customers of third-party payers and MCOs, e.g., employers and labor unions) on the demand side. In government health care schemes, the electorate are on both sides at once. In addition to their supply function, physicians also may influence demand through their opinions and recommendations concerning the need for cooperative pharmaceutical care systems.

Medication use systems are not a product, at least at present. They are an idea, a goal, that may be realized in many forms. Therefore, adoption of them is not as simple as with other innovations. Widespread adoption of medications use systems would depend on decisions by both the supply side and the demand side.

The supply side is much more developed than the demand side. Pharmaceutical societies have adopted pharmaceutical care as a goal. Early questions have been answered about how the theory of pharmaceutical care could be realized in community pharmacy, especially whether pharmacists could provide the care, whether physicians and patients would accept the changes and cooperate in care, and whether care could be cost-effective.

A number of realizations of the theory have been shown in research studies to be feasible, safe, effective, and efficient (see Chapter 9). Pharmaceutical care practices exist in the United States and many other nations. However, the rate of adoption is too slow to keep pace with other changes in health care finance and delivery. These reports do not seem to influence most policy makers as they consider expanding access to prescription medicines.

One reason that these clinically successful practices have not spread is that managed care dominates the marketplace but rarely pays a provider for providing pharmaceutical care. Pharmaceutical care is usually — disingenuously — presumed to be included in physicians' and pharmacists' services.* Managed care pays pharmacists as if they were retail merchants, on the basis of sales (prescriptions filled). Professional services from pharmacists are either assumed to be included in the price (as with physicians) or held to be unnecessary, because the physician is presumed to provide care. This argument in the status quo begs the question of how to promote change.

Demand (desire plus payment) for pharmaceutical care, in turn, depends on the existence of real medications management systems in managed care, i.e., a way for managed care to evaluate the quality of medications use among its members. This is the main sticking point at present. The point is that lack of demand is stalling the adoption of pharmaceutical care, at present, well below the level needed to become self-sustaining.

Adoption of Medications Use Systems

Chapter 6 introduced the theory of diffusion of innovation (DoI) for new drug therapies. The theory proposes that certain issues are relevant in predicting the speed of adoption of a new idea or product. The model seems useful for understanding the issues that might be salient to stakeholders' adoption of medicine use systems.

---

* The argument that pharmaceutical care is already included in professional service is disingenuous in view of the data presented Chapters 2 and 3.

TABLE 14.1

Adoption Issues Depend on Perspective

Adoption Issue	Supply Side (Pharmacy and Medicine)	Demand Side (Patients and Payers)
Recognition of need	Declining status (autonomy) and income per unit of service; questionable future success (pharmacy especially)	PDRMs are prevalent; need to increase quality and access to care and reduce expenditures
Risk of change	A pharmaceutical care project depends on many people with differing identities and priorities; it may fail, resulting in further loss of prestige and income; investment may not be recovered; physicians fear responsibilities for actions they did not control	Pharmaceutical care cooperative systems are inconsistent with conventional notions about structure of health care, professional roles, and ideas of accountability; medications management systems are inconsistent with some concepts of professional autonomy
Advantages	If project succeeds, professional power (status and income) may rise; technology would become a tool rather than a threat	Increased safety, effectiveness, and efficiency of health care; possible net decrease in costs

Application of DoI theory to MUSs introduces an interesting complication. Usually, DoI assumes that a supply already exists. In other words, it presumes a push strategy by the innovators. For example, enough photocopiers, personal computers, cell phones, electric cars, etc., exist to allow trial and adoption decisions by consumers. In the instance of MUS, however, diffusion and adoption by both potential suppliers and purchasers have to go on concurrently, and there are three to four stakeholder groups. Furthermore, although the basic issues may be similar for all groups, the same arguments will not persuade pharmacists, patients, physicians, and payers. Table 14.1 summarizes some examples of this point.

This may explain, in part, why pharmacy has been unable to convince society of its view. Obtaining such acceptance is too much to expect, even from a professional association. Certainly it is too much to expect from a small group of innovative pharmacists who are busy enough with the technical elements of establishing a new practice. Therefore, it is important to recognize that the acceptance of pharmaceutical care cannot be left to a few innovative professionals who try it first, or even professional leaders in medicine and pharmacy. *Investment capital is needed to create more workable prototypes.*

The background for the supply side of this discussion is in Chapters 8 to 11 and elsewhere.[8,9] The following sections introduce and briefly summarize some remaining demand side issues.

Recognition of Unmet Need or Problem

The needs involved in a demand for medications use systems were described in Chapter 2. The fundamental obstacle in the adoption of MUSs, however, is that preventable drug-related morbidities (PDRMs) remain largely invisible to most stakeholders, in particular clinicians. Even after publication of the Adverse Drug Event Prevention Study (ADEPS),[1] even after publication of *To Err Is Human*,[2] people still denied the problem (see below).

Managers rely on their information systems or clinicians to identify problems of this prevalence and significance. If the database does not include many reports of PDRM, then the problem must be "out there" in somebody else's organization. The reason that managed care databases do not show PDRM events is because they are not set up to find them. For example, in one study only 18% of drug-related admissions (determined by medical audit) had been coded as such in hospital records by the admitting physicians.[10] If this is typical, then the prevalence of PDRMs would not be visible in medical records. Routine hospital and managed care epidemiology would miss it, even though specific research projects would find it.

Professionals and managed care executives may be aware of those research studies. It is not unusual, however, to hear practitioners and managers deny the problem, especially in their practice or organization. Like the NIMBY (not in my back yard) defense, this is the NIMP defense — not in my practice/program. They may place the problems reported in the research literature "out there," in teaching hospitals, or in another less fortunate and (implicitly) less well managed population. They may criticize details of research methodology. Practitioners and managers focus on solving the problems they see, not problems reported in other populations.

The public may be aware that problems occur in drug therapy, as in other aspects of medical care. It lacks specific knowledge about causes and preventives. Medication use is a technical field, usually left to professionals. Denial and other defense mechanisms ("My doctor and pharmacist know what is best for me") may operate to reduce anxiety about the danger of necessary medical treatment, so one hears, "Our members do not demand better medication use systems."

The NIMP argument can be tested. A group practice or an MCO can evaluate the quality of medications use in its own population by using indicators. Some process indicators, such as frequency of medications use, therapeutic duplication, and duration of therapy, are available from prescription reimbursement records. Performance indicators such as those used in Chapter 11 require a bit more data. They may require clinical data and prescription data to be matched by patient and merged. Many MCOs in the United States and other countries have that capability or can develop it.

Advantages of MUSs over the Status Quo

Examples of research suggesting that MUSs are effective and efficient were summarized in Chapter 9. These studies certainly are encouraging, especially because they tend to confirm plausible theories predicting outcome improvement through systems development. The empirical and theoretical support for MUSs is at least as strong as it is for widely accepted practices, for example, some surgical procedures. Some skepticism may be explained simply by the fact that pharmaceutical care practices are not common or easy to find (which brings us right back to adoption kinetics again). A possible double standard for evidence notwithstanding, the evidence for MUSs is somewhat fragmented and incomplete.

The classical next step would be large-scale randomized, controlled evaluations. Many people have called for such studies to "prove" the worth of medications management. The following paragraphs describe some major problems with this strategy.

Scientific research is the bedrock of professional self-legitimization and progress in health care. It has many proud accomplishments throughout history that continue today. The speed of scientific progress, however, depends on resources. Scientific truth can take decades or centuries, depending on how much interest (and money) the problem can attract.

Large-scale randomized controlled trials of MUSs would have three major problems: expense, design, and generalizability. The expense of randomized controlled trials (RCTs) to evaluate patient care systems is well known and should not require elaboration. Medications management has received little funding, relative to the cost consequences of PDRM or the cost of doing the needed studies. This surely results in part from the invisibility of PDRM described in the preceding section. Perhaps the recently heightened interest in medical safety (e.g., following the publication of the IOM reports) will attract more attention.

Research design problems concern myriads of decisions (e.g., about the details of the interventions, inclusion and exclusion criteria, process and outcome measures). The science of medications management is not fully developed. Although passionate opinions about the "right way to do it" are plentiful, clear empirical support from comparative studies is nonexistent. The worry is that a study might succeed or fail based on unrecognized details, which might not be repeated on replication or fuller implementation. This is somewhat related to the problem of generalizability.

Scientific studies like RCTs, if carried out correctly, may be generalizable if the intervention being studied is standardized, e.g., a drug product or specific medical procedure. Generalization may be further justified if the sample represents the population with respect to variables that may affect outcomes, e.g., age, sex, diagnosis. The U.S. health care system, however, is a mélange of health care programs, none of which are like the highly regulated or single-payer programs of Canada and Europe. Even after a large-scale, successful RCT, a program may not accept that the problems, solutions, or results would apply to its members (see NIMP, above). A local medications management program, such as the one described in Chapter 11, therefore might not be generalizable. Its results, however, would apply to the program within which it was done.

Chapter 11 described a realistic alternative, or perhaps complement, to a massive randomized controlled trial. MCOs, insurance companies, and other groups representing large patient populations could implement quality improvement (QI) programs. These would, first, identify problems that actually exist in the population rather than in the research literature. Then the MCO could proceed to solve the problems. This gradual approach might find workable solutions to real problems much more efficiently than a few grand studies.

Perceived Risk of Change

The most frequently mentioned risks are financial and social feasibility and social acceptability. This is related to the NIMP phenomenon mentioned above. If one does not accept the problem statement, i.e., the prevalence of costly and injurious PDRMs, it would be difficult to see how a program or practice could recover its additional expenditures. Also, if one did not accept the problem statement, then the comfort of a particular constituency would seem more important. Worries about unfavorable reactions might include provider refusal to cooperate, payer refusal to pay, objections to potential changes in professional responsibilities and relationships, and statements to the effect that "Our members (or customers) do not demand medications management." To suspicious professionals, a proposal for a system may seem to be an increase in the intrusion of managed care into professional decision making. To managed care, it may appear as a professional's way of avoiding guidelines.

There is an implicit "don't ask, don't tell" philosophy about outcomes in some organizations. At some point, someone may ask, "What if we find all these problems, but then we can't fix them. What then?" (This may belong with the learning disabilities, below, because it begs the question of what a health care program is obliged to know about its effectiveness.)

The greatest risk of change is, of course, risking failure by trying something new and untested. A MUS project might carry the additional social risk to middle managers because it is outside the conventional wisdom of pharmacy benefit management (as described in Chapters 6, 12, and 13).

The risks of the new program would have to be evaluated in the context of the risks of PDRMs and their consequences. Therefore, the use of process, outcome, or combined performance indicators may be essential for the initiation of MUS development programs.

A high prevalence of questionable medications use processes, or of PDRMs, especially when accompanied by large avoidable costs, should elevate management discussions beyond conventional wisdom and broaden them beyond component cost management. The risk of change might then seem small compared to the risk of the status quo.

Another potential area of risk is providers' cooperation with each other or with MCOs. Suffice it to say, many disagreements and sources of tension may exist in almost every nation or health care program. Most health professionals have experienced economic and professional pressure from managed care, including denials of service and delays in payment. For their part, most managed care programs have experienced resistance and "gaming" (including outright fraud) from providers.

Likewise, changes outside the provider community have intensified pre-existing boundary conflicts within and between professions. As Chapter 5 illustrated, the basic functions of medications use are now up for grabs. If nurse practitioners can now provide primary care, with limited prescribing privileges, can pharmacists be far behind? For their part, pharmacists have willy-nilly become unpaid, unofficial health insurance police, enforcing managed care and health insurance polices, telling patients and prescribers what a third-party payer will and will not cover, and enforcing formularies into which neither the pharmacist nor the prescriber had input, and from which they have little recourse. As one physician said about his experience before a pharmacist was added to his group practice, "When the pharmacist was on the telephone, my first thought was, 'Oh, what did I do wrong now?'" Often, the point of the call is not an important clinical issue, but a (professionally) trivial one, e.g., a choice between two equivalent products, one in the formulary and one not.

This environment is not ideal for professional "buy-in" to a cooperative MUS, especially one that had been developed elsewhere, e.g., one that was successfully tested in a large research project. The environment may result in large part, however, from micromanagement attempts to minimize component costs like expenditures for office visits and the prescription benefit in isolation from patient outcomes and total costs of care.

The relationships needed for a cooperative MUS may, in some situations, need to be developed gradually, along with the systems themselves. A local-level QI approach such as the example described in Chapter 11 may be an effective and realistic (data-driven) way for managed care, physicians, pharmacists, and patients to work together, solving specific types of DRMs, gradually developing new systems and the new relationships needed to make them work.

The environment may also put managed care executives in a defensive posture (see Chapter 5). A defensive posture may make it difficult to let go of the "old way," tacit admission that it was not as safe or effective as one has been insisting it was.

The way forward is first to critically analyze the validity of the conventional wisdom. Chapter 3 showed that PDRMs have complex causes, and Chapter 6 showed that prescribing restrictions are not the answer. It concluded that prescribing restriction activities should lose their presumption of effectiveness and that MCOs should evaluate the consequences of their existing medications use policies with respect to outcomes and total costs of care.

MCOs hold prescribers to evidence-based standards of prescribing. They expect providers to change the way they practice, to conform to the evidence. By the same token, unless this is merely an exercise of market power, the managed care industry should hold itself to the same standard. If it does not, payers, private accreditation bodies, and government agencies should hold them to it.

Compatibility of the Innovation with Current Values, Norms, Beliefs, and Procedures

As mentioned above, pharmaceutical care is an official goal of many pharmaceutical societies worldwide. Pharmaceutical care is totally consistent with the norms and values of pharmacy, nursing, and medicine, with one possible exception. Some physicians and pharmacists are accustomed to isolated practice. They may have developed negative stereotypes and may either not value interprofessional cooperation or not believe that it is possible. Some professional organizations may be preoccupied with maintaining or expanding professional power and boundaries. They would need to see the benefits to patients and ultimately to all professions that could result from interprofessional cooperation.

Superficially, medications management is a major departure from current procedures and norms. Managers responsible for medications management are routinely assigned to operate restrictive formularies with DUE programs to enforce compliance. Pharmacy benefit managers may define quality of drug use too narrowly, as conformity to prescribing guidelines. The basic structure of pharmacy benefits management is component cost control, quite far from systems development as the term is used in this book. (See Chapters 5 and 6.) For example, the scenario in Chapter 11 may seem utopian, in part, because Dr. Theriz was willing to propose a program that did not emphasize drug cost minimization.

On a more fundamental level, medications management is highly consistent with values and beliefs about quality that are held by nearly all stakeholders. The fundamental principle of professional ethics (beneficence and nonmaleficence) is "First, do no harm." The ideals of QI are familiar and respected by most professionals and managers, and objections tend to be about procedural details rather than to oppose the quality mandate.

Competition on Quality

Price has often been a transient basis of competition in new markets. Managed care justified its existence in large part with a promise to reduce health care costs. Certainly market conditions created by government and then by managed care have changed medications use, e.g., through the rise of mail-order and mass-merchandising pharmacies. This may have increased efficiency in some parts of drug distribution, but there is no reason to believe that component cost management has improved outcomes or reduced total costs of care. Further reduction in expenditures for pharmacy will produce proportionately smaller reductions in pharmacy cost at proportionately greater loss of quality and resistance from patients and professionals.

Some American MCOs may voluntarily move away from component cost management toward managing quality and total cost of care per member per month (PMPM). This is a classic shift in a maturing market, made perhaps even more likely by mounting evidence that today's cheap care is tomorrow's hospitalization or chronically ill patient.

Emerging Concept of Value

Another part of the maturing market is a definition of value that is changing from a short-term emphasis on acquisition cost to a longer-term life cycle cost that includes the value of outcomes, in other words, from units of professional services and products per dollar to the number of successfully treated cases per dollar.

New Accreditation Standards for Medications Use

The National Committee on Quality Assurance (NCQA) Health Plan Employer Data and Information Set (HEDIS) has established standards for MCOs. The stated objectives of HEDIS are to give purchasers and consumers the information they need to make decisions based on value rather than simply cost:

- To provide tools for quality and value determinations
- To use standardized performance measures
- To provide information needed to reliably compare the performance of managed health care plans
- To evaluate quality of different health plans along a variety of important dimensions

For these voluntary standards to have any effect, however, purchasers and consumers must understand and accept the value of quality standards.

The HEDIS 3.0 performance domains include much more than medications use. They include:

- Effectiveness of care
- Access and availability of care
- Satisfaction
- Health plan and stability
- Use of services
- Cost of care
- Informed health care choices
- Health plan descriptive information

Some HEDIS 3.0 performance measures are related to drug therapy. More seem likely:

- First trimester prenatal care
- Treating children's ear infections
- Beta-blocker treatment after a heart attack
- Aspirin treatment after a heart attack

- Use of appropriate medications for asthmatic patients
- Antibiotics for HIV-related pneumonia

Quality standards in community practice have been developing quietly for years, although their emergence may come as a surprise to many community pharmacists and physicians. Chapter 5 briefly reviewed the expanding scope of the Joint Commission on Accreditation of Healthcare Organizations (JCAHO). JCAHO already accredits community practices as part of their hospital, long-term-care, home care, and mental health facility programs. The Joint Commission standards for pharmacies are written in the language of QI, and in essence, a pharmacy must have a QI program to be accredited. For example, the JCAHO Home Care Pharmacy Standards include:

1. The leaders establish a planned, systematic, organization wide approach to process design and performance measurement, analysis, and improvement.

...

3. Data are collected to monitor the stability of existing processes, identify opportunities [and] changes that will lead to improvement, and sustain improvement.*

Possibilities for the Future

Present efforts in QI and performance evaluation do not extend as far as they can. The trend in health care over many years (see Chapter 4) has been toward increased standards and improved quality. Some reasonable possibilities for the future include:

- National performance databases.
- More outcome-based indicators. HEDIS is already introducing the idea of "rotating" indicators to avoid the syndrome of "studying for the test."
- More statistical process control.
- Report cards for providers so that MCOs can more closely approximate their ability to add value.
- New responsibility and accountability for some providers, especially pharmacists.

Complexity: The Ease of Understanding and Using the Innovation

As Chapter 3 pointed out, the reality of medications use is complicated. The initial appearance of system descriptions and explanations may appear to

* From Comprehensive Accreditation Manual for Long-Term Care Pharmacies. © 1998 by the Joint Commission on Accreditation of Health Care Organizations, Chapter 4.

complicate matters because they encompass more aspects than simple, process-based explanations. The systems view is, however, actually a way to simplify a complex reality.

Operationally, Chapters 10 and 11 show how the complexity of systems can be routinized and regularized. A pharmaceutical care system (PCS) can be expressed as a series of steps, and necessary information can be organized according to the five principles of medications use and the taxonomy of drug therapy problems.

An indicator-driven FOCUS-PDCA procedure requires some training of quality circle members and requires expert facilitation. According to Deming's philosophy, quality circles should be comprised of workers who do not need a theoretical understanding of the process they are improving. In our experience, the expertise of the facilitator should include a thorough understanding of the theory of medications use and of group processes in QI.

Most physicians should be able to participate in pharmaceutical care systems with little additional training. Many pharmacists today received extensive clinical education and training, but those in high-volume dispensing practices would have to mentally shift gears.

The usual reimbursement basis for pharmacy is the number of prescriptions filled. This would be completely inappropriate for a pharmaceutical care system. Professional fee systems do exist, however, and could be adapted to pharmaceutical care. Pharmacy practice management would have to change. Practice managers would need to develop a performance-based evaluation system based on quality indicators. These would be analogous to the example in Chapter 11, except that practice management might rely on process indicators, for example, the process component of performance indicators, such as those described in Chapter 11.

Divisibility: Required Degree of Commitment

Theoretically, MUSs are not divisible. Patients at risk of PDRMs should require intact systems that address all of the five principles listed in Chapter 8. According to systems theory and the analysis described in Chapter 3, many types of errors and system failures cause PDRM; therefore, many components must be in place to prevent it. If the innovation being considered were a complete MUS, especially one developed elsewhere and presented as an "off the shelf" product, then an answer to the divisibility question would be clear.

This may have been an obstacle to system development: creating a combined PCS-MMS might appear worlds more complicated than creating a prescribing improvement or compliance improvement program.

If, however, the innovation were the institution of a QI program for medications management — for example, a FOCUS-PDCA process based on process or performance indicators as described in Chapter 11 — the assessment of the divisibility issue would be a bit different. Developing indicators requires some time and talent. Instituting existing indicators would require some database manipulation and some computer programming. The FOCUS process has to be carried out in its entirety to produce any effect. None of these, happily, represents a major, irreversible commitment by an MCO. The PDCA process also must be carried out completely and consistently over time. Implementing an improvement, especially an MMS-PCS, might require considerable commitment. However, by the time an MCO got to this point, it would be very well informed about the need for (value of) the improvement.

Communicability of Results

A large, comprehensive demonstration project in an MCO would be extremely valuable for accelerating adoption of medications management systems. Such a project would be worthy of major funding by the federal government or by a foundation with a commitment to quality improvement in health care, for example, the Pew Foundation or the Robert Wood Johnson Foundation.

In the United States, more perhaps than any other country, problems with communicability could significantly retard the diffusion of medications management locally developed within an MCO as a QI project. An effective PCS-MMS might represent a competitive advantage to an MCO, especially if the cost of PDRM is as large as it appears to be. The money not spent on preventing and correcting PDRM and on consequences such as lawsuits could be used to lower premiums, increase access, etc. Unfortunately, some MCOs might consider detailed information about the experience to be proprietary. In public programs, however, especially single-payer programs, if MUSs were found to be successful, they would be communicated throughout the system.

Summary of the DoI Analysis

NIMP and other forms of skepticism about the PDRM problem appear to be at the root of the marketing problem. The NIMP assumption that one's particular program or practice has a much lower than average prevalence of PDRM seems unjustifiable and irresponsible, especially because of the modest investment required to test it. This defense is so durable, however, that it may be a system learning disability (see below).

Performance indicators are the key to breaking the logjam. Professional and patient advocacy organizations should work harder to publicize the problem (as the IOM has done.) The ultimate source of demand for medications management is not MCOs; it is organized purchasers of health coverage, e.g., employers, labor unions, government programs, and individual persons. They should use accreditation standards like those of NCQA to select an MCO and should then hold them accountable for value targets, not cost alone.

This may require considerable initial energy from patient advocacy groups and human resource departments, because they would be demanding services that their present MCOs may not offer. Likewise, MCOs who outsource (contract for) pharmacy benefit management should demand more than drug cost minimization. If purchasers insist on assessing the value received for their health care expenditures and if MCOs evaluate the performance of their medications use processes, the logjam may be broken.

At least with respect to drug therapy, accreditation standards requiring QI cycles are much more than boxes to tick off on an accreditation survey. It seems very likely, based on the numbers given in earlier chapters, that quality of medications use often is free, and in many cases, profitable.

Returning to the theme of the marketplace, this discussion assumed that the supply side had developed more than the demand side, and it addressed the latter much more than the former. It would be a sad irony, indeed, if managed care began to demand MUSs and health care professionals declined the challenge.

System Learning Disabilities: Psychological Barriers to System Improvement

The preceding section discussed issues in adoption mainly as issues of fact and reason. Not all of the obstacles to the adoption of a new idea are rational, however. There may also be an overlay of irrationality throughout the adoption process (or rationality that is too tightly constrained). We cannot offer any proof that managers and professionals use irrational defenses against change, but our experience has certainly suggested that they do. After all, they are only human.

In his book, *The Fifth Discipline,* Peter Senge[15] listed a number of "systems learning disabilities" — patterns of inappropriate response to complex problems. He suggests these responses may interfere with spontaneous (or even planned) system improvements. Many are variations of recognized psychological ego defenses such as identification, projection, and denial. He phrases them as follows.

Denial, Justification of Status Quo

This defense might in some cases be very similar to the NIMP defense, described above. It is also known as "circle the wagons." It may be the most self-explanatory and familiar. It also may be people's first line of defense. Some examples from my personal experience are:

"We don't have that problem here."

"Things are not really as bad as they may seem."

"It's just those muckrakers (researchers, activists, professors, ...) again."

"The research is flawed."

"You can show anything with statistics."

"Things will get better by themselves."

"These things will never change."

"I Am My Job (Profession ...)"

In some ways, this is related to assessing the risks of adopting an innovation. If a person defines himself in terms of his job, work group, profession, etc., he may use ego defenses against criticism of the job. Evidence of poor performance can be minimized as a mere unfortunate aberration, error, or "unintended consequence."

This defense seems to proceed as follows: "To admit this problem would find fault with me or my profession. Since we are basically good people, we would not allow this problem to exist; therefore, the evidence is wrong or biased, or shows an unfortunate exception to normally excellent performance. There is no problem, or it's somebody else's fault, or it's the best we can hope for."

An alternative perspective is to see one's job objectively, e.g., in terms of its immediate objectives and purpose. Assessment and problem solving can be facilitated if a person can separate himself from his job, identify with the value or purpose of the job instead of its process, and admit the possibility of human failure.

The Root Cause Is "Out There"

This defense is basically a form of blaming or scapegoating. It does not necessarily emphasize simple explanations for problems as much as explanations that involve other people, or factors beyond the person's control. For example, Odedina et al. found this contrast when they asked community pharmacists to describe their efforts to change their practices toward participation in a pharmaceutical care system. Pharmacists who reported progress tended to speak of problems they had identified and resolved, or which remained to be resolved. Pharmacists who had done little described barriers to pharmaceutical care, none of which included themselves.[12,13]

For another example, we gave pharmacists process indicator data. The pharmacists were quality circle panelists in a quality improvement exercise. The data showed that some asthmatic patients might have been misusing their asthma medicines for many months, in a way that might indicate significantly worsening asthma and could lead to crisis and even death.

(Panelists were selected from four different pharmacies and knew that their pharmacy had contributed to the aggregated data.) The panelists were guided through an exercise (nominal group process) intended to identify possible root causes of the data.

The panelists preferred the following explanations for these indicators: the indicators may not be valid; some pharmaceutical manufacturers promote medications misuse; some physicians lack correct drug knowledge and prescribe inappropriately; some health insurers' policies encourage medicine misuse; some patients have incorrect beliefs or inappropriate attitudes; pharmacy corporate policy does not encourage, and local pharmacy management discourages, pharmacists from advising patients about proper medications use. The panel did not mention the values, beliefs, and behaviors of pharmacists until after they were specifically asked if these might contribute to the problem, about 2 h into the exercise.

An alternative to this defense is:

- Identify core problem and alternative solutions.
- Do not wait for other people or systems to change.
- Do what *you* can to improve outcomes, including, when possible, convening and reorganizing other contributory elements.

Proactive Reaction

Proactive reaction is inadequate decision making under the pressure of a nonexistent emergency, choosing an immediate, expedient solution as if it were the only remaining choice. In systems language, *actions* are distinguished from *responses* and *reactions*.[14] Actions are proactive — autonomous and chosen by the system. A response follows the recognition of a problem or other external stimulus but is not determined by the problem or stimulus. The system still has some alternatives to choose among. A reaction also follows an external stimulus, but it is determined by it. All but one, or a very few, alternative responses would have been foreclosed by circumstances, and the system would be forced to carry out the remaining choice.

Acquiescence, Adjusting Expectations, Accepting the Unsatisfactory

This is the error of ignoring a problem until it is bad enough to merit attention. Sometimes, the problem will have become much more difficult or expensive to solve, or may have become insoluble. This is similar in some ways to denial and can reenforce denial as an inappropriate defense. Acquiescence does not require one to deny the problem, just to accept it. It also leads to reactive panic solutions.

The classic parable is Senge's "boiled frog."[15] A frog was placed in a pot of cool water. He was comfortable and did not jump out. The heat was turned on under the pot, and the temperature of the water began to rise. The frog noticed this, and briefly considered jumping out of the pot. But he didn't really dislike being in the pot. He thought, "The devil you know is better than the devil you don't." The water became warm. He was no longer comfortable, but he could stand it. He thought that he would jump out when things got bad enough. Frogs are cold blooded, so as the water continued to warm, the frog became sleepy and finally passed out. Thus, he was boiled by his own acquiescence. The correction is obvious. Decide what is needed or right, and do not accept less in the name of being realistic. The *plan* to improve things needs to be realistic. The *goal* of improvement should never be based on what appears to be achievable at the moment.

Fixation on Events

This is the phenomenon of seeing trees but not a forest, of seeing concrete details but not relationships. It may lead to solving superficial problems, sometimes essentially the same problem again and again. Gary Larsen drew a wonderful cartoon of a person standing on the sidewalk examining a broken piano stool. He is focusing on an event. He has not thought about root causes and has not even looked to see where the stool fell from. He does not see the piano falling after the stool.

A better alternative is to follow a systematic method for finding and evaluating common features among problems, then addressing underlying causes:

- Interpret events with reference to the objectives of the system.
- Look for relationships among process and structural elements and seek underlying (root) causes.

Delusion of Self-Correcting Experience

People learn best from experience, but this does not automatically lead to improvements. Learning is severely impaired if people cannot observe consequences, compare experience with expectation, and accept responsibility for part of any discrepancy. The scientific method may lead to the truth, but sometimes it takes years of trial and error.

The difficulties in learning about the outcomes of medications use are that DRMs often manifest as a new medical problem. Patients who notice a DRM may consult their doctor. Therefore, some professionals, e.g., pharmacists, may not be in a position to see many DRMs. Most patients do not have DRMs, and even physicians and nurse practitioners may not consider this potential cause of adverse outcomes. For example, in one study only about 18% of hospital admissions that were identified by researchers as caused by DRMs had been recorded as such by the patient's doctor. About

1% of non-DRMs had been miscoded by the doctor as a DRM.[10] MCOs see the big picture but cannot recognize the magnitude of the problem because few DRMs are coded as such.

Myth of the Management (Health Care) Team

Effective team members cooperate and coordinate the delivery of health care. In addition, effective teamwork requires the courage to be uncertain, to question, and to disagree with teammates. Teamwork requires a balancing of one's own objectives with those of others. There are many important areas of possible disagreement involving, for example, effectiveness vs. safety, lack of a clear therapeutic objective or end point, a therapeutic plan vs. a therapeutic reality. To some, the physician is the "quarterback" in American football, issuing orders to be carried out. Some team members, knowing that they will not get the ball, may not run very hard.

A much more realistic metaphor for a pharmaceutical care team, however, is basketball or soccer, where the "game" of drug therapy is fluid and somewhat unpredictable, and everyone may have a unique contribution at any moment.

Summary: Performance Indicators Are Crucial

To function properly, markets require timely, specific and accurate information. By providing timely, specific, and accurate information about a particular system, performance indicators can help to identify needed change. For example, denial of a problem is more difficult when data describe specific problems in one's program specifically, especially if benchmarks are available. When a significant problem is seen to be widespread, indicator data make some explanations untenable, e.g., focusing on events and placing the problem "out there." Frequently occurring problems involve too many people to use blame as a response. Indicators may focus attention on problem recognition and resolution. They might create market conditions favorable to the construction of medication use systems.

References

1. Institute of Medicine, *Crossing the Quality Chasm: A New Health System for the 21st Century*, National Academy Press, Washington, D.C., 2001.
2. Berwick, D.M., A user's manual for the IOM's Quality Chasm Report, *Health Aff.*, 21, 80, 2002.

3. Larsen, M.S., *The Rise of Professionalism,* University of California Press, Berkeley, CA, 1977.
4. Hepler, C.D., Pharmacy as a clinical profession, *Am. J. Hosp. Pharm.,* 42, 1298, 1985.
5. Hall, R.H., Professionalization and bureaucratization, *Am. Sociol. Rev.,* 33, 92, 1968.
6. Hall, R.H., Some organizational considerations in the professional-organizational relationship, *Adm. Sci. Q.,* 12, 461, 1967.
7. Illich, I., *Medical Nemesis: The Expropriation of Health,* Pantheon Books, New York, 1976.
8. Hepler, C.D., The future of pharmacy: pharmaceutical care, *Am. Pharm.,* NS30, 583, 1990.
9. Hepler, C.D., Unresolved issues in the future of pharmacy, *Am. J. Hosp. Pharm.,* 45, 1071, 1988.
10. Bero, L.A., Lipton, H.L., and Bird, J.A., Characterization of geriatric drug-related hospital readmissions, *Med. Care,* 29, 989, 1991.
11. Kohn, L.T., Corrigan, J.T., and Donaldson, M.S., *To Err Is Human: Building a Safer Health System,* National Academy Press, Washington, D.C., 2000.
12. Odedina, F.T., Segal, R., and Hepler, C.D., Providing pharmaceutical care in community practice: differences between providers and non-providers of pharmaceutical care, *J. Soc. Adm. Pharm.,* 12, 170, 1995.
13. Odedina, F.T. et al., Changing pharmacists' practice pattern: pharmacists' implementation of pharmaceutical care factors, *J. Soc. Adm. Pharm.,* 13, 74, 1996.
14. Schoderbek, P.P., Schoderbek, C.G., and Kefalas, A.G., *Management Systems: Conceptual Considerations,* 3rd ed., Business Publications, Inc., Plano, TX, 1985.
15. Senge, P.M., *The Fifth Discipline — The Art and Practice of the Learning Organization,* Doubleday, New York.

15

Finding a Way Toward Medications Use Systems

Even if you're on the right track, you'll get run over if you just sit there.

Will Rogers

The "story" developed in this book so far should provoke two serious concerns. The primary concern is, of course, the problem of preventable treatment failures and adverse outcomes of drug therapy, described in Chapter 2. The legitimate use of approved medicines frequently results in preventable drug-related morbidity (PDRM). PDRM may manifest as emergency room visits, hospitalizations, hospital transfers to intensive care, or death. Estimates by various methods and in various populations suggest that PDRM may be prevalent and costly, on a par with heart disease or cancer as a cause of hospital admission. It is a leading cause of death in hospitalized patients. Many nations in the industrialized world have this problem.

Clearly, the health care delivery system should provide necessary drug therapy correctly. This is a quality issue, not merely a safety issue. Improvements in the quality of drug therapy would not only avoid suffering, unnecessary health care, and death, but also make health care much more efficient by avoiding the costs associated with PDRM.

In Phillip Crosby's famous phrase, "Quality is free." In health care, however, too many people still believe that quality can improve only with increased cost or decreased access (the so-called iron triangle). Tell that to Toyota. The issue is confusing because the truth of the iron triangle depends on how one defines quality. The iron triangle may have been true with old ideas that process and structure quality were whatever doctors said they were. That kind of quality now looks like luxury, not quality. It is probably not true with modern ideas of outcome-related quality. (See Chapter 5.) Toyota did not believe in the iron triangle. As the story goes, Toyota and other Japanese automobile manufacturers did not realize that the American automobile industry was largely ignoring QI principles as advocated by Deming and others. Toyota listened. Its cars got better every year, in terms of outcome utility, not cup holders. Value went up much faster than price.

The rest, as they say, is history. We need a Toyota in medications management, not to say health care in general.[1]

That brings us to the secondary problem, society's nonresponse to the primary problem of PDRM prevalence. Despite many reports over many years, the response of providers and organizations has been slow and inadequate.

Chapter 3 proposed a provider- and patient-level model for medications use. That model was intended to describe the generation and prevention of PDRM, the "shadow" of the medications use process. It proposed a theory of preventability and argued that the causes of PDRM constitute system failures. Error, patient noncompliance, and other simple explanations are incomplete at best. Chapter 14 described the diffusion of information about medication use and described the organizational level from an educational and marketing perspective. This chapter will continue to explore causes of both problems from an organizational and environmental perspective. It will propose some changes in the organization and environment of health care that may promote the development of medications use systems.

Improving the safety and effectiveness of medications use will require changes on patient, provider, organizational, and environmental levels. It may ultimately depend on grassroots support. Purchasers, consumers (patients), and providers must insist on safer systems.

Organizational and Environmental Context of PDRM

The problem of preventable injury and death from medications use must be understood as a part of the larger problem of health care quality in America. The two recent reports by the Institute of Medicine's (IOM) Committee on the Quality of Health Care in America have now propelled health care quality into broad public awareness. The first IOM report, *To Err Is Human*, reframed medical injury from a rare result of bad products, bad care, or bad luck. It recognized it as a "chronic threat to public health, as lethal as breast cancer, motor vehicle accidents, or AIDS."[2] A year and a half later, the IOM released *Crossing the Quality Chasm*. It calls for improvements in six dimensions of health care performance: safety, effectiveness, patient centeredness, timeliness, efficiency, and equity. It asserts that those improvements cannot be achieved within the existing system of care. The IOM found that "in its current form, … American health care is incapable of providing the public with the quality health care it expects and deserves." The second report provides a rationale and a framework for the redesign of the U.S. health care system.[3]

Lack of Response

Despite mounting evidence, PDRM and other health care quality problems continue. This nonresponse problem, a lack of effective measures to correct the primary problem, is obvious from the literature. Many institutions have responded to specific events, but change, especially in the way we deliver drug therapy, has been glacially slow. The IOM commented, "What is perhaps most disturbing is the absence of real progress toward restructuring health care systems to address both quality and cost concerns."[3]

The lack of effective responses cannot be explained by a lack of awareness. The two recent IOM reports may have increased public awareness, but the studies cited in *To Err Is Human* had been previously published, some many years ago. The committee found "more than 70 publications in leading peer-reviewed journals [that] documented serious quality shortcomings."[3] Studies showing PDRM have been available for a decade or more from the Harvard Medical Practice Study and others, especially those from the Adverse Drug Event Prevention Study (ADEPS).[4] The ADEPS has lead the way in demonstrating the problem in hospitals and in proposing solutions.[5] News stories have exposed horrific examples. The public has been outraged, but little has been done to change the use of medicines, in hospitals or, especially, in ambulatory care.

Severe quality problems in American health care should not have surprised the leadership of American medical, pharmacy, nursing, or managed care establishments. The fact that the IOM has written these reports may be, in a manner of speaking, as important as what it had to say. The two reports may represent an intellectual sea change. Until recently, it seemed unimaginable that the Institute, one of four prestigious national academies, with strong traditions in basic medical science, would publicly recognize the limitations of the biomedical paradigm and turn to social science to provide the solution. There has been, and will continue to be, a backlash. Expert knowledge of systems theory, however, may rapidly move from the margin to the mainstream.

The IOM has clearly called on Americans to reconstruct our health care delivery system. It said, "In its current forms, habits, and environment, American health care is incapable of providing the public with the quality health care it expects and deserves." Further, "Trying harder will not work. Changing systems of care will."[3] This is a partial explanation for the nonresponse. The basic nonsystem has to change, but in our pluralistic society, no single entity has the authority or the resources to do that. We have, in effect, turned large parts of the health care enterprise over to market forces, but the market has not, until now, rewarded quality improvement (QI) in health care. In fact, the market often penalizes quality. One can see why some people have advocated federal law as a means of change, in particular federal drug law. Federal drug law has the necessary scope, but as Chapter 5 described, federal drug law and regulations can influence only product purity, potency, and commercial claims about effectiveness. Tighter federal drug laws would be able, in theory, to keep some drugs with safety problems off the market, but this might deprive patients of access to necessary therapies. It cannot, in any case, make medications *use* safer and more effective unless Congress were willing, for example, to provide the Food and Drug Administration

(FDA) with authority to encourage and require safer systems as a condition for marketing certain drug products. (See Chapter 5.)

Various constituencies — patients, providers, organizations, payers, managed care networks, accreditors, regulators, and legislators — have tried various solutions, most of them ineffective, such as the prescribing influence programs described in Chapter 6. Lack of technique to improve medications use, however, cannot be a complete explanation for the nonresponse problem. The concepts and tools necessary to construct a medications use system (a pharmaceutical care system within a medicines management system) are adaptations of familiar quality improvement tools (Chapters 7 to 11).

The poverty of even crude systems approaches cannot be fully explained by legitimate ignorance of how to begin. Like the primary problem of PDRM, the nonresponse is a systems problem. As with specific quality examples, blame, scapegoating, and simplistic solutions will not be effective and may actually make matters worse. A defensive posture does not promote needed change.

Chapter 1 used the case of Katherine LaStima to introduce the idea of system failure. It described a classic example of patient injury involving the use — or in that case, the nonuse — of medications. Katherine had a continuing undertreatment of her asthma. It was, in some ways, a micro analogy to our macro nonresponse problem. The discussion showed that all of the system levels contributed to her death and could have contributed to preventing it: any of her direct caregivers — Katherine and her parents, her pharmacist and physician — could have prevented it. In addition, the local hospital, her insurance company, even the boards of pharmacy and medicine in the Commonwealth of Massachusetts, could have contributed to preventing her death. Blaming any of them, however, would surely set them into defensive mode. Then changing their behavior rules and policies would be more difficult.

For about 5 years now, we have been using that story as a teaching tool. Every group of students and professionals who have heard it included people who were outraged and wanted to blame somebody, especially the pharmacist, because he was the last professional to see Katherine and should have had the knowledge and means to resolve her undertreatment. Others take a more traditional route, holding her doctor responsible for everything.

Likewise, different observers of the quality chasm and the PDRM problem may tend to focus on the importance of one or two causes. The key to understanding, however, is to recognize that the causes are systemic. At any level — patients, providers, organizations, or environment — multiple causes interact and, since this is a persistent problem, interlock. Furthermore, causes at any level interact and interlock with causes at other levels. Good people are intellectually invested in the way things are now and make their living from it. This is the proverbial can of worms.

Problems with medications use are embedded within the health care system. Solving them would be easier if improvements were also going on in the larger health care system. Joseph Newhouse has offered several reasons for the quality chasm, including consumer inability to judge quality and their willingness to accept poor quality; technological innovations that arrive faster than professionals can learn to use them safely; payment arrangements, such as the need for administered pricing and the difficulties of fine-tuning it; difficulty in appraising and rewarding provider quality; and a public sector with competing objectives.[6]

The causes and resolution of the persistently malfunctioning drug use process are not documented in the health care literature. I offer the following interacting and interlocking causes:

- People who take medicines (or administer them to family members) without fully understanding how to do that safely and effectively
- People who do not know what to expect from their health professionals and how to get it
- People who do not accept a share of responsibility for their own medications use
- Professionals who succumb to production pressure (time and interruptions), who prescribe and dispense medicines without adequate knowledge, without adequately informing patients about how to use them, and without specific plans to monitor outcomes
- Professionals and consumers who accept poor quality care and harmful rules
- Medications use policies that do not improve patient care outcomes yet persist year after year
- Managed care networks that use raw market power to force behavior and get what they want
- Payment arrangements that do not reward, and often punish, quality improvement
- National drug laws that regulate drug products through the limited theory of drugs as commercial products rather than as complicated and potentially dangerous instrumental technologies
- Pharmaceutical manufacturers who accept present medication use methods, despite the experience of withdrawing safe and effective drug products that failed in the unsafe and ineffective medications marketplace
- Curricula in health professions schools that are virtually silent about medication use, even though medications are the most common form of therapy, and PDRMs rank with asthma, cancer, and diabetes as causes of hospital admission
- Public health education that virtually ignores the safe use of medications, especially compared to the volume of direct-to-consumer drug advertising and enthusiastic "pill for every ill" stories in the popular press

- Legislators who protect the managed care industry from the consequences of its policies
- Employers, governments, labor organizations, etc., who purchase care without understanding or evaluating the quality or the consequences of what they pay for

Admittedly, much medications use does not fit this gloomy list. Millions of patients and thousands of professionals surely perform their roles correctly, most of the time. But each of these behaviors arguably occurs often enough to contribute to the prevalence of PDRM. We should be as willing to ask about these behaviors as to ask why unsafe automobiles are made, sold, registered, and driven; why unsafe nuclear generators are not shut down; why airlines order pilots to fly when they are fatigued; and why sea captains keep to routes and schedules that endanger crew, cargo, ship, and the environment.[7] Drug catastrophes are much less dramatic than an airplane crash, but they kill and injure many more people every year.

Managed Care

Managed care — in a very broad sense, including American business models, government programs like the Veterans Administration, and single-payer schemes such as the National Health Service of the U.K. — now wields considerable influence over professional decision making in medications use. Any problem analysis or solution set must recognize its power. By the same token, managed care is a common thread that ties together almost every one of the causes listed above. Managed care can influence every one to some degree. Managed care organizations (MCOs) accordingly should be more sensitive to the overall effect that their industry has on practice. Individual MCOs should be accountable for the overall performance of their systems and the quality of care they provide. Successful strategies to improve medications use must involve managed care.

Some MCOs and providers may voluntarily move toward medicines management. Others may require regulations that mandate regular system performance assessments and patient outcome assessments. Government programs that are not subject to regulations would have a duty to require the same from themselves and from their paymasters, providers, trust holders, and other contractors.

Managed care was an exciting idea. As described in Chapter 12, once upon a time, 20 years ago or more, managed care was going to replace the "cottage industry" of American health care with organized delivery systems. (The term HMO came into popular use in the Nixon years.) Each organized delivery system would be capable of producing rational, evidence-based decisions and controlling quality of care.

Managed care's other mandate, in addition to improving outcomes, was to get control of input costs. America was spending 10% of its gross domestic product on health care, but our leaders did not think America was getting its money's worth. Health insurance premiums were rising, and employers were worried about international competitiveness. Somebody in the automobile industry complained that his company spent more on health care insurance premiums than it did on steel. There was a flurry of health reform activity.

Things did not work out quite that way. Managed care became big business. Like any good business, managed care had to charm investors, merge, divest, spin off, advertise, compete, and above all sell.[8] It replaced an admittedly imperfect and inefficient cottage industry with what Kassirer called "the morality of the marketplace."[9] It became part of the health care infrastructure, a cost of delivering care. Ten years ago, however, even Alan Enthoven, one of managed care's leading theorists, wrote that managed care was failing to control costs.[10] A recent article in *Managed Care Quarterly* entitled "Who Lost Cost Containment? A Roster for Recrimination" said that "the battle to contain medical costs certainly has not been won. It has returned as the most significant health care issue facing the nation.... [C]ost containment via managed care has largely failed. Obviously new methods need to be identified and tested."[11]

The broad topic of managed care's failure or success is beyond the scope of this book (and my expertise). Clearly, however, some managed care programs have failed in their mission to provide cost-effective drug therapy, seemingly when they focused on cost control instead of quality of care. Inexpensive drug therapy is a good idea, but the evidence shows that component cost control, as an end in itself, sometimes hurts people and therefore can be really expensive in the longer run. Correcting medical failure usually costs a lot more than it would have to prevent failures.

Further, some trends in managed care networks may be in the wrong direction. Some activities that would improve medications use, such as taking more time with patients to discuss drug therapy, are being squeezed out by an emphasis on component cost minimization. The substitute for negotiation and education is often coercion, which creates a climate of profound hostility and mistrust. Some managed care networks seem to have a tiger by the tail. They have alienated their members and providers, and now their costs are rising. Could it be that cost and quality in health care support each other, when the money is spent to get defined outcomes?

Managed care is a central part of the problem, not the problem itself. The managed care industry is not evil or greedy. It employs hundreds of thousands of dedicated people. But, according to some accounts, the industry includes some companies that are predatory, at best, by business standards, if not criminal.[8] Some pharmacy benefit management companies (PBMs) operate policies, like promoting products of certain manufacturers, that belie their claims of promoting rational therapeutics and evidence-based medicine. Some managed care networks seem, at best, unresponsive to decent dictates of patient care. The good companies seem unable or unwilling to police the bad ones. The good people distance themselves from the exploiters, but the exploiters do not seem to notice.

In our pluralistic society, health care delivery and finance take many forms. Many managed care organizations seem to have it right. They try to control costs by improving quality. Kaiser Permanente, in many regions, and the Group Health Cooperative in the Northwest have pharmacy systems that are widely recognized as evidence based, patient centered, and QI oriented. Many others surely exist. If the managed care pharmacy can follow their examples — even improve upon them — it can become part of the solution, and progress can occur rapidly.

ERISA: A Shield for Employers and Managed Care?

Regulation of MCOs in the United States is made difficult by the provisions of a little-known law entitled Employee Retirement Income Security Act of 1974 (ERISA). ERISA was enacted to protect employees covered by employer pension plans from abuse by plan managers. As interpreted by the U.S. Supreme Court and lower courts, it has been used to block health care reform at the state level. Employee benefit plans, including health care, "are now asserting their rights to be completely free of state regulation of health care financing."[12]

In the United States, damages for tort liability and for breach of contract are a penalty that may be paid by professionals and other providers when someone can prove that he was denied care or injured by substandard products or services. The effectiveness of the tort system in promoting quality improvement is complicated, a matter of some debate. However, according to Brennan and Berwick,

> If the reach of ERISA continues to expand, it may well be that HMO liability will decline.... This in turn will mean that liability for medical negligence will continue to attach to the individual practitioner [and] that managed care organizations ... will be essentially immune from liability.... ERISA thus retards the sort of liability that could nationally give rise to improvements in the health care system as a whole.... [S]everal other courts have now decided that utilization management liability is preempted by ERISA.[12]

Utilization management is such a bland phrase that an example is necessary. Brennan and Berwick recount the case of Mr. K. Mr. K.'s doctor had recommended an emergency cardiac procedure. His employee health plan, however, had a precertification requirement for that procedure. It denied precertification for Mr. K. and required a second opinion. The second opinion concurred that Mr. K. was at high risk of sudden death. The health plan continued to delay precertification over several months. Mr. K.'s heart meanwhile deteriorated to the extent that he was no longer a candidate for the originally recommended surgery. He died of the precise ailment that had been diagnosed but not promptly treated 7 months earlier. Under ERISA, a court found Mr. K.'s health plan immune from money damages.[12]

So-called "patient's bill of rights" legislation was originally directed in part at correcting the impact of ERISA on health care reform. The debate was considerably distorted by rhetoric, for example, by slogans about giving money to lawyers instead of patients. Some original proposals to eliminate the ERISA exemptions were watered down.

The right to sue for damages is, for well or ill, part of the American justice system. While other approaches, e.g., compulsory arbitration, might promote quality more efficiently, ERISA seems to simply remove tort liability as a negative incentive without providing an alternative. Over the years, sovereign immunity has never seemed salutary, even for the "king."

Getting the Problem and Solutions in the Open

Patients, practitioners, managers, purchasers, and regulators all have essential contributions to improving the outcomes of drug therapy. However, many are stuck in a logjam of denial of the problem and responsibility, production pressures, and narrow focus. To give mainstream pharmacy due credit, pharmacy organizations in the United States, U.K., and some other industrialized nations recognized the problem over 10 years ago. Over the past decade or so, they formulated a part of the solution under the labels of clinical pharmacy, pharmaceutical care, and comprehensive drug therapy management.

The PDRM problem may be invisible to senior leadership, and the ideas of medications use systems (MUSs) are unfamiliar to the majority of providers and payers. In particular, few real MUSs are available for potential adopters to observe and build upon. The theory of diffusion of innovation (DoI) was applied in Chapter 14 as a possible explanation of how knowledge of MUSs might spread and may also explain part of its slow diffusion. A large, comprehensive demonstration project in an MCO would be worthy of funding by a federal agency or a foundation interested in health care quality. Performance indicators also would be crucial for initiating the adoption process in MCOs.

Health services research surely can help. Without published research, for example, the IOM reports and this book would be extended editorials rather than interpretations of fact. Federal and private research priorities, however, do not reflect the social and economic significance of PDRM. Federal programs and major foundations spend billions of dollars on areas that are less important to public health than medications use, but relatively little on research that would lead toward improved medication use systems. The published research studies mentioned in Chapter 9 were usually done on tiny budgets. Too few of those studies used expensive, state-of-the-art randomized, blinded designs. Consequently, many are dismissed even though their critics offer no solutions with better evidence.[24] Admittedly, many would require replication and confirmation However, even if some studies are individually unpersuasive, taken together, they justify allocation of adequate research funds.

Pharmacists and physicians in many countries have improved the use of medications, but with very little success in proportion to the intelligence and energy that they put into it. They study their practices and design, implement, and study improvements. Often they help their patients and reduce total costs for a managed care organization or insurance company. *Their* costs go up, however, and they cannot sustain the program. They publish their results and, for all practical purposes, watch their reports gather dust. The problem and promising solutions have been publicized, but little happens. The problem is bigger than a few pioneers can resolve.

Managed Care Is an Essential Part of the Solution

One way to create adaptive health care delivery systems might be to let them grow spontaneously. We have tried this approach. Many of the problems of managed care are to be expected in a young industry that grew spontaneously and too fast in an underregulated market. Perhaps the creators of managed care imagined that somehow professional ethics (as imperfect as they may be) would govern the industry. Another example of the result of unregulated growth is commerce on the World Wide Web. Few people, however, would want to buy health care on eBay® (not for themselves, anyway).

Another way to develop a large adaptive system is to plan, design, and engineer one. NASA is an example. America is lucky to have a framework already in place — managed care — in which we can design, test, improve, and perhaps perfect an adaptive health care system. Some centralized organizational structure is necessary, by definition, to create the kind of health care system that the IOM envisions.

A middle ground is to design parts of a system and to grow the system spontaneously within an environment of tax incentives, laws, regulations, and standards intended to promote growth in desired directions. This is more or less the way that growth in the rest of American business is managed. Managed care is part of the problem, and it has to be part of the solution. Managed care pharmacy has the opportunity to lead the way for pharmacy and to be at the cutting edge of health care systems redesign.

A Vision of Medication Use on the "High Plateau"

If patients, providers, and organizations are to move medications use out of the quality chasm, we need to know what the higher ground would look like. The following headings summarize how a redesigned medications use system for ambulatory care under the IOM's proposed "new rules" for redesigning health care processes might compare to the existing medications use process and its implicit "rules." The new rules are supposed to be interrelated, and it makes no sense to discuss them in isolation, so the discussion under each new rule connects in some way to other rules. See also Donald Berwick's simplified "user's manual" for *Crossing the Quality Chasm*.[13]

Rule 1: Care Is Based on Continuous Healing Relationships

Old

Care is episodic, based on visits, and a prescription is an isolated part of one episode. Patients see pharmacists as the retail end of a chain of drug distribution. Patients shop for prescription prices. Visits with pharmacists for advice about medication use, and payments to the pharmacist, are usually tied to a prescription transaction. Patient advice and counseling use leaflets (patient package inserts) with brief encounters on the telephone and when a prescription is dispensed. The content of leaflets is drug oriented, as opposed to patient oriented.

New

Care is continuous, even for acute diseases. (See Brodie et al. definition of pharmaceutical care in Chapter 8.) Pharmacists develop individual therapeutic relationships with patients (see Chapter 4). Prescribing is integrated with medications use throughout the duration of therapy. Therapy is routinely monitored. Physicians and clinical nurse practitioners are busy diagnosing and initiating therapy. Pharmacists and nurses are efficient as co-therapists, especially as a team. The pharmacist or nurse co-therapist has responsibility under protocol or collaborative practice agreements throughout the duration of therapy to authorize refills, adjust doses, and refer patients to their prescriber. (See rules 6, 8, and 10.) Patients know when therapy should be professionally monitored and expect monitoring and co-therapist services (see Chapters 4 and 8). Visits with ambulatory care pharmacists for monitoring and advice are scheduled according to patient need regardless of prescription refill cycle. (Prescriptions may be provided through a separate channel.) Information about drugs is integrated with other care. The provider group practice offers integrated information and support in various media to suit the needs of the patient, including 24-h emergency line, e-mail, Internet, CD, and fax services. Centralized patient-level drug information services are available, usually included as part of the care plan. The pharmacist receives a copy of each institutional discharge summary and provides a current drug history when each patient is admitted to an institution.

Rule 2: Care Is Customized according to Patients' Needs and Values

Old

Professional and, increasingly, *business* autonomy dictate care. Most payment plans use transaction-based direct prescribing controls, e.g., restrictive formularies. Drug of choice applies to every transaction without regard to patient need. Exceptions to the norm, e.g., nonformulary drugs, cost the prescriber extra time and inconvenience and may be expensive for the patient, regardless of patient circumstance. Drug utilization evaluation (DUE) is usually based on therapeutic agent only. It is used to enforce formulary choices and does not evaluate dose, duration, or suitability to patient need. Prescribers learn that DUE means "don't use, ever." (Pharmacist is used as an unpaid agent of the payment plan to enforce uniformity *within* the plan. Drugs of choice, however, vary widely *among* plans because only a few networks actually base drugs of choice on clinical evidence. Some base them on their own buying practices, rebates, and other nonclinical issues.)

New

Patient needs drive care. Variation among patients is expected based on need, culture, psychology, etc. Most payment plans use indirect prescribing controls (education and cooperative practice) and evaluate prescribing based on efficient achievement of patient outcomes by a practice group over time, using outcome-linked process indicators. Pharmacists assist in adjusting and customizing regimens. Media and content of advice and information on medication use are customized to the patient. (See discussion of new rule 1.)

Rule 3: The Patient Is the Source of Control

Old

Payment system considers quality-of-life objectives as secondary to clinical objectives. The prescriber has sole responsibility for therapeutic decisions, including drug choice, despite strong influence by the insured's payment plan. Pharmacist has a disincentive to discourage unnecessary drug use.

New

Quality of life is a primary objective of therapy. Patients are better informed and are given the opportunity to actively participate in decisions about their own care, including drug therapy and available alternatives. The prescriber or co-therapist takes time to educate patients about therapy to reduce demand for unnecessary and inappropriate prescriptions.

Rule 4: Shared Knowledge and Free Flow of Information

Old

There is little sharing of information between physician, pharmacist, and patient. The pharmacist and patient often lack sufficient knowledge to intelligently coordinate or facilitate therapy. The desired standard for patient behavior is compliance or adherence. Patients rarely see their records. Some payment plans discourage or prohibit providers from discussing drugs or services that are not covered by the plan.

New

Information is shared frequently and automatically among physician, pharmacist, and patient over secure electronic network. Patients normally have access to a copy of their records. Pharmacist and patient normally have sufficient knowledge to intelligently coordinate or facilitate therapy and are expected to do so, consistent with collaborative practice agreements and patient's abilities. The desired standard for patient behavior is concordance (essentially, active participation based on informed consent). Payment plans are open about coverage provisions and encourage providers to discuss drugs or services that are not covered by the plan. (See discussion of new rule 9.)

Rule 5: Decision Making Is Based on Evidence

Old

Decision making is based on subjective beliefs. Professional autonomy is framed as a professional prerogative rather than a necessity to meet individual patient need. Some payment plans promote evidence-based prescribing, but the scope of evidence usually ignores patient-specific factors. Many plans use their business autonomy to restrict prescribing without a clinical evidence base. Evidence-based *medications use*, e.g., necessary monitoring and management of therapy, receives very little attention compared to prescribing. Few standards exist for medications use.

Payment plans and provider organizations do not require evidence as a basis for their own business practices and exempt themselves from evaluation. Operations of restrictive formularies, prescription caps, and exclusion from coverage of certain conditions are often arbitrary. Patients and professionals "game" these rules to the extent possible and necessary.

New

Professional decisions and provider and payer practices are all subject to evidence and evaluation. Controls on medications use are patient oriented, with promotion of best practices as appropriate for individual patients or specific patient populations. When possible, performance evaluation according to evidence addresses cost-effectiveness of medications use. Evidence links process and outcome by means of medication use performance indicators. Quality improvement is a norm.

Rule 6: Safety Is a System Property

Old

DRMs are largely invisible except in research. They are seen as being caused by error. Error is seen as personal failure, e.g., of competence or caution, consistent with an environment in which "*Health System* is a misnomer."[3] Personal blame, litigation, and secret settlements are ineffective for improving the system. (See Chapters 1 and 3.) "Defensive" medicine and pharmacy are common. Physicians in private practice have authority and responsibility without regard to scope of competence; delegation of authority to co-therapists is discouraged, even to medical specialists. Safety (avoiding harm) is isolated from effectiveness (achieving good). Systems are discouraged by the payer, and legal focus is on the individual provider. (See rule 10.)

New

DRMs are monitored in a medications management system (MMS). They are seen as being caused by system failure. (See Chapter 3.) Root cause analysis leads to improvement. Safety and effectiveness are seen as complementary and equal goals of quality improvement. Systems are understood to be essential for safe and effective medications use.

Rule 7: Transparency Is Necessary

Old

Patients may not be fully informed of their needs and the choices available to them; potential risks and benefits of therapy; and what they should do (if able) to assist in their therapy. (So, they are usually expected to follow directions rather than participate in their therapy. See old rule 4.) Some payment plans discourage providers from disclosing alternatives that the plan does not cover. Managed care and payment plan requirements are often burdensome to patients; utilization management may create adversarial relationships. Patients may mistrust, and professionals may resent, managed care attempts to educate or advise the patient. Drug advice from the pharmacist is a passive "offer to counsel," sometimes disguised by a clerk's request to "sign here" on a waiver written in fine print. Pharmacists may conceal availability of professional services and even their performance of necessary services (stealth pharmacy). Payment and managed care infrastructure is poorly regulated and subject to business rather than professional rules. Managed care and the payment plan are often unaccountable to the patient or public under business laws and ERISA (see above).

New

Patients (or caregivers) are normally fully informed of their needs and the choices available to them; potential risks and benefits of therapy; and what they should do (if able) to assist in their therapy. Managed care is a partner in educating patients. Drug advice from the pharmacist is active and suited to the patient's need. Pharmacists actively recommend their professional services and are visible performing co-therapist functions. The payment and managed care infrastructure is regulated, accountable under rules compatible with professional duties and ethics. Managed care and the payment plan are not immune from any normal requirement for professional accountability.

Rule 8: Needs Are Anticipated

Old

The medication use process is fragmentary, informal, and unorganized. It has little means to recognize and resolve most drug therapy problems before they become DRMs, or to recognize PDRMs as preventable or drug related. Drug distribution is often "carved out" of health care and, for most community pharmacists, is the only source of payment for professional services. Pharmaceutical care (seeking and correcting drug therapy problems) is discouraged: "one price fits all" payment for prescriptions constitutes a "quality tax" on superior performers. Most medication use arrangements are haphazard and have no means of identifying recurring problems and process or structure (design) failures, and therefore no means of anticipating problems.

New

The medication use system is planned and organized (see Chapters 7 to 11). The MUS is built to recognize and resolve most drug therapy problems before they become DRMs, and recognize recurrent PDRMs. Drug distribution is integrated with the health care system, but is not the major focus of pharmacy practice. Pharmaceutical care (Chapter 10) is required, and superior performers are systematically identified and rewarded. Medication management systems (see Chapters 7 and 11) identify and correct recurring problems and process or structure (design) failures.

Rule 9: Continuous Decrease in Waste

Old

The major (if not only) economic objective of most payment plans is input (component) cost reduction. Prudent buying, utilization management, and demand management are main strategies. Coercion (restrictions, limitations, denial of coverage) is often the first and only method. The payment plan is organized by budget (accounting) categories instead of patients and providers, and the goal is to meet budget targets rather than optimize or minimize expenditures on care.

New

The goal of managed care is management of total expenditures, the same as that under the old rules, but the methods have changed to patient-oriented outcome optimization strategies. Instead of controlling separate budgets (carve-outs), providers assist in optimizing patient care. Demand management and utilization management are accomplished through education of patients and providers. Incentives are used for providers and patients to use resources efficiently. Mechanisms such as provider accounts and member accounts provide needed flexibility to meet specific patient needs. Coercion (denial) is a last resort, and used only when the disagreement involves significant waste or danger to the patient or to public health. Medication use is managed by the same outcome efficiency strategy. Evaluation of efficiency, with feedback to providers, is carried out routinely. Interpatient variation in utilization is expected. The tug-of-war between provider recommendations and payer restrictions is a historical curiosity.

Rule 10: Cooperation among Clinicians

Old

Medical care is understood as physician care. Medications use systems are optional, or discouraged by the payment plan. Pharmacist care from the community pharmacy is poorly coordinated with physician and hospital care. Managed care and the payer framework do not encourage the system or connection or cooperation of providers; in addition, the payment plan (emphasis on component cost) is often adversarial and discourages managed care leadership to systems and coordination of care across providers or sites of care.

New

Medical care and health care are understood as cooperative activities. Cooperation is encouraged as a priority, e.g., condition of preferred provider status. Every provider has a stake in patient outcome. The managed care system and payment plan provide incentives to pharmacists and physicians who enter into collaborative drug therapy management agreements (in compliance with state regulations). Managed care and payer plans encourage systems through collaborative practice arrangements and pharmacist–physician partnerships, supported by drug therapy protocols, that contribute to the pharmaceutical care system (see Chapter 11). Emphasis is on outcomes, coordination across providers, and sites and occasions of care. Managed care operates medication management systems (see Chapters 8 and 11.) To promote systems, managed care organizations have integrated pharmacy benefits into all aspects of care (carve-outs have been eliminated because they discourage systems integration). Pharmacy benefits are evaluated according to their contribution to patient outcome and total cost of care.

Moving Forward

Model-T Era

By analogy to the automotive transportation system, drug therapy is still in the Model T era, with few and poor roads and inadequate standards for driving. However, there is one major exception to the analogy: the roads of medications use are unpaved, but people are not driving cute little 20-horsepower cars on them. The vehicles for medication use — drug products — are like 300-horsepower behemoths. And although these powerful technologies have been well tested in carefully controlled trials, once they leave the test track, they frequently run into things, go off the road, or get stuck in a ditch.

The analogy to automobile travel is useful in many ways. Most fundamentally, we should recognize the relationship between the value of motor vehicles and the quality of the system in which they are used. Cars and trucks were less intrinsically valuable in the muddy road era than they are today, because the infrastructure limited their safety and effectiveness in improving the quality of people's lives. The same is true for drug products today.

In the horse-and-buggy era, today's network of regulated highways, driving rules, and vehicle standards would have been hard to imagine, just as true medications use systems are hard to imagine today. Somehow, industry and political leaders were able to recognize that a weak infrastructure can limit the true value of a technology, while a strong infrastructure can enhance it. Developed nations improved the infrastructure for automobile use. Then the process took off, for as the system improved, the value of the products increased. More value lead to better technology, higher prices, and more profits. The process became almost self-sustaining. The industry has needed stimulation from outside, in the form of regulation and market changes (e.g., automobile safety standards, reduction of tariff protection). It benefited tremendously from the infrastructure changes it had resisted.

In contrast, improving the infrastructure of drug therapy appears itself to be bogged down. Manufacturers, regulators, policy makers, and many professionals seem to minimize the unique significance of drug therapy in health care. Instead, they treat drug products as products to be bought or sold. The clearest examples of this are the so-called carve-outs of the prescription benefit of health insurance. Health insurance programs routinely assign to prescription benefit managers the responsibility of minimizing expenditures for drug products, independently of patient outcomes or overall program costs. This ignores evidence that drug use cannot be limited independently of the overall care program without harming outcomes. Many people think about drug products as "magic bullets" or "two-edged swords" that, sufficient unto themselves, either help or harm.

Somehow, automobiles escaped the "magic bullet" fantasy that the technology could be made sufficient unto itself. Fortunately, the automobile transportation system did not seek to carve out expenditures for concrete and traffic lights. Automobile and fuel manufacturers did not insist on profiting directly from infrastructure improvements, and did not complain that people might use another brand on the roads that they had helped to pay for. Somehow, the industry recognized that improvements would benefit many people, including manufacturers, users, and suppliers.

Margaret Coye has also used an automotive analogy, but in a somewhat different way. She has pointed out that producing safer and more cost-effective automobiles suddenly became much more attractive to American automakers when Toyota provided a business case for them. She points out that managed care lacks that business case for quality improvement.[1] Managed care will not discover a business case for quality because of imports. But America can find a way to make the case. The domination of the American automobile industry's "unsafe at any speed" gas hogs ultimately went away because the American consumer got tired of low quality. The Corvair and Pinto went away because consumer advocates raised hell about them. The IOM report is polite drawing room conversation compared to what is possible.

Change at Every Level

The focus of this section is to describe briefly how patients can protect themselves from the dangers of medication-related injury, and how each level of the drug therapy "nonsystem" can promote change and prepare for change. Every level of the medications use process and the health care enterprise will have a part in creating a self-regulating medications use system within an adaptive health care system. In some countries, including the United States, health care delivery is pluralistic and market driven. Regulation and market forces acting on MCOs will influence the timing and direction of change. In other countries with single-payer systems, government policy will drive change. Even in single-payer systems, medicines management systems may initially have to be constructed on the basis of local initiative, around patients, practice groups, and provider groups.

Patients and professionals are the front-line participants in drug therapy. They could promote development of medications use systems if they could intensify grassroots efforts to develop cooperative systems. Although the evidence indicates the need for increased pharmacist participation in medication use, pharmaceutical care is not about pharmacists or doctors. It is about patients. All participants in drug therapy need to understand drug therapy as a system and to look for weaknesses in the specific system that they or their patients are in. Individuals can do a great deal to construct or strengthen these specific medications use systems.

Chapter 8 presented three models of pharmaceutical care: five principles of medications use, the relationships model (initiator–facilitator–co-therapist), and flow diagrams. Patients and professionals can use each of these simple checklists to organize their thinking about the specific system that they or their patients are in. For example, a patient or caregiver should think about whether his care satisfies each of the five principles, and use the relationships model to ask who is responsible for the three basic functions, and how well they are being carried out. Pharmacists, physicians, and patients could use these models to understand and improve the specific circumstances of their care and to take steps to improve them.

Patients

Crossing the Quality Chasm repeatedly states that the patient is the center of the health care system, even "the source of control."[3] The Joint Commission on Accreditation of Healthcare Organizations (JCAHO), in launching its Speak Up campaign, noted the nearly 100,000 deaths from medical error described in *To Err Is Human*. It recommends that patients "participate in all decisions about [their] treatment" and declares, "You are the center of the health care team."*

The National Council on Patient Information and Education (NCPIE) advises that "seeking and sharing information about medicine-taking, and talking with your health care professionals before starting any new medicine, are healthy behaviors that will give us [*sic*] peace of mind."*

Public awareness of the problem of PDRM is inadequate. Recall that Chapter 2 suggested that the prevalence of hospital admissions caused by PDRM ranks on a par with cancer, and ahead of heart attacks, diabetes, and asthma (to mention a few benchmarks). However, research funding and activity, professional education, and public awareness campaigns are quite limited, pathetically disproportionate to the magnitude of the problem.

Further, most people lack the ability to direct their own care, nor would most want to. As David Angaran put it, when people get on an airplane, they should know where they want to go. They may know some ways they *do not* want to get there. After that, it is up to the pilot. The JCAHO Speak Up program advises patients to "make sure you're getting the right treatments and medications." It does not say how patients are supposed to do that.

Many people may actually know more about air travel than they do about using medicines. Most of us do not want to know about it until we have a problem. Few high schools or colleges offer courses in basic knowledge for consumers about how drugs work (and do not work). Many useful books and newsletters on drug therapy are available for patients and, especially, family caregivers.

A good example is *USP DI Volume II: Advice for the Patient*. It is published by the United States Pharmacopeia, a private nonprofit organization that sets standards for drug purity and monitors for adverse effects. *USP DI Volume II* provides patient-oriented drug information in lay language. Its simplified monographs correspond directly to the listings in *USP DI Volume I: Drug Information for the Health Care Professional*. Drug monographs include

---

* http://www.jcaho.org/news+room/news+release+archives/npsg.htm

common U.S. and Canadian brand names, a description, advice "before using this medicine," proper use, precautions, and side effects. Information about unapproved (off-label) uses is also provided. Additionally, pronunciations and special considerations such as age, allergies, and use in pregnancy and when breast-feeding are included. It is available on CD and in a printed version from Micromedex (http://www.micromedex.com/products/uspdi/). Many libraries and pharmacies have a copy available. It is also available online from the National Library of Medicine Medline Plus® Service at http://www.nlm.nih.gov/medlineplus/druginformation.html.

Consumer understanding of medications use has three essential foundations: First, remember that drug therapy often involves the twin perils of adverse effects and treatment failure. Medicines have the power to cure and to harm, so neither blind obedience nor blind opposition is a safe course. It is a pity, for example, when an asthmatic patient does not use an inhaled steroid because he is afraid of steroids, but does not discuss this decision with his doctor or pharmacist. Likewise, it is a pity when someone overuses ibuprofen because it is over-the-counter (OTC) and therefore "safe."

Second, the safety and effectiveness of therapy depend on the match between the drug, the therapeutic objective, and the manner of use (dose, frequency, duration). Terms like *good drugs* and *bad drugs* may sell books, but they do not provide a useful way to think about therapy. Even though they may look like jelly beans, and even though one has taken them every day for a year, drug products are nonetheless very complex technologies in a cute wrapper. They are neither good nor bad, safe nor unsafe. It is certainly true that some drugs are easier to use correctly than others. Every drug legally on the market in the United States and the U.K., however, has been proven in rigorous trials to be safe and effective — *when used for the indications tested and when used in the exact manner tested.*

The risks of drug therapy depend greatly on prescribing the right drug at the right dose for the right indication, but also on how well the therapy is *managed*. Patients should know if they are taking a medication (like digoxin, warfarin, and nonsteroidal anti-inflammatory drugs) that is known to require especially careful management, and they should know how and when it should be monitored (more about this below).

Drug therapy should never become a matter of lifestyle, any more than surgery should. Below are listed example justifications for inappropriate medication taking:

- "I don't take drugs."
- "I only take natural herbal medicines."
- "If two are good, four should be terrific."
- "I just went off my diet, so I'll double my dose of diabetes medicine."
- "I feel better, so I'll stop taking the medicine."
- "I don't know what it's for, but the doctor (TV) said it is wonderful."

Third, patients do not need to know much about medicine, pharmacy, or nursing to improve their chances of success. For example, a patient with asthma does not need a deep understanding of asthma to know that he should avoid drugs like aspirin and beta-blockers. His doctor or pharmacist should have given him a list of drugs to avoid. It would be a good idea to put the list on the refrigerator door or bathroom mirror. Before that patient takes a new medicine, he should ask his doctor or pharmacist if the medication is like aspirin or a beta-blocker.

He does not need a medical background to learn that it is dangerous to overuse his "rescue" inhaler and to underuse his "preventer." When he or his asthmatic child wants to overuse the rescue medication, he needs to know what to do. The point is that people often can make their therapy safer and more effective by informing themselves about what to expect from their therapies, what to watch out for, and what to do if they suspect a problem.

In health care today, a patient's participation in managing his therapy may take some considerable effort. People may expect too little medicines management from their physicians and pharmacists, and often, that is what they receive. People have a right to necessary services, and if those services are not offered, they should be requested. If a patient is too young, old, or ill to assert those rights, he should have somebody to help him or find another provider. In a society that is ostensibly consumer oriented and market driven, this situation seems ironic, but there it is.

The average time of a routine medical office visit is short, often less than 10 min. The time that patients are allowed to speak without interruption during an office visit is measured in seconds. For example, Beckman and Frankel analyzed tape recordings of office visits with primary care physicians. About 70% of patients' initial statements of health concerns were interrupted by physicians. The average time before the first interruption was 18 sec.[14]

Many people may leave their doctor's office with some of the same unanswered questions that they went in with. For example, Tuckett et al. interviewed 100 patients immediately after an office visit with their doctor. Seventy-five people reported that they had questions or concerns that they had not voiced to the doctor. Reasons given were fear of humiliation, that the visit was too hurried to clearly formulate questions, and that other people were waiting to see the doctor.[15]

Kimberlin et al.[25] interviewed elderly patients about their current, chronic therapy. Over 50% of patients had questions or perceived problems that they had not mentioned to providers: main themes included the purpose of the medicines, their duration, how treatment effectiveness was determined, and symptoms experienced due to medication.

Corporately owned pharmacies (e.g., chain, mail-order, mass merchandiser, and supermarket pharmacies) now have the dominant share of the retail prescription market. Usually, in America, one walks past food, beach balls, and motor oil displays before finding the pharmacy. It may be difficult to believe that health care professionals actually practice in such a commercial environment, but sometimes they do. Others, unfortunately, are little more than they appear.

Many independent pharmacies feel that these giants set the rules. Perhaps they do. Many people seem to expect faster and cheaper prescription service, perhaps from mail-order services or even drive-thru prescription windows. Perhaps it is not surprising, therefore, that some patients (and family caregivers) tend to think about pharmacy in commercial, product-oriented terms. Then, if there is a "pill for every ill," the patient may not realize that he needs help using the medicine. Many have the traditional view of the physician as the complete health professional and expect too little from their pharmacist. The pharmacist, however, may be accessible when the physician is not.

Pharmacists are busy filling prescriptions, but they are usually happy to discuss the safe use of medicines with their patients. In fact, most state laws oblige the pharmacist to speak to patients who say they have a question. Some pharmacists say that they are seldom asked for advice. There may be two ready explanations for that: people may not know when they need advice, and they may not think that pharmacists have time to speak to them.

Over-the-Counter Medicines

Over-the-counter status does not mean that a medicine is safe for everyone to use under all conditions (see Chapter 4). Following is a list of important points:

- OTC medicines may have significant side effects. For example, allergy medicines like diphenhydramine (Benadryl®), chlorpheniramine (Chlor-trimeton®), and other antihistamines can cause significant drowsiness in some people, especially if used with alcohol. Side-effect and other warnings on OTC labels are not "boilerplate."
- Some OTC medicines can be contraindicated for patients with certain diseases. For example, people with hypertension or diabetes should avoid phenylpropanolamine and pseudoephedrine (Sudafed®). People should read and heed warnings of disease contraindications on OTC packages.
- OTCs are often not as effective as prescription medicines. For example, asthma almost always requires professional attention and should not be treated with OTC medicines.
- OTCs can interact with each other and with prescription medicines. A patient who regularly uses an OTC should ask his pharmacist to enter it into the medication profile along with prescription medicines. A patient who is taking more than one OTC should read the ingredients and ask his doctor or pharmacist if he has any questions. For example, Pepto-Bismol® contains salicylates, similar to aspirin and many other pain medications. Medicine containing salicylates

probably should not be taken with ibuprofen, other OTC or prescription nonsteroidal anti-inflammatory medicines, or anticoagulants (blood thinners). Many popular OTC medicines contain more than one active ingredient. A patient who takes many combination products may be getting too much of some of the ingredients. The words *plus* or *formula* on a label should be red flags.
- Some OTCs can be habit forming. Strong, long-lasting nasal decongestants can cause "rebound" nasal congestion if they are used too often or for too long.

Prescription Medicines

A patient should not allow the "business" that owns the pharmacy to interfere with his or her need for information about medicines. For example, a pharmacy assistant or clerk may not encourage a patient to seek advice from the pharmacist. Sometimes a busy pharmacy clerk will say "sign here" when a patient is picking up a prescription, without asking whether the patient has any questions for the pharmacist. When this happens, the patient should take a minute to read the fine print on the form. He is *not* just signing that he picked up the prescription. He is also agreeing that he has no questions about how to use it and that he is declining the pharmacist's offer to counsel.

A concerned patient should insist on understandable information from his doctor or community pharmacist. Most pharmacies give out patient information leaflets, but a patient may have trouble understanding which parts of it apply to his situation. It is a good idea for the patient to go over the patient leaflet with a pharmacist or doctor, using a highlighter to indicate the most important points, and to ask questions until he understands.

If admitted to a hospital or nursing home, the patient or family caregiver should ask to speak to the hospital pharmacist, to ask what services to expect and to request that the pharmacist and doctor work together to provide safe and effective drug therapy.

To take care of themselves, people taking medicines can do a "review of systems," using the principles of pharmaceutical care in Chapter 8. For example, a patient should make sure that he is receiving appropriate responses to the symptoms that bother him and that he knows how to participate in managing his drug therapy (see the ten questions below). Especially if he is taking medicines for a chronic condition, he should learn whether (and how) the therapy should be routinely monitored.

Surveys show that many people select a pharmacy based on convenience and price rather than quality of professional service. Some people expect to run into a pharmacy to pick up their prescription while double-parked or waiting for a bus. Some look for drive-thru service. Most patients need all the help they can get in taking their medications wisely, so they may be risking their health if they assume that the doctor is always right, always on top of things, and that the pharmacy is just a medication store.

Furthermore, all pharmacies are not equal. Most may be more or less equivalent in their basic drug distribution functions. These are well regulated, and accurate dispensing and labeling is a core value of every pharmacist (at least every pharmacist who deserves to have a license). Pharmacists and pharmacies vary greatly, however, in their patient care functions. Patients should choose a pharmacist based on professional services, such as willingness to cooperate actively with their doctor to help them manage medicines, especially chronic medicines. They should choose a pharmacist who will routinely do the following every time he or she dispenses a prescription:

- Ask the patient about drug allergies, sensitivities, and chronic diseases that might affect drug safety.
- Review the patient's medication record for duplication or possible drug interactions.
- Provide individualized patient instruction on how to properly take the medication (see below).
- Ask for and answer questions about the medicine.
- Pay attention to when a patient refills — or does not refill — his prescriptions.
- Work with the patient and physician to monitor the long-term effectiveness of therapy.

Some pharmacists also provide limited patient testing, such as cholesterol screening, glucose monitoring, and blood pressure checks. A few offer therapeutic drug monitoring (blood levels), either independently or cooperatively with other practitioners.

Patients also should understand some basic issues about health insurance, especially the use of prescription carve-outs. They should know (or find out) whether their insurance company or MCO might be discouraging their doctor and pharmacist from providing a drug they happen to need. A few American MCOs discourage physicians from even mentioning therapeutic options that the insurance does not cover. A patient with any doubt should ask if his MCO has a "don't tell" rule.

Finally, every person who is taking medicines should be willing to accept the appropriate amount of responsibility for his own care. Here are four general rules for safe and effective medications use that patients can follow:

1. Allow enough time in the pharmacy to get their questions answered and the advice they need.
2. Tell the pharmacist about *all* of their current medications, even if they buy some of them elsewhere and even if some are herbal remedies or nutriceuticals (see Chapter 5).
3. Ask their doctor or pharmacist about symptoms that could be side effects.

4. Cooperate with their doctor and pharmacist in tracking problems. Sometimes, for example, a doctor or pharmacist might ask a patient to keep a diary of drug taking and self-testing, e.g., for blood glucose in diabetes or blood pressure.

Specifically, a well-informed patient would be able to answer the following ten questions:

1. What are the names of my medicines?
2. How much of each should I take, and when?
3. What should each medicine do for me?
4. How can I tell if each medicine is working as intended?
5. When should I notice that it is working?
6. What are the most important problems of these medicines? Are there any tests that I need in order to avoid problems?
7. What should I do if I thought I was having a problem with a medicine?
8. What should I do if I miss a dose of my medicine?
9. Did I tell my doctor and pharmacist about every medicine I'm taking? Including nonprescription medicines and herbs? Should I avoid any of them now?
10. Is alcohol safe to take with my medicines?

This sounds like a lot of work. Surely it is, but it is clear by now that using medications safely can be as important as the safety of the products themselves. It is not safe to play Russian roulette with medicines.

A Final Note for Patients

If the patient, doctor, and pharmacist do everything "right," the patient will, in effect, have emulated the essential parts of the research protocols that got the drug cleared for marketing in the first place. (See Chapter 5.) The patient will be "cured"; his disease or its symptoms will be controlled. Congratulations will be in order. The team will have reached the limit of what drugs can do. Simply, they can *cure*, but they cannot *heal*.

Scientific medicine, pharmaceutical manufacturers, and the FDA are not in the healing business, despite what TV ads and press releases may imply. Anybody who says otherwise may have snake oil in the trunk of his car. Caring professionals can help immensely, but healing is up to the patient, and, if you like, to God. Drugs or herbal remedies may have helped a patient to fend off panic attacks or depression, quit smoking, control asthma, lower lipids, or drop blood pressure. Healing requires re-entry into wellness and often, new ideas and behaviors. Sometimes they are easy to learn, but sometimes patients have more to do than medications can do for them. It is important that patients and professionals remember that.

What Should Physicians and Pharmacists Do?

Almost every patient who was injured by an adverse effect or a treatment failure involving a medicine got that medicine from a pharmacist on a prescription from a physician. Both pharmacists and physicians are the first line of professional defense against injury. Or, to put it the other way, pharmacists and physicians (including office nurses and physician's assistants) share immediate responsibility for PDRM in community practice.

The key to improving medications use in community and hospital practice is pharmaceutical care — cooperative efforts to find and correct drug therapy problems before they injure patients. Cooperation is essential because pharmacists and physicians have complementary knowledge, skill, and accessibility. However, in community practice, especially, pharmaceutical care is in its infancy.

Although physicians and pharmacists are subject to professional standards of practice, there are few standards for drug therapy per se. There is no clear expectation that physicians, pharmacists, nurses, and patients should cooperate in medication use or how they are expected to cooperate. Some physicians insist that they alone should decide all aspects of drug therapy. Custom and conventional wisdom support that. Some judges have said, in effect, that a pharmacist's efforts to cooperate in drug therapy would constitute interference in the doctor–patient relationship. This would have, as lawyers say, a "chilling effect" on efforts to change the nonsystem.

A busy physician is accustomed, however, to working with office staff and hospital staff (nurses, physician's assistants, etc.) and with supporting professionals (social workers, physical therapists, dieticians, etc.). The existence of community-acquired PDRM shows that physicians also need the help of a pharmacological co-therapist. A pharmacist would be ideal.

Pharmacists are trusted by patients, accessible, educated in pharmacology, and skilled in taking medication histories. They maintain medication profiles and refill records, and know how to stay up-to-date with new drug products. They can carry out informative drug use reviews to track prescribing, so that a practice can improve itself. They can provide unbiased drug information and in-service education. And, finally, they do not diagnose or practice medicine, so practice boundaries are actually much clearer than with medical specialist consultants.

Some medical and pharmaceutical societies are preoccupied with protecting their professional turf (privileges, fees) in the new environment. Meanwhile, patients are injured by an obsolete and ineffective method of providing drug therapy. This obsolete method is no longer merely an accidental carryover from a simpler time. It is being enforced, perhaps with the best of intentions, by managed care reimbursement policies. These policies are not subject to the ethical standards of health care professions, and as described above, managed care is often immune from the consequences of those policies. Obviously, pharmacy, medicine, and nursing should be making common cause to elevate the quality of medications use by creating cooperative systems and the regulatory changes necessary to make them the standard of care.

Concerns about the possibility of professional interference (whether pharmacists "practicing medicine" or physicians "practicing pharmacy") may be common at first, but they usually reflect uncertainty about a new relationship. They can be addressed by collaborative practice agreements.

Regarding pharmaceutical care, begin with the premise that pharmacy benefits management and carve-outs tend to misdirect attention toward prescribing instead of medications management. Even a generally effective and appropriate prescriber may feel bombarded by hospitals and MCOs with messages to change his prescribing, often to follow guidelines that he did not help to write and may disagree with. Worse, different plans have different formularies. Usually, it is the pharmacist who calls with the annoying information that a patient is in insurance plan Y, which insists on ranitidine, not cimetadine (these are very similar drugs used for ulcers and gastrointestinal reflux). The *previous* patient was in insurance plan X, which insists on cimetadine, not ranitidine. This not only may direct the physicians' attention toward prescribing and away from medicines management (or just drive him crazy), but also may greatly complicate the relationship between physicians and pharmacists.

Physicians, pharmacists, and nurses are the products of their educations, which by and large were inadequate preparation for cooperative drug therapy management. Physicians should recognize this and recognize the need to develop better arrangements for their patients. If they did, they might feel a stronger need for pharmacists or nurse practitioners who are willing and able to provide cooperative drug therapy management services. They could work with that colleague to develop efficient practice arrangements, so that cooperation becomes routine.

To do that with community pharmacists in the modern day of complicated insurance coverage, physicians and pharmacists should develop agreements about what services (e.g., patient drug histories, therapeutic monitoring, drug therapy evaluations) the pharmacist is prepared to provide in a routine, predictable, and professionally responsible manner, and how to handle routine necessities efficiently, such as prescribed drug products excluded from insurance and generic dispensing. If a dispensing pharmacist is too busy in the pharmacy, a consulting contract can be drawn up in which the pharmacist can provide drug therapy services a few hours each day in the physician's office.

Pharmacists as Part of the Solution

Pharmacists are an essential resource for improving the outcomes of drug therapy. For a variety of reasons, however, the traditional medications use process is not set up to use pharmacists, especially community pharmacists, to their full potential. Even some pharmacists do not recognize their great potential to improve people's lives by improving medications use.

Nevertheless, participation in pharmaceutical care may represent an important opportunity for pharmacists in many nations. It may even be essential for the survival of pharmacy as a profession.[16–19] Most pharmacists can contribute to each of the three functions of pharmaceutical care, especially as co-therapists and facilitators. Pharmacists may also play an important role as initiators for minor ailments, guiding patient self-care for self-limiting diseases and referring patients to medical practitioners when necessary.

Pharmacists can effect some valuable improvements just by changing their participation in drug therapy, especially by asking patients more questions that would identify DTPs and by communicating important information about specific patients to physicians. Their immediate objective, however, should be to develop and extend cooperative relationships with physicians and nurses. One place to start was mentioned above — find a way to organize the many questions and contacts from the pharmacy that physicians see as clinically unimportant, e.g., questions about covered drugs and generic dispensing, so that clinically important questions can get the attention they need.

Perhaps physicians will initiate discussions with a pharmacist, as happened in Chapter 11. Perhaps the pharmacist has to call on physicians and offer to develop collaborative practice agreements. A pharmacist who visits a general practitioner with a specific proposal for efficient cooperation is often welcomed with interest and an open mind about what the pharmacist has to offer. One service that many physicians can appreciate immediately is a drug profile or history for some "problem" patients and an offer to help improve their therapy.

In a talk to the community pharmacy section of the International Pharmaceutical Federation, Dr. Larry G. Rooks of the University of Florida's Family Practice Department said, "Because of the ever-increasing complexity of pharmaceutical options and the need to properly select and monitor those pharmaceutical options, a well-trained clinical pharmacist focused on the drug use process is a necessity in outpatient clinical practice."* Dr. Rooks routinely cooperates with pharmacists, and expects a pharmacist to bring three functions to a collaborative practice. The clinical pharmacist should be:

1. An advisor who knows drugs and knows the patient as well as the physician does, but not a pharmacology professor or drug policeman
2. A consultant who will write his recommendations and take responsibility for them
3. A colleague who will be there whenever needed, not only during business hours

Pharmacists especially should recognize each patient's specific arrangements for drug therapy, and do what they can to systematize them. The list

* Rooks, L.G., *How Do We Change the Drug Use Process? A Physician's Perspective on Pharmaceutical Care.* Community Pharmacists Section, International Pharmaceutical Federation, Jerusalem, September 5, 1996.

of DTPs in Chapter 10 is the basis of pharmaceutical care from a pharmacist's perspective. The principles of pharmaceutical care have the same function on a more macro level. For example, if a patient has an untreated indication or a problem obtaining a needed therapy, the pharmacist may be the best — perhaps the only — person to notice this and either resolve it or refer it. Examples earlier in the book illustrated this point.

Some pharmacists doubt their ability to participate in pharmaceutical care. Some assume that it would take too much time. In fact, there are many examples of severe drug therapy problems that a pharmacist can detect and resolve (or refer) in a few minutes.

MCOs are reluctant to pay pharmacists for patient care services beyond dispensing. While a few pharmacists cannot change this by themselves, they should not acquiesce or react by withholding necessary services. Pharmacists should not become the "boiled frogs" of health care reform (see Chapter 14). Certainly every practice has many patients like Katherine LaStima and Donald Ashwell. If a pharmacist ignores them, the consequences are truly catastrophic, not only for the patient, but also for the doctor, the pharmacist, and society. Pharmacists must ethically provide the care their patients need. Period. Then they have a right to bill for medically necessary services, especially if provided in concert with the patient's physician. They can bill the patient or the third-party payer. If their bills are ignored, they can undertake collection procedures, sometimes in small claims court. It is not an easy road, but it seems to be the only proper road.

Managed Care

Managed care organizations, including providers and third-party payers who "manage" expenditures, now greatly influence the structure and process of health care in many nations. They have a major part of the responsibility for either allowing medications misuse to continue or reforming the system. Many of the examples of "old rules" and "new rules" above involved managed care policies, and it is not necessary to belabor those points further. In order for managed care to become part of the solution instead of part of the problem, many MCOs will have to change their policies in three major ways.

First, MCOs occupy *the* strategic position for creating medications use systems, especially for creating performance databases. They are in the best position to collect and organize relevant data, to develop or collect guidelines and performance indicators, to use them to evaluate performance and identify and resolve problems, and to follow up on the solutions. They can establish program-wide performance benchmarks (Chapters 7 and 11). Four steps will get managed care pharmacy moving toward the kinds of systems that the IOM has said are necessary:

1. Replace prescribing with medication use as a management objective.

   The use of medications includes prescribing, dispensing, consumption, and outcomes. It can fail to produce its objective because of misuse, underuse, or overuse. Taking the lead in managing all aspects of the medication use process is the basis of pharmaceutical care.

Crossing the Quality Chasm says it this way: "The purpose of the health care system is to reduce continually the burden of illness, injury, and disability, and to improve the health status and function of the people of the United States."[3] Its first recommendation for change is that all health care organizations, professional groups, and purchasers should adopt this as their explicit purpose. Managed care pharmacy cannot respond to this recommendation if it continues to confine its scope to managing prescribing and drug expenditures.

2. Assess the quality of medication use: identify recurring problems among members.

   Although outcomes of drug therapy are prevalent in America and perhaps throughout the industrialized world, organizations that do not look for PDRM do not find much of it. Then, sometimes, they can claim that the whole problem is exaggerated or place the problem "out there," in other unfortunate populations, but not in their organizations. (See Chapter 14.)

   Drug use evaluation should be expanded to encompass all steps in the medication use process. Most so-called drug use evaluations do not evaluate drug use — most do not even include dosage, just choice of agent. As usually carried out, DUE cannot detect nontreatment at all, and does a poor job of detecting underdosage, overdosage and other problems.

   Some useful process indicators for medication use are widely available now, e.g., from the National Committee for Quality Assurance (NCQA) and its Health Plan Employer Data and Information Set (HEDIS), the Joint Commission on Accreditation of Healthcare Organizations, and the SCRIPT project. Process indicators, however, are only a start. The quality of medication use cannot be adequately assessed using process indicators or similar intermediate measures. Quality assessment must increasingly take into account the outcomes of therapy. Earlier chapters of this book describe a new type of process–outcome indicator that has been used to screen population databases such as managed care records. Results can then be used in interprofessional quality circles at many system levels — managed care organization clinic, hospital, or practice group.

3. Carry out QI activities at the MCO level.

   Quality improvement is already familiar to many program managers. It just is not done often enough for the right reasons (internal motives, as opposed to external motives such as accreditation). When it is done for internal use, it can have some surprising results.

4. Use market power to encourage change.

   Standards are a tool for modifying the marketplace. Suppose an MCO carried out steps 1 through 3 above. Suppose that it discovered recurring, severe problems in the way its members used medications, and it found that it was paying for thousands of emergency department visits and hospitalizations because heart failure was often not being treated correctly. The MCO performed a root cause analysis that showed two main reasons: (1) physicians sometimes did not prescribe according to guidelines or renew a patient's discharge prescriptions; and (2) patients sometimes stopped taking their prescribed medications. Sometimes neither the pharmacist nor the physician intervened to find out why. It might be in the MCO's best interest to use its influence to effect change and to follow up with indicators to find out if the intervention was working. Once it found an intervention that seemed to work in most circumstances, could it not target the outlier patients, physicians, and pharmacists with appropriate incentives?

Second, insurance payers and network model MCOs should leave direct patient care to the provider level. (Staff model HMOs should expect interpatient variability in utilization and allow providers to cater to it.) MCOs have a major opportunity to develop systems and to improve care, e.g., through evidence-based guidelines and by operating MMS systems. Rarely should they preempt decision making about specific patients. Some MCOs, for example, regional health authorities in the U.K., operate formulary and DUE systems actively, but only at the group practice level, not the patient level. The idea of a PCS nested inside an MMS is a theory with empirical support. In the area of medications use there is no evidence that strictly *enforcing* guidelines, patient by patient, has improved outcomes. Considerable evidence suggests that it is detrimental. However important their influence will be for advancing medicines management systems, MCOs belong in the *environment* of a pharmaceutical care system.

Third, MCOs should hold their own operations to the standard that they demand of providers: consistency with evidence. The bulk of evidence suggests that MCOs should reallocate resources now spent on prescribing restrictions. The funds should instead be spent to provide quality control and improvement (MMS) functions.

Purchasers

The consumers of health care, individual people, rarely pay directly for services received and are seldom well organized as payers. Government and employers are the largest actual purchaser of health care. These powerful purchasers have changed the American market for health care in some ways that they had intended, but surely also in some they did not. Some purchasers, in trying to control the costs of health care, are actually getting *less* than they pay for. The business community should recognize that its power over health care delivery in the United States extends well beyond the ability to control expenditures. It now shares influence over the organization and quality of care. This influence should bring a sense of important new responsibilities, not only to their employees but also to the public.

For example, when an MCO contracts to provide care, it is a *business* transaction. MCOs are not bound by professional ethics. This puts the onus of *caveat emptor* squarely on the business that purchases care or coverage from third parties. A contract that calls only for reductions in drug expenditures may be a poor bargain.

There is a right way to manage the prescription benefit and a wrong way (see Chapter 6). The wrong way may deny needed care and may increase sick days and total costs of care per employee. There are no laws requiring that a pharmacy benefit management company (PBM) know the effect of its policies on overall quality of care or total costs of care. The PBM may, as a part of its business, establish prescription limits, require that providers use a restrictive formulary of less expensive drug products, without regard to the effect on employee sick days, and make side deals with drug manufacturers to promote one manufacturer's drug products over another. Often, however, performance is defined only in terms of controlling the drug budget. As long as the drug budget is reduced, the PBM will have met its contractual obligations.

Sick days, physician office costs, hospital costs, etc., are rarely a basis for evaluating the performance of the PBM. The problem is not, by the way, limited to separate contracts with PBMs or even to privately owned PBMs. Many in-house PBM departments of large MCOs and most state Medicaid agencies operate and are evaluated on the same basis.

American business and government purchasers should consider the effect of their purchasing power on the welfare of employees and beneficiaries, and on the overall state of health care delivery in America. (The argument is similar to environmental pollution and energy use arguments.) If organized purchasers use their market power mainly to lower the cost of health care, instead of insisting on value for money, then we should expect proposals for government regulation to rebalance cost and quality.

Accreditors and Regulators: Quality Standards

An organization may legally operate without meeting the standards of voluntary accreditation. In addition, an organization that has met legal requirements may voluntarily submit itself to more exacting standards and review. Accreditation is recognition that the organization has met those higher standards. Accreditation may greatly influence an organization's ability to sell its products. Obviously, most people would prefer to go to an accredited school or hospital (see Chapter 5). For a variety of reasons, accreditation, e.g., by NCQA, has not had the effect on managed care organizations that accreditation by Joint Commission has had on hospitals and other health care providers. It may just be a matter of time until competition based on quality really becomes predominant. But perhaps we cannot afford to wait.

In contrast, a license is governmental permission to engage in certain activities. Licensure and compliance with regulations are legally mandatory. Many businesses and occupations require one or more licenses to operate.

Regulatory boards exist for the purpose of protecting the public health. They operate at the interface between business and public interest. Their standards are intended to modify the marketplace, to make it serve public interests, e.g., an interest in safety, as well as private business interests.

Health care market imperfections are well recognized. *Crossing the Quality Chasm* includes many examples of provider disincentives caused by toxic payment plans. Certainly these are a major problem in medications use. In most managed care plans, if physicians and pharmacists cooperated to improve the safety and effectiveness of drug therapy in a population, they would bear the additional expense of doing so, what has been called a quality tax. Suppose the program cost an additional $10 per physician office visit.

Suppose further that the theory presented in this book were correct, and that the average savings from reduced physician office visits, emergency department visits, hospitalizations, and other treatments to correct PDRMs averaged $20 per physician office visit. This would be a good deal for the patients, who suffer less injury from drug therapy, and a great deal for the MCO, which saves perhaps $50 to $60 annually per patient. Unfortunately, it is an economic raw deal for the innovative pharmacists and physicians. They are paying a quality tax of $10 per office visit so that the MCO can save $20.

The issue is not whether they can afford it, although most providers have experienced shrinking revenues per patient. The issue is the inequity and the negative incentive for superior production. The payment plan (insurance company, MCO), which took no risk, would reap the financial benefits.

Severe market imperfections at the MCO level are also well documented.[1] Protection from legal liability under ERISA was mentioned above. Most other markets have required regulations to protect the public welfare, and it should be no surprise that the managed care marketplace may require the same.

Of course, regulators, including professional boards of pharmacy and medicine, are subject to political pressure from the industries and professions they regulate. Interprofessional turf battles are often fought with the weapon of professional regulation. However, there may be some useful overlap between these sometimes competing objectives.

Both pharmacists and physicians share immediate responsibility for PDRM in community practice and should work together. If pharmacists propose new standards for pharmacy, intended to ameliorate this problem, physicians should support them (or at least not resist), and vice versa. Resistance would be especially untenable if the proposals were to increase standards of practice. Concerns about professional interference in the new relationship should be addressed by collaborative practice agreements.

Professional Practice

If the market (i.e., purchasers and payers) does not demand pharmaceutical care and medications management, an alternative pathway would involve professional standards. Specifically, professional standards should require that physicians, pharmacists, and nurses cooperate in patient care and evaluate the quality of medications use. Since we have argued so far that purchasers and MCOs hold the key to better medications use, proposing new professional standards may seem like overkill. However, the present structure of health care delivery contains an important discontinuity and disincentive, as described above.

Professional standards should continue to move from an emphasis on structure to an emphasis on outcome. Each practice should be obliged to show evidence of an active, regular, continuous process of self-evaluation, problem detection, problem resolution, and follow-up, both for individual patients and for the practices as a whole. The scope of such standards should include formal, cooperative practice agreements between providers (as needed), patient assessments, and professional performance reviews.[20]

Improved professional standards may be more difficult to enforce than managed care standards, because there are so many more practices. However, professionals might be able to accept such regulations once they understand their intent. Professional standards might be much easier to enact. If all providers were required to operate pharmaceutical care programs or QI programs on their own patients' outcomes, the quality tax on those doing the right thing might be ameliorated or eliminated.

Managed Care Organizations

New quality standards are needed to move some MCOs into medicines management and to assist purchasers to make purchase decisions based on quality and efficiency. Minimum standards should require managed care organizations to evaluate the safety and effectiveness of drug therapy, using established quality improvement methods. Specifically, standards should require that MCOs:

1. Identify, document, and resolve specific, recurring patient problems in medications use, such as those described earlier:
   - By actively seeking out sentinel events
   - By monitoring selected medications use indicators and comparing them to accepted treatment guidelines developed by other bodies
2. Assess system performance and identify recurring systematic problems, e.g., using the five principles in Chapter 8.

3. Implement reasonable solutions.
4. Follow up solutions, e.g., with the same indicators used to discover them, to assess their effectiveness in addressing the problem.
5. Describe and document the process (patient and system assessments, problems found, actions taken, and follow-up) in permanent records that are subject to review.

Standards should mandate systematic reviews of the patient care process, but not specify details for specific diseases. This level of specificity may be impractical, perhaps even counterproductive. Such regulations, initially at least, should be significantly simpler and more flexible than is common today. Many detailed structure and process standards could be relaxed if MCOs were responsible for operating QI systems that were capable of detecting major problems in medications use.

An Incrementalist's Concerns

Theory and evidence strongly suggest that MUSs would revolutionize the quality of medications use and reduce our "second drug problem" by at least an order of magnitude. It would not be a panacea, however. Nadler and Hibino recommend that systems redesign always consider the "solution after next."[21] In other words, we should ask what problems would arise if the recommended solution were actually implemented. In the instance of MUSs, the next set of problems would depend on how MUSs were implemented.

A company with enough resources could develop a medications use system as a product and sell it. The company would, presumably, put energy into marketing and solve many of the diffusion-of-innovation problems that are unresolved at present. That would speed change in the right direction. The problems in that scenario might come from unexpected consequences of innovation. Some high-tech "fixes" have created new problems almost as bad as the ones they were meant to fix. To some extent, that is what an unbridled enthusiasm for market forces and "getting out of the way of business" seems to have done to managed care.

In particular, we should be wary of an uncritical enthusiasm for adopting an off-the-shelf MUS before it has been thoroughly tested in the real world. Even relatively simple computer software may have too many possible combinations of system states to test them all, as any computer user has learned. Sometimes, when the program operates dangerous equipment, the outcomes of a computer malfunction can be horrific.[22] In addition, the human–computer interface and the procedures to be carried out by people are subject to variation of unknown significance.

Incompletely tested innovation has caused horrific accidents.[7,22] Steven Casey recounts an example from the war in the Pacific.[22] In retrospect, this one is more amusing than horrific, because no one was killed or injured.

An American airfield on a Pacific island had come under attack by enemy airplanes. It was essential that the fliers get their aircraft into the air immediately, because both aircraft and people would otherwise be easy targets for destruction. One unfortunate pilot, Dan, was the last to reach the small group of P-47 Thunderbolts. Dan was an experienced P-47 pilot, and he climbed into the cockpit of a brand new airplane, just arrived, ready to get into the air and defend the base. The enemy fighters were fast approaching and had opened fire. As Dan frantically reached for the ignition switch and starter, he realized that the entire cockpit had been redesigned. Not only could he not find the ignition switch, he could not recognize the familiar instrument display that he needed to fly the plane, let alone fight in it.

As bombs began to fall at the far end of the airfield, Dan frantically began to press at the unfamiliar switches. One proved to be the ignition switch, and another proved to be the starter. Time for taking off, however, had run out. Dan took the best action he could. He pulled out the throttle and taxied the Thunderbolt around the airfield at high speed, zigging and zagging to make it a difficult target. He kept that up until the other (airborne) aircraft had chased away the enemy. Dan wondered why someone back in the Pentagon had ordered a complete cockpit redesign in the middle of a war, or why delivery did not include a checkout for every Thunderbolt pilot on the base.

The medications use system described in Chapters 8 to 11 would be considerably larger than a new, computerized order entry, drug distribution, and documentation system. If a complete MUS were designed, tested, and implemented, it might create the equivalent of Dan's problem, except that people might actually be hurt. The evidence pointing to the need for MUSs is convincing. However, many details have yet to be worked out.

A more conservative, perhaps safer, incremental approach would be to implement performance indicators in specific MCOs or other programs and submit the data to quality circles. This approach would improve medications use incrementally, with solutions that were easier to adopt locally. Theoretically, the result would look something like the template described in Chapters 8 to 11. An incremental approach would fit solutions to real problems, might be safer and easier for providers to learn, and might lead to extremely important variations on the theme. The innovator of such a service product, however, might find it more difficult to promote than an off-the-shelf software product.

Research is needed to support systems design and implementation, especially through the incremental, local approach. In particular, we need to know more about:

- How to carry out medications use quality circles, for example, how much QI and medications use theory the panels should understand before taking up root cause analysis and designing solutions
- How to accumulate medications use experience within and among organizations to maximize its value for systems improvement while minimizing liability exposure
- How to effect systems change among professionals
- How to balance human and machine performance
- How to educate patients for greater participation in care (e.g., as described earlier in this chapter)

Safety and Quality Are Different

The subject of this book has touched on human error only in passing, in Chapter 3 as part of a theory of how DRMs happen. Authors like Reason, Perrow, and Casey have written extensively about error from complementary viewpoints. The publications of the Harvard Medical Practice Study, the Adverse Drug Event Prevention Study, and *To Err Is Human,* the first IOM report, have thoroughly addressed medical error. Researchers like Ken Barker, Michael Cohen,[26] and others have discussed and dissected pharmacists' and nurses' dispensing and administration errors in great detail, and many pharmacy corporations have volumes of private knowledge about it. Listing this work would be a project of its own.

This book was meant to draw sometimes blurry distinction between error prevention and quality improvement. Quality improvement includes error prevention, but the absence of errors cannot, by itself, provide acceptable quality. True, the first rule is "Do no harm," but people practice health professions to remove the harm of disease, not to avoid error. Patients consult a health professional and literally (sometimes) put their lives in another's hands to *remove* harm, not to avoid new harm. The safest aircraft stays on the ground (except in Dan's case). The safest ship is tied up in port, empty. The safest medicine is still in the bottle. The danger of complete immersion in safety is that it would eventually deny benefits. Federal drug law is a clear example, but other, even more important examples occur thousands of times every hour in health care.

This book has been about quality improvement in medications use. Probably no *useful* medications use system can be foolproof, meaning error-proof. Anybody can have a bad day, misread the best-labeled bottle, fail to recognize an obvious DTP. One of Deming's principles is that systems cannot rely on inspections to maintain quality. Errors must be prevented, and work in the science of error prevention must continue. It can only make MUSs safer. But error prevention will never cure anybody.

Conclusion

Real improvement in medications use is possible only by changing how the delivery of drug therapy is organized, provided, regulated, and financed, and how individuals behave in specific cases.

The PDRM problem will continue until the changes occur on every level. The basic assumptions, concepts, and arrangements for providing drug therapy must change. This should involve major changes in the role of pharmacists or, failing that, creation of new specialties in medicine and nursing. PDRMs are not pharmacy's problem alone, but pharmacists, more than any other group, have a huge stake in the problem and are ideally suited to contribute to its solution. Pharmacists can and should play an important role in bringing medications use systems into existence. Pharmacists are accessible, trusted professionals with extensive education in drug therapy. They are strategically located in the medications use process. Therefore, pharmacists have an opportunity to play a major part in developing a safer and more cost-effective system of drug therapy. However, they are often overlooked.

By means of specific changes in how they practice, pharmacists can influence physicians' and patients' ideas and expectations. In light of a modern pharmacist's potential contribution to health care, it is clear that consumers and managers expect too little participation by pharmacists in medications use, community pharmacists especially. For their part, many pharmacists seem to expect a great deal from themselves, but sometimes these expectations are limited to dispensing efficiency and accuracy. This view is short sighted. It reflects a marketplace that treats drug products as if they were merchandise to be purchased as cheaply as possible, even if it means that necessary point-of-sale services are depreciated.

Recommendations

In summary, here are some recommendations to improve the environment and structure of medications use, especially in community practice:

1. Increase funding for research, development, and demonstration projects involving the prevalence, causes, and prevention of PDRMs. This should be explicitly included in all responses to the proposals made by the IOM for research funding in this area.
2. Increase and broaden public awareness and understanding of the general problem of PDRM.
3. Teach patients how to cooperate in making every medications use system work more safely and effectively for them.
4. Teach health professional students more about the realities of safe medications use, for example, how to cooperate in managing therapy.

5. Develop and test more methods to assess PDRM prevalence in specific populations, e.g., among members of a managed care plan. Performance measures for medications use are necessary for patients, providers, and managers to recognize problems locally, e.g., in the management of a health program.
6. Develop and demonstrate practical ways to correct recurring problems in medications use.
7. Adopt provider standards that reflect such practical understanding.
   a. Encourage and require managed care programs to develop clinically significant indicators for overall patterns of drug use, to evaluate the effectiveness of present prescribing and component cost control programs, and to consider outcome-oriented controls. For example, MCOs should keep track of patients who are repeatedly admitted for diseases that should not require frequent rehospitalizations.
   b. Encourage and require managed care organizations to evaluate their medications use policies and to develop data-driven outcome improvement programs based on the Shewhart cycle: plan, do, check, act.
   c. Encourage and require hospitals to identify people at high risk of preventable injury, such as those repeatedly admitted or seen in emergency departments for diseases that should be controllable.
8. Adopt professional practice standards that reflect a practical understanding of PDRM causes and preventives.
   a. Standards of practice for medicine and pharmacy must encourage formal, voluntary pharmacist–physician cooperation in drug therapy management (collaborative practice agreements). Physicians should accept that they cannot manage drug therapy alone — if for no other reason, because modern medicine demands so much else from them. Boards of medicine could encourage this, at least collaborative practice agreements among physicians and pharmacists.
   b. Standards of practice for pharmacists should explicitly require documenting care and periodic identification and resolution of recurring problems in medications use. Pharmacists should take a share of responsibility for the outcomes of drug therapy — not just for accurate dispensing and an offer to counsel. Pharmacists should identify high-risk patients and regularly review their therapy in cooperation with their doctors. Pharmacists could document such reviews and their follow-up in a permanent record, in an updated version of what is now required for nursing home patients.

9. Educate the public to expect increased participation of pharmacists in medicines management and their insurance to pay for it when provided. Patients and family caregivers can participate more in the management of their own drug therapy. They should expect to cooperate more and expect their doctor and pharmacist to cooperate more. Patients should expect their pharmacist to be able to assist in drug therapy, should be willing to pay for it, and should demand health insurance that covers this care. The mass media could present information on how consumers can understand and cooperate in their therapy.

The facts of PDRM suggest that, with medications use at least, quality is free. Billions of dollars, pounds, and euros have to be spent each year to correct or ameliorate PDRMs. These expenditures are pure waste. A hospital stay caused by PDRM may transfer dollars, but it does not transfer wealth — it decreases it. Improved medications use systems are not an optional luxury. To a large extent, preventing PDRM would be analogous to public hygiene programs like immunizations or safe drinking water. The money spent on cleaning up after a PDRM should instead be spent on prevention. Even if all of the wasted money were spent to prevent the problem, society would benefit.

The PDRM problem has a theoretical explanation that is supported by some encouraging empirical evidence. We do not know everything that we need to know about how to manage medications use in the real world. Regulations mandating the details of medications use systems would be premature. However, we already know enough to begin. We must contruct a medications use system that allows physicians and pharmacists to apply what they know to patient care. To quote Robert Rakel, one of the pioneers of the American Family Practice movement,

> It has been said that more mistakes in medicine are made by those who do not care than by those who do not know.[23]

Can the same be said of our entire health care enterprise?

Health care accreditation agencies are moving toward requirements for systematic quality improvement programs that may lead to managing for outcomes in MCOs and provider organizations like hospitals and nursing facilities. Indicators of medications use problems are included, but perhaps not emphasized as much as the problem deserves. This top-down approach is necessary to achieve change and should be accelerated by public and political pressure.

The health professions should lead the change and work harder against a status quo that injures the very people who they have promised to help. By doing so, they could constitute a grassroots or bottom-up complement to top-down changes in managed care. If cooperative pharmaceutical care became part of the standard of health care, the prevalence of many common kinds of PDRM might be substantially reduced. Professional regulations that required participation in pharmaceutical care and other medicines-related QI programs would reduce the quality tax that is today required of pharmacists and physicians who wish to implement such programs. They would eliminate many obstacles to the wider implementation of pharmaceutical care practices, which would in turn make drug therapy safer and more cost-effective.

Boards of pharmacy and medicine, in particular, should share the lead in promoting such regulations. This would be entirely consistent with their mandate to promote public health and welfare. It would clarify pharmacy's and medicine's potential for cooperation in support of safe and effective drug therapy. It would demonstrate both professions' commitment to patient safety and pharmaceutical care as more than rhetoric. Widely adopted measures of medications use quality could eventually lead to quality benchmarks for medications use.

Every change has its detractors. Even planning how to lower arsenic levels in America's drinking water is too expensive for some people. The economic interests involved in health care are huge — let us say they represent more than 10% of America's gross domestic product. Some businesses live on insurance carve-outs and component cost management. Change will not be easy. The daily papers provide many informative stories about improving standards, examples from airlines to zoos. A pattern emerges, which we should expect to see in medications use as well:

- Change begins when leaders push for better standards to protect the public and to lower the "quality tax" on superior producers.
- Conservatives then complain that they cannot afford the higher standards or that the cost of higher quality will "harm the economy."
- Then, if the higher standards have been adopted, some marginal operators are forced either to improve or to leave the industry. But there is no catastrophic rise in prices or drop in sales. Finally, most people understand that "a rising tide lifts all boats."

References

1. Coye, M.J., No Toyotas in health care: why medical care has not evolved to meet patients' needs, *Health Aff. (Millwood)*, 20, 44, 2001.
2. Kohn, L.T., Corrigan, J.T., and Donaldson, M.S., *To Err Is Human: Building a Safer Health System,* National Academy Press, Washington, D.C., 2000.
3. Institute of Medicine, *Crossing the Quality Chasm: A New Health System for the 21st Century,* National Academy Press, Washington, D.C., 2001.
4. Leape, L.L. et al., The nature of adverse events in hospitalized patients: results of the Harvard Medical Practice Study II, *N. Engl. J. Med.*, 324, 377, 1991.

5. Cullen, D.J. et al., Prevention of adverse drug events: a decade of progress in patient safety, *J. Clin. Anesth.*,12, 600, 2000.
6. Newhouse, J.P., Why is there a quality chasm? *Health Aff. (Millwood)*, 21, 13, 2002.
7. Perrow, C., *Normal Accidents: Living with High-Risk Technologies*, Princeton University Press, Princeton, NJ, 1999.
8. Anders, G., *Health against Wealth: HMOs and the Breakdown of Medical Trust*, Houghton, Mifflin, Boston, MA, 1996.
9. Kassirer, J.P., Managed care and the morality of the marketplace, *N. Engl. J. Med.*, 333, 50, 1995.
10. Enthoven, A.C., Why managed care has failed to contain health costs, *Health Aff. (Millwood)*, 12, 27, 1993.
11. Hurley, R. and Rawlings, R.B., Who lost cost containment? A roster for recrimination, *Manag. Care Q.*, 9, 23, 2001.
12. Brennan, T.A. and Berwick, D.M., *New Rules: Regulation, Markets and the Quality of American Health Care*, 1st ed., Jossey-Bass Publishers, San Franciso, 1996.
13. Berwick, D.M., A user's manual for the IOM's Quality Chasm Report, *Health Aff.*, 21, 80, 2002.
14. Beckman, H.B. et al., The doctor-patient relationship and malpractice: lessons from plaintiff depositions, *Arch. Intern. Med.*, 154, 1365, 1994.
15. Tuckett, D., Boulton, C.O., and Williams, A., *Meetings between Experts: An Approach to Sharing Ideas in Medical Consultations*, Routledge Kegan & Paul, London, 1986.
16. Parish, P.A., What future for pharmacy practice? *Pharm. J.*, 234, 209, 1985.
17. Hepler, C.D., Unresolved issues in the future of pharmacy, *Am. J. Hosp. Pharm.*, 45, 1071, 1988.
18. Hepler, C.D. and Strand, L.M., Opportunities and responsibilities in pharmaceutical care, *Am. J. Hosp. Pharm.*, 47, 533, 1990.
19. Brown, P., Are pharmacists necessary? *Scrip*, no. 24, May 3, 1994.
20. Hepler, C.D., Regulating for outcomes as a systems response to the problem of drug-related morbidity, *J. Am. Pharm. Assoc.*, 41, 108, 2001.
21. Nadler, G. and Hibino, S., *Breakthrough Thinking*, St. Martin's Press, New York, 1990.
22. Casey, S., *Set Phasers on Stun, and Other Tales of Design, Technology and Human Error*, 2nd ed., Agean Publishing Co., Santa Barbara, CA, 1998.
23. Rakel, R.E., Compassion and the art of family medicine: from Osler to Oprah, *J. Am. Board Fam. Pract.*, 13, 440, 2000.
24. Strom, B.L. and Hennessy, S., Pharmacist care and clinical outcomes for patients with reactive airways disease, *JAMA*, 288, 1642, 2002.
25. Kimberlin, C.L. et al., Effects of an education program for community pharmacists on detecting drug-related problems in elderly patients, *Med. Care*, 31, 451, 1993.
26. Cohen, M., Ed., *Medication Errors: Causes, Prevention, and Risk Management*, 1st ed., Jones & Bartlett, Sudbury, MA, 1999.

Glossary

Accreditation Official or formal recognition that a health care organization, e.g., a hospital, HMO, or PPO, has met predetermined standards. Examples of organizations that accredit managed care plans are the National Committee for Quality Assurance (NCQA), the Joint Commission on Accreditation of Healthcare Organizations (JCAHO), and the Utilization Review Accreditation Commission (URAC).

Active error An error that is sufficient to cause injury, especially immediate injury.

Active failure See *active error.*

Actual DTP See *DTP.*

Adaptive system A system that can change its procedures or structures according to changing conditions, consistent with its purpose. See *system.* As defined here, all systems are capable of first-order adaptation. *First-order adaptation* manages preestablished processes, based on feedback, to reach an external objective. *Second-order adaptation* can change processes (methods) to reach an external objective. *Third-order adaptation* is reflective — it can change the objectives themselves to reach a greater goal or change goals to reach greater values. See *teleological.*

ADE See *adverse drug event.*

Adherence See *compliance.*

ADR See *adverse drug reaction.*

Adverse drug event (ADE) Patient injury caused by the drug itself or by an error in how the drug is used (p. 40).

Adverse drug reaction (ADR) Any noxious and unintended effect caused by the drug itself. By far, the most widely recognized adverse outcome from drug therapy.

Adverse event A patient injury caused by medical management (p. 19).

Average wholesale price (AWP) A standard price, commonly used in pharmacy contracting for setting reimbursement rates for prescriptions. The AWP is generally determined by pharmaceutical manufacturers and rarely reflects the actual acquisition cost of a pharmaceutical to the pharmacy. Most pharmacies accept a payment for a pharmaceutical product that is discounted from the AWP, such as AWP less 10%.

Belief Subjective knowledge, interpretation of evidence. As distinguished from knowledge, a belief may not be as fully supportable by evidence.

Capitation Payment plan in which a per capita amount is paid to a provider for a group of specified health services, regardless of quantity rendered. The total amount paid depends on the number of persons covered at the time — per covered life, per member, per member per month (PMPM). It does not depend on whether services were provided for a particular member or the amount of service provided. A capitation rate may be set for all members, or it can be adjusted for the age and gender of the member based on actuarial projections of health utilization.

Carve-out Exclusion of specific covered services, e.g., pharmacy and mental health, from a capitation agreement. A provider may be reimbursed for the service on another basis, e.g., fee-for-service, or the excluded service may be provided by another provider. Carve-outs allow payers to create a separate health benefits package and assume greater control of their costs.

Change agent A person (not a member of the network) who influences the attitudes or behaviors of network members about an innovation, usually in a direction deemed desirable by a *change agency* (p. 172).

Clinical impression A professional's opinion regarding the cause of a patient's problem; the result of a professional assessment of clinical data about the patient; loosely, a diagnosis, except that a clinical impression may be more tentative, less conclusive than a diagnosis.

Clinical practice guidelines A systematically developed description of desirable care decisions and processes for specific clinical circumstances in a typical patient (p. 198). An *evidence-based guideline*, developed through a formal consultative process, incorporates clinical evidence, expert opinion, and professional judgment. It may focus on disease prevention, diagnosis, or treatment. The primary function is to guide practitioners in delivering appropriate evidence-based care for patients.

Closed panel Physicians who belong to a medical group that serves only the patients of a given HMO, e.g., in a staff or group model HMO.

Co-insurance A cost-sharing requirement by a health plan that specifies the insured patient will assume a portion or percentage of the costs of covered services. For example, under Medicare Part B, the beneficiary pays a co-insurance of 20% of allowed charges.

Many HMOs provide 100% insurance (no co-insurance) for an annual checkup provided "in network."

Co-therapist Professional who can cooperate with initiators and facilitators in providing and managing drug therapy after it has been initiated (p. 223).

Compliance Conformity to instructions, in particular medication-taking behavior that conforms to prescriber's directions for use. Also called *adherence*. See also *concordance*.

Concordance A patient's informed consent to therapy, based on understanding of the therapeutic objectives, negotiation, acceptance, and commitment to therapy (p. 222).

Copayment A cost-sharing arrangement in which a managed care organization member pays a specified flat amount for a specific service (such as $10 for an office visit or $20 for each brand name prescription drug). Most MCOs now have two-tier or three-tier cost-sharing (copayment) formulas for prescription drugs.

Credibility (of information or of an informant) Quality, capability, or power to elicit belief; the degree to which information is likely to influence a recipient's beliefs. *Competence credibility* is the degree of respect for an informant's knowledge and judgment in a matter; *trust credibility* is the degree of respect for an informant's trustworthiness in a matter, especially with regard to conflict between accuracy and self-interest (p. 173).

Criteria for appropriate prescribing Aspects or dimensions that should be considered as a basis for prescribing assessments. Criteria for prescribing appropriateness should logically depend on the function of prescribing in health care (p. 158).

Database A collection of data, organized for rapid retrieval.

Deductible An amount subtracted from the first payment made on behalf of an insured person, that is, the amount that an insured person must pay before benefits become payable.

Delphi panel A group of people, chosen for expertise in a subject area, who communicate anonymously, in writing, with a moderator. The moderator may compile and summarize the comments, revise a document to incorporate suggestions, etc., and then resubmits the material to panel members until they reach consensus. In essence, a Delphi panel is a committee that works without actually meeting.

Diffusion of innovation (DoI) Diffusion is the process of communicating an innovation among the people in a social network or group via various media, over time. *Diffusion rate* is the number of adoptions per unit time, often measured either by asking people questions about their stage of adoption or by observing adoption behavior (p. 171).

Disease An abnormality or derangement of structure or physiology; a professional interpretation of a person's (patient's) account of illness experience and additional information, e.g., from physical examination or laboratory tests. Disease is a professional's *secondary* perception of the primary illness experience.

Disease management A program aimed at the improvement of medical practices in specific diseases. Comprehensive programs that address all of the needs of their members rather than focusing on the management of specific medical conditions are called *health management*. Drug therapy aspects of health management programs have sometimes been referred to as *pharmaceutical care.*

DoI See *diffusion of innovation.*

Dominated In decision analysis, an alternative is *dominated* when another alternative is superior on all dimensions considered in the analysis, e.g., cheaper and more beneficial.

DRP See *drug-related problem.*

Drug cap (prescription cap) A limit on the number of prescriptions or quantity of drug per prescription. Drug caps are used by some payment plans to influence patient behavior or to shift costs.

Drug-related morbidity (DRM) An unintended patient injury with a scientifically plausible relationship either to (a) drug therapy or (b) an untreated indication for drug therapy. See *relationship* and *injury.* DRMs include significant adverse or toxic effects of drugs (ADEs and major ADRs), treatment failures, and occasions when a valid indication was not treated. DRMs do not include DTPs or minor (technical) ADRs. For example, oozing of blood after brushing teeth is technically an ADR, but not a DRM; however, it is a DTP.

Drug-related problem (1) A drug therapy problem, i.e., an event in the process of drug therapy (see *drug therapy problem*). (2) An adverse drug event or drug-related morbidity, i.e., an outcome of drug therapy (p. 47).

Drug therapy problem (DTP) Any circumstance that a competent professional would judge to be inconsistent with achieving a therapeutic objective, but which does not itself constitute injury (p. 37); an observable latent injury *before* it has become a manifest injury (p. 274). A *potential* or *theoretical* DTP is a discrepancy between a patient's actual drug regimen and a treatment guideline, usual dose, or other therapeutic generalization. An *actual* DTP requires a theoretical DTP and a corresponding physical manifestation, e.g., symptom or laboratory test (p. 274).

Drug therapy process See *medications use process.*

Drug use evaluation (DUE) (1) A structured, ongoing, authorized quality assurance process designed to promote safe, appropriate, and effective drug use (American Society of Health-System Pharmacists). (2) An evaluation of prescribing appropriateness according to explicit criteria.

Drug use review See *drug use evaluation.*

Drug utilization review (DUR) Review of an insured population's drug utilization with the goal of determining how to reduce the cost of utilization. DURs may be used by PBMs to ensure appropriateness of drug therapy (as a quality assurance activity) or to assure compliance with a formulary. The term is often used interchangeably with the second definition of drug use evaluation, but utilization review usually refers to costs. See *drug use evaluation.*

DTP See *drug therapy problem.*

DUE/DUR See *drug use evaluation.*

Effectiveness Beneficial effects, e.g., of a drug product, in actual use in everyday conditions (p. 139).

Efficacy Beneficial effects, e.g., of a drug product, under ideal conditions (e.g., a controlled clinical trial) (p. 139).

Efficiency The ratio of input to output, for example, (a) the cost per treated case, or (b) the degree to which the care has the desired effect with respect to the resources expended (p. 107).

Equifinality The ability of a system to reach the same output by different processes or pathways (p. 233).

Error (1) An act or condition of ignorant, imprudent, or accidental deviation from a code, truth, or accuracy; implies a standard for judging deviation. (2) "A generic term to encompass all those occasions in which a planned sequence of mental or physical activities fails to achieve its intended outcome, and when these failures cannot be attributed to the intervention of some chance agency" (James Reason).

Evoked set The collection of alternative therapies that come into a prescriber's mind in response to a clinical impression or therapeutic objective (p. 165).

Facilitator A nonprofessional person who assists with drug therapy, e.g., the patient himself, family caregivers; similarly, facilitative services may be performed by professional aides (p. 224).

Fee-for-service (FFS) Payment for health care goods and services based on the number of units provided, e.g., payment per visit, prescription, hospital day.

FFS See *fee-for-service.*

FOCUS A five-step quality improvement process: find, organize, clarify, understand, and select (see Chapter 11).

Formative evaluation An evaluation for the purpose of identifying opportunities for improvement. See *summative evaluation*.

Formulary A list (compendium) of therapeutic agents used in a practice setting, payment plan, or managed care population to influence prescribing and dispensing: (1) a simple list (drug list) of drug products approved for use in a health care organization or for payment by a third party; (2) a continually updated list of therapeutic recommendations, including but not limited to drug products and dosage forms, produced by a representative committee of professionals, as part of a prescribing management system, with provisions for a prescriber to obtain nonformulary drugs.

Formularies may be *open* (educational) or *closed* (restrictive). Open formularies allow many drug products, and those that are not listed are generally available and reimbursed. Closed formularies contain fewer drug products. Other terminology used for describing formularies are *positive*, meaning that listed drug products are explicitly approved for coverage or reimbursement, and *negative*, meaning that listed drugs are explicitly excluded, which is often a method used for Medicaid formularies (p. 180).

A special type of negative formulary is used under *generic dispensing* policies to list drug products that may not be substituted with a product from another manufacturer, usually because of bioavailability concerns.

Four bads Bad drugs, bad prescribing, bad patients, and bad luck (common oversimplification of the causes of DRM).

Gatekeeper A primary care provider (PCP) who is responsible for determining what services a patient can access and when. The PCP is involved in overseeing and coordinating all aspects of a patient's medical care, including specialty care referral or hospital admission.

Generic dispensing A policy that allows the dispensing of a different brand (or a nonbranded drug product) when a trademark name was used in the original prescription order. The drug product dispensed should be exactly the same chemical entity in the same dosage form. Differences in salt form (e.g., sulfate vs. hydrochloride, sodium vs. potassium) are usually ignored.

See *therapeutic interchange*.

Generic drug name A nonproprietary common name for a drug, for example, a U.S. adopted name (USAN), USP-NF official name, international nonproprietary name (INN), or British approved name (BAN). Generic names are not trademark and do not designate a specific brand (manufacturer, licensee, distributor, etc.).

Group model HMO In a pure group model HMO, the HMO contracts with a multispecialty physician group practice to provide all physician services to HMO members. Physicians and other PCPs are employed by the group practice and not by the HMO. The medical group may also be responsible for paying or contracting with hospitals and other providers. Physicians in the group practice share facilities, equipment, medical records, and support staff. The physician group practice may contract with the HMO on an all-inclusive capitation basis to provide physician services to HMO members.

Health maintenance organization An organized health care system that is responsible for both the financing and delivery of a broad range of comprehensive health services to an enrolled population. HMOs generally offer prepaid, comprehensive health coverage for both hospital and physician services. Most HMOs are paid monthly capitation rates by payers, e.g., employers and insurance companies, and contract with health care providers, e.g., physicians, hospitals, and other health professionals. The several types of HMO models include group model, individual practice association, network model and staff model. The members of an HMO are required to use participating providers for all health services. HMOs tend to be the most restrictive type of managed care plan because they restrict the providers and benefits.

Health Plan Employer Data and Information Set (HEDIS) A set of performance measures for managed care plans, designed to ensure that purchasers and consumers have the information they need to reliably compare the performance of MCOs. The measures in HEDIS are related to many significant public health issues such as cancer, heart disease, smoking, asthma, diabetes, mental health, controlling high blood pressure, and menopause. HEDIS is a project of NCQA (see *National Committee for Quality Assurance*).

Heterophilous information source An informant who is seen as different from the person whom he is informing (recipient) in some significant way, especially with respect to basic beliefs and values (p. 171).

HMO See *health maintenance organization.*

Holism A view that comprehends interactions within and among whole organisms (or equivalent nonliving systems); the doctrine (assumption) that the whole may be more than the sum of its parts because of interactions among components.

Homophilous information source An informant who is seen as similar to the recipient (e.g., potential adopter) in most significant ways, especially as having compatible beliefs and values (p. 171).

HQOL See *health-related quality of life.*

Illness A person's subjective experience of being unwell; the subjective somatic and psychological counterpart of disease (p. 90).

Incidence The number of new cases in a population per unit time. A measure of the frequency with which an event, such as a new case of illness, occurs in a population over a period of time. The denominator is the population at risk; the numerator is the number of new cases occurring during a given time period.

Independent practice association (IPA) An association of physicians that contracts with an HMO to provide physician services to HMO members. The physicians are members of the IPA, which is a legal entity, but they remain individual practitioners and retain their separate offices and identities. IPA physicians will often see patients from many HMOs as well as PPO members or even patients that are covered by traditional indemnity insurance. Most HMOs compensate their IPAs on an all-inclusive physician capitation basis. The IPA then compensates its participating providers on either a fee-for-service basis or a combination of fee-for-service and primary care capitation.

Indicator An observation or measurement that reflects an underlying condition; a measure thought to be highly correlated with such a condition; a highly significant, nearly conclusive, sign or symptom. For example, a PDRM indicator suggests the presence or absence of an actual PDRM. Collectively, PDRM indicators reflect important aspects of overall drug therapy system performance.

Indicator positive/negative The value of an indicator is often dichotomous. A *positive indicator* (e.g., positive clinical sign or laboratory test) satisfies the definition of the indicator; a *negative indicator* does not. Collectively, the proportion of indicator positives may reflect an aspect of overall system performance.

Initiator A professional with legal authority to prescribe a needed regimen. Examples are general practice and primary care specialist physicians, physician's assistants, clinical nurse practitioners, dentists, podiatrists, and pharmacists who have prescribing authority, or for OTC medications (p. 223).

Injury (in the context of a drug-related injury) A severe, dangerous, or disabling clinical outcome that was not correctable or that required significant additional resources to correct, e.g., emergency treatment, hospitalization.

Knowledge-based (KB) action Nonroutine, consciously controlled problem-solving activity, for example, the result of reasoning, speculation, and feedback (trial and error) (p. 43).

Lapse A memory or perceptual error between planning and execution (p. 13).

Latent condition Latent error.

Latent error Latent failure.

Latent failure A system operation or design defect that permits latent injury to persist (pp. 39, 62).

Latent injury A propensity or predisposition for injury that occurs in a patient during the processes of care. Latent injury is an attribute of a patient at a particular time. Some latent injuries may be recognizable and correctable at a subsequent time during therapy (p. 31).

Latent outcome Latent injury.

Managed care organization (MCO) A method of organizing the finance and provision of care delivery so that payers and insurers can influence providers and suppliers. An MCO may contract with purchasers (e.g., employers; labor unions; business coalitions; federal, state, and provincial governments; and individuals) to provide health care to people (members) in defined populations, providing and paying for health care services that organize payers, insurers, providers, and suppliers. Although it is widely regarded as an American model, the health care systems of many countries use various forms of managed care (p. 308).

MCO See *managed care organization.*

Medicaid A federally aided, state-administered program that provides medical benefits for certain indigent or low-income persons in need of health and medical care. Each state determines its own standards for qualification. Subject to broad federal guidelines, states determine the benefits covered, program eligibility, rates of payment for providers, and methods of administering the program.

Medicare A U.S. health insurance program for people aged 65 and over, for persons eligible for social security disability payments for 2 years or longer, and for certain workers and their dependents who need kidney transplantation or dialysis. The program is open to all disabled elderly regardless of financial status. It consists of two separate but coordinated programs: hospital insurance (Part A) and supplementary medical insurance (Part B). Payroll taxes are deposited in special federal trust funds to meet the expenses incurred by the insured.

Medications management system A controller for a group of medications use processes and pharmaceutical care systems, intended to evaluate, maintain, and improve the quality of medications use in a patient group, e.g., all patients in a practice or an insurance program (pp. 226, 285).

Medications use The process of patient assessment, therapeutic planning (SOAP), prescribing, dispensing, and consumption or administration of medications.

Medications use process People, objects, decisions, and procedures that interact to provide drug therapy to individual patients, often without explicit therapeutic objectives, planned monitoring, and formal cooperation.

Medications use system A collective term for a *pharmaceutical care system* operated within a *medications management system* (see Chapters 10 and 11).

Mistake A *knowledge-based* error in judgment while planning an action, e.g., misapplication of knowledge or production of an inappropriate conclusion.

National Committee for Quality Assurance (NCQA) A nonprofit organization created by employers to improve patient care quality and health plan performance in partnership with managed care plans, purchasers, consumers, and the public sector.

Network model HMO An HMO that contracts with more than one physician group, sometimes with single or multispecialty groups, as well as hospitals and other health care providers. Network HMOs may be either closed or open panel. (In contrast, group model plans contract with a single panel; staff and group model plans use closed panels.)

Opinion leader A member of a social group, e.g., network or clique, who is frequently mentioned as a source of information, especially about innovations.

Optimal The most favorable amount or degree, especially of an input, with respect to given criteria. For example, the optimal selling price of a product with respect to revenues would not maximize price, but would maximize revenue.

Outcome The stable (not necessarily permanent) result of complex causes or forces; a stable change in a patient's condition resulting from antecedent care (Donabedian). A patient's outcome is often difficult to define precisely, especially in chronic diseases (p. 118).

Patient satisfaction Fulfillment of a need or want, or a person's subjective evaluation of that fulfillment (p. 128).

PBM See *pharmacy benefit management company.*

PDCA cycle PDCA stands for *plan, do, check, act*. The basic cycle of *quality improvement*; it is also known as a Shewhart cycle or a Deming cycle.

Performance indicator A quantitative criterion measurement, often based on a guideline; for example, the percentage of patients with a given disease whose treatment corresponded to a treatment guideline (p. 227).

Pharmaceutical care Responsible, cooperative provision of drug therapy for the purpose of achieving definite outcomes intended to improve a patient's quality of life. It includes the determination of the drug needs for a given individual and the provision not only of the drug required but also the necessary services (before, during, or after treatment) to assure optimally safe and effective therapy. It includes a feedback mechanism as a means of facilitating continuity of care by those who provide it (pp. 218, 263).

Pharmaceutical care system Elements (people, objects, decisions, and procedures) that directly interact *within a defined structure* to provide *pharmaceutical care* to individual patients, i.e., one patient at a time; the structure includes explicit therapeutic objectives, planned monitoring, and formal cooperation.

Pharmacy benefit management company (PBM) An organization that manages drug and dispensing costs and provides related administrative services, usually to an MCO. Ideally, a PBM applies managed care principles to prescription drug programs to promote optimal, cost-effective drug use for a positive impact on the total cost of care (p. 323).

Point-of-service plan (POS) A health plan benefit in which patients can select various providers or delivery systems when care is needed. Patients who use nonaffiliated providers may pay a larger share of expenses.

Population The total number of members of a group, e.g., inhabitants of an area or country. Population may also refer to people similar to those in a sample, not necessarily the total population of people.

Positive predictive value A measure of the predictive value of an indicator; the proportion of indicator positives (e.g., reported by a screening or surveillance system) that are true cases.

Potential DTP A circumstance in the process of therapy in which the patient has a theoretical DTP but no corresponding manifest problem (p. 275).

PPO See *preferred provider organization.*

Preferred provider organization A combination of hospitals and physicians that agrees to provide specific health care services for a discounted or negotiated payment, excluding co-insurance or deductibles paid by members.

Prevalence The number of cases (individuals with a disease or condition) in a population at a certain point in time; the number or proportion of cases, events, or conditions in a given population. *Period prevalence* is the number of people with a particular disease present in a population over a period of time.

Preventable Avoidable; a foreseeable consequence of a recognized and controllable cause.

Preventable drug-related morbidity, adverse drug event, etc. A *preventable drug-related morbidity, adverse drug event*, etc., follow a recognizably significant premonitory event, e.g., a DTP, that should have revealed the underlying cause of eventual injury, when the cause could have been controlled without sacrificing the therapeutic objective. The formal elements for preventability are (1) a recognizable DTP; (2) the foreseeability of the DRM, given the occurrence of the DTP; (3) an identifiable cause of the DTP and DRM; and (4) the ability to control that cause without foregoing the therapeutic objective (p. 21).

Prior authorization A formal process requiring a provider to obtain payment approval for particular services or procedures before they are done. This is usually required for services that are expensive or overused.

Process A sequence of operations intended to transform an input into an output; part of a system.

Profiling The practice of gathering data about utilization (e.g., prescribing) by individual physicians and comparing them to a norm, e.g., expected prescribing patterns within select therapeutic categories for medications or other services. Profiling focuses on the patterns of an individual prescriber's care rather than the provider's specific clinical decisions for an individual patient.

Quality improvement (QI) A systematic process of quality measurement, often with quality indicators; deliberate changes in structure or process; and feedback (monitoring). See *PDCA cycle*. The objectives of QI are to reduce variability in quality and to improve average (median) quality. Also called total quality management (TQM) and continuous quality improvement (CQI) (see Chapters 8 and 11).

Quality indicator A quantitative measure that can be used to monitor and evaluate the quality of clinical and support functions that significantly affect patient outcomes (p. 120).

Random variation Transient fluctuations in an indicator caused by (or attributed to) unrecognized, usually short-lived, events that do not affect performance over time. In a stable and high-quality system, random events are not considered to be related to quality.

Relationship (as in drug related) An event R in a patient is *related* to a drug D if: (1) D is a recognized cause of R, based on prior studies or valid theory; (2) R followed administration of D within a theoretically expected time interval; (3) other necessary contributing factors were present; and (4) no other attribution for R is more likely. Note that drug-related events are organized about patients rather than drugs. The evidence required for *relationship* is less stringent than for *cause*.

Reliability Consistency or reproducibility of measurement. It is a measurement of the ratio of true variation to total (observed) variation (p. 205).

Risk (financial) Financial risk is the chance of monetary loss. HMOs that accept fixed-premium and capitation contracts are at risk for all of the care provided to its patient members regardless of the cost of care. Physicians who accept capitation are at risk because they will not receive additional payments if their patients consume large amounts of health resources such as hospitalizations or large pharmacy expenditures. In HMOs, the patient is at risk only for copayments and the cost of excluded services.

Rule-based (RB) action A problem-solving activity selected from personal generalizations, formulas, and policies, somewhat more automatically than KB actions.

Sensitivity (decision analysis) The extent to which a calculated value or a decision would depend on the assumptions used in a decision analysis.

Sensitivity (indicator) The proportion of people with a condition, e.g., a PDRM, who also have a positive indicator for the condition (p. 207).

Sentinel event An outcome or other important occurrence (usually adverse) that does not occur in the presence of adequate care.

Skill-based (SB) actions Highly routine activities performed in familiar circumstances, not under careful conscious control; psychomotor activities; colloquially, a habitual response to a familiar stimulus.

Slip An error of execution.

SOAP A format for problem-oriented medical records. The acronym stands for *subjective* and *objective* data acquisition, data *assessment* or *analysis*, and production of a therapeutic *plan* (p. 276).

Special variation Fluctuations in an indicator caused by (or attributed to) changes in system structure or process. See *random variation* (p. 293).

Specificity (indicator) The proportion of people without a condition, e.g., PDRM, who also have a *negative* indicator for the condition.

Staff model HMO An HMO that employs the physicians and most of the other providers who offer care to members. Staff providers are typically paid a salary and may also receive bonuses or other types of incentive payments based on their performance. A staff HMO employs physicians representing most of the common specialties needed to provide care to its members.

Standard A minimum level of acceptable performance or a maximum level of unacceptable performance. Level can be, e.g., a proportion or frequency from a sample.

Structure The type, number, and characteristics of resources, including physical facilities, written policies and procedures, and qualifications of staff (p. 122).

Summative evaluation An evaluation for the purpose of classifying or grading.

System paradigm A perspective, or unifying view of reality, that emphasizes purpose, dynamic (interactive) relationships, holism, cooperation, or coordination of elements and self-control. See *holism*, *system*, and *teleological* (p. 228).

System failure An occasion in which a planned sequence of discrete interdependent decisions and actions, carried out by many individuals and directed at a common objective, fails to achieve its intended outcome, when the outcome had been achievable (p. 49).

System (1) A set of interdependent human or material elements interacting to achieve a common aim (IOM). (2) An organized collection of potentially interacting elements capable of self-control toward common purposes.

A specific system is defined by its environment, purpose, inputs, outputs, transformations (processes), and control subsystem (command signal, comparator, and feedback) (pp. 229, 232).

Teleological Able to seek one or more objectives; purposeful.

Theoretical DTP See *DTP.*

Therapeutic failure See *treatment failure.*

Therapeutic interchange A policy that permits the dispensing of chemically different drugs that are considered to be therapeutically equivalent to the drug actually ordered. Therapeutically equivalent drugs are chemically dissimilar but produce essentially the same therapeutic outcome and have similar toxicity profiles. See *generic dispensing.*

Therapeutic objective The intended culmination of a therapeutic plan, e.g., cure, control of disease, relief of symptoms, improvement of quality of life (p. 277).

Therapeutic plan Means to achieve the therapeutic objective. It should include a scheduled follow-up to assess whether the plan is succeeding (p. 277).

Treatment failure An occasion when drug therapy was attempted but did not reach a realistic, intended outcome (therapeutic objective) in a reasonable interval of time.

Trigger An event that causes a latent injury to become an actual, manifest injury, e.g., another error or happenstance, usually one that would not be expected to cause injury by itself.

Validity Measurement validity addresses the fundamental issue of whether a measure reflects whatever it was intended to measure, including its accuracy or bias (pp. 206, 291).

Violation A deliberate deviation from operating procedures, codes of practice, and rules necessary to operate a potentially hazardous system safely and effectively. Violations may be unintentional (where they overlap with errors), well-intentioned shortcuts, or intentional sabotage. Violations depend on social norms and rules (p. 45).

Index

A

Abbreviated new drug application, 132
Academic detailing, 179
Access to care
- arbitrary limitations, 102
- cost and, 98–99
- definition of, 99
- financial, 100–103, 220
- levels of, 220
- physical, 99–100, 103
- quality and, 98–99
- statistics regarding, 101

Accountability, 6
Accreditation standards
- definition of, 392, 403
- description of, 350–351, 353
- development of, 399
- managed care organizations effect, 392–395
- professional practice, 394, 399
- providers, 399

Active errors, 37, 60–61, 403
Active failures, 37
Active problem solving
- decision rules, 166–168
- description of, 165–166

Adaptive potential, 176
Adaptive system, 233, 403
Adoption
- environment issues associated with, 176
- influencing of, 172–173
- innovation knowledge, 173–175
- issues that influence, 175–176
- product issues associated with, 175
- stages of, 173–175
- willingness for, 176–177

Adulteration, 133
Adverse Drug Event Prevention Study, 363
Adverse drug events
- adverse drug reaction vs., 40
- attitudes toward, 30
- definition of, 40, 61, 403
- drug withdrawals caused by, 142
- historical view of, 30
- preventable, 62

Adverse drug reaction
- adverse drug event vs., 40
- definition of, 13, 39, 61, 403
- description of, 241
- drug-related morbidity caused by, 59
- drug withdrawals caused by, 142
- FDA reporting of, 140
- incidence of, 1, 13
- inpatient, 23
- manifestation of, 59
- medical record review of, 13–15
- mortality caused by, 1, 13
- prevalence of, 13
- preventability of, 13–15, 59
- severity of, 39–40
- World Health Organization definition of, 13, 39

Adverse effects, 19
Adverse outcomes
- adverse drug reaction, *see* Adverse drug reaction
- attitudes toward, 29–31
- definition of, 39
- foreseeability of, 56–57
- medication use process as cause of, 33–35
- severity of, 39–40

Advertising, 136
Affinity diagram, 294–296
Alternative medicine, 91
American College of Surgeons, 119
American Society of Health-System Pharmacists, 325–326
ANDA, *see* Abbreviated new drug application
Antibiotics, 77, 169
Aspirin, 137
Assessments
- definition of, 277
- prescribing, 160–162
- quality of care, *see* Quality assessments

Assumptions, preventability based on, 58–59
Attention deficit hyperactivity disorder, 77

Autonomy, 45
Average wholesale price, 403–404

B

Beliefs, 166, 349–351, 404
Biopsychosocial paradigm, 242
Blame, 6, 46, 355
Boards of pharmacy, 401

C

Capitation, 111, 311–313, 404
Care, *see* Health care; Pharmaceutical care
Carve-outs, 323–325, 376–377, 384, 387, 404
Cerivastatin, 143–144
Change agency, 172
Change agent, 172, 404
Churchman's rule, 235
Cimetidine, 137
Clinical impression, 165, 404
Clinical practice guidelines
  definition of, 404
  description of, 333–334
  health maintenance organization use of, 334–335
Clinical research
  review of, 253–260
  validity of, 126
Clinical trials
  drug safety vs., 140
  new drug, 132–133
  protocols for, 12
  randomized, 132, 346
Clique, 171
Closed-panel health maintenance organization, 312, 404
Clozapine, 144
Coercion, 375–376
Co-insurance, 404–405
Command signal, 235
Community practice, 5
Comparator, 235
Compensatory decision rules, 167–168
Competence, 86
Competence credibility, 173, 405
Compliance, 405, *see also* Noncompliance
Concordance, 405
Confidence interval, 303
Consumer(s), *see also* Patient(s)
  cost shifting to, 188
  focus of, 129–130
  medications use understood by, 380
  professional relationship with, 84–85, 87
Consumerism, 84
Consumer movement, 129
Consumer price index, 104
Content validity, 207
Controlled Substances Act, 136
Copayments of managed care organizations
  pharmacy benefit management companies effect on, 328–329
  reasons for, 328
  tiered, 328–329
Cost(s)
  common ground for decision making, 114–116
  development, 104
  efficiency assessments, 107–110
  framework for evaluating, 105–106
  minimization of, 187
  overpricing concerns, 105
  sensitivity analysis, 113–114
  statistics regarding, 103–104
  studies, 106–107
  summary overview of, 147
Cost-benefit analysis, 106, 109
Cost-effectiveness analysis, 106, 109, 152–154
Cost management, 9, 349
Cost minimization study, 106–107
Cost of illness study, 106–107
Cost shifting, 103
Cost utility study, 106
Co-therapists, 223–224, 231, 263–265, 374, 405
Covenants, 85
Credibility
  competence, 173, 405
  definition of, 405
  safety, 173
  trust, 405
Criteria for appropriate prescribing, *see* Prescribing, appropriateness criteria for
Criterion validity, 207
Critical mass, 177
Crohn's disease, 150
Culture, 87
Cutaneous T-cell lymphoma, 150

D

Database, 198, 405
DEA, *see* Drug Enforcement Administration
Decision making, 163, 373

Decision rules
compensatory, 167–168
definition of, 166–167
description of, 112, 170
noncompensatory, 167
Deductible, 327–328, 405
Delphi panel, 209–212, 405
Deming cycle, 297–305, 352, 412
Design failure, 52
Dialog, professional
data validity and reliability, 279
description of, 278–279
example of, 279–283
schematic diagram of, 278
Dietary Supplement and Health Education Act of 1994, 137
Diffusion of innovation, 171, 173, 178, 343, 353–354, 369, 405
Diffusion rate, 405
Disease
classifying of, 88–89
definition of, 88, 242, 406
illness vs., 88
models of, 91–92
Disease management
definition of, 8, 406
programs of, 333–334
Distributive justice, 160
Documentation
pharmaceutical care steps, 277
reasons for, 276
SOAP notes, 276–277, 281, 415
summary overview of, 281
therapeutic objectives, 266–267, 276
Dominated, 406
DRM, *see* Drug-related morbidity
Drug(s), *see also* Nonprescription drugs; Over-the-counter drugs; Prescription(s)
advances in, 4
approval process for, 99–100
as instruments, 79
clinical trials of, 12
commerce uses of, 79
development of, 99, 104
"difficult," 146
elderly use of, 317–318
expenditures for, 4, 105
financial access to, 100–103, 220
Food, Drug, and Cosmetic Act definition of, 132
hypersensitivity, 36
licensing requirements, 11
new, *see* New drug
off-label use of, 12, 135, 138–139
patient access to, 220
pharmacy stocking of, 221
physical access to, 99–100, 103
prescribing of, *see* Prescribing restrictions
risks of, 12
safety of, *see* Drug safety
unapproved uses of, 99–100, 135, 139
unsafe, 134–135
worthless, 133–134
Drug abuse, 2
Drug caps, 329–331, 406
Drug choice model, 164
Drug consumption, 231
Drug distribution, 375
Drug effectiveness
definition of, 131, 138, 140, 407
evaluation of, 140
Drug efficacy, 131, 407
Drug Enforcement Administration
Controlled Substances Act, 136
function of, 136
nonprescription drugs, 136–137
nutriceuticals, 137–138
Drug formulary, *see* Formulary
Drug industry, 4
Drug laws, 363
Drug licensing, 131, 220
Drug lists, 181
Drug marketing
description of, 132, 139
drug effectiveness evaluations after, 140
regulation of, 11–12
Drug monographs, 379–380
Drug product
adoption of, *see* Adoption
dispensing of, 270
Food and Drug Administration approval of, 132
marketing of, 132, 139
paradigm of, 240–241
postmarketing surveillance of, 145
premarket testing of, 145
quality of, 131–133
withdrawal of, 140–146
Drug regimen, 158
Drug-related admissions, 14
Drug-related adverse patient events, 42
Drug-related deaths
costs of, 22
studies of, 19–20
Drug-related morbidity
causes of
adverse drug reaction, 59
happenstance events, 36–37
human error, 32, 42–47, *see also* Error

    - nonprescription drugs, 222–223
    - nontreatment, 40
    - overview of, 31–33
    - patient medication use, 58–59
    - simplistic approach, 32
    - system failure, *see* System failure
    - systems failure, 34–35
  - costs of, 22
  - definition of, 42, 61, 406
  - drug therapy problem and, 47
  - elements of, 42
  - health care provision and, 25
  - manifestation of, 357–358
  - medications management system monitoring of, 374
  - medication use process view of, 36–37
  - preventable, *see* Preventable drug-related morbidity
  - public inquiries, 46–47
- Drug safety
  - benefits of, 32
  - clinical trials vs., 140
  - definition of, 138
  - description of, 380
  - evaluation of, 140
- Drug therapy
  - change in, 377–378
  - costs of
    - common ground for decision making, 114–116
    - development, 104
    - efficiency assessments, 107–110
    - framework for evaluating, 105–106
    - overpricing concerns, 105
    - sensitivity analysis, 113–114
    - statistics regarding, 103–104
    - studies, 106–107
  - definition of, 39
  - description of, 285
  - effectiveness of, 380
  - elements of, 75
  - environment that supports, 9
  - functions of, 75, 263
  - inappropriate, 380–381
  - infrastructure improvements for, 377
  - management of, 272–273, 380
  - monitoring of, 221
  - objective of, 11
  - outcomes of, 166, 390
  - paradigms of, 240–243
  - participants in, 377
  - perspectives of, 88–89
  - pharmacist's participation in, 388
  - process of, 224–225
  - purpose of, 158–159
  - reasons for, 1
  - risks of, 12, 380
  - safety of, 380
  - satisfaction with, 129
  - steps involved in, 272–273
  - systematic management approach to, 67–69
- Drug therapy problem
  - actual, 274–275
  - cause of, 55, 365–366
  - classification of, 49–51, 269, 273–274
  - criteria for preventability, 49–51
  - definition of, 38, 47, 62, 273, 406
  - drug-related morbidity and, 47
  - error complemented by, 47–48
  - example of, 48
  - health-related quality of life and, 82, 90
  - overt nature of, 47
  - potential, 267, 271–272, 275, 413
  - prevalence of, 245
  - preventable drug-related morbidities caused by, 219
  - recognition of, 369–370
  - recognizability of, 55–56, 209
  - risk accumulation, 229
  - studies of, 63–67
  - theoretical, 274–275
  - types of, 48
- Drug use evaluation
  - definition of, 123, 406–407
  - description of, 79, 155, 339
  - enforcement uses of, 183, 185
  - explicit criteria use by, 122
  - managed care organizations, 390
  - patient-oriented, 183
  - prescribing assessments, 124
  - principles of, 372
  - product-oriented, 155–156
  - retrospective, 157
  - scope of, 123–124
  - uses of, 183, 185
- Drug utilization reviews, 331–332, 407
- DTP, *see* Drug therapy problem
- DUE, *see* Drug use evaluation

E

- Education
  - patient, 270, 374, 381, 400
  - prescribing influenced by, 178–180
  - public health, 365
- Educational formularies, 179

Effectiveness
  definition of, 131, 138, 140, 407
  evaluation of, 140
Efficacy, 131, 407
Efficiency
  calculation of, 109–110
  definition of, 107, 407
  therapeutic alternatives, 111–113
  variations in, 107–109
Elderly
  hospitalization studies, 18
  prescription drug use by, 317–318
Elimination by aspects, 167
Emergency department visits, for preventable drug-related morbidity
  costs of, 23
  studies of, 18
Empiric antibiotic prescribing, 77, 169
Employee Retirement Income Security Act, 368–369, 393
Equifinality, 233, 407
Equitability, 160
ERISA, *see* Employee Retirement Income Security Act
Error, *see also* Human error
  active, 37, 60–61, 403
  critique of, 45–47
  definition of, 42–43, 407
  detection of, 51
  drug therapy problem as complement to, 47–48
  Institute of Medicine definition of, 43
  insufficiency of, 45
  lapses as, 43
  latent injury caused by, 37
  medication, 43
  mistakes as, 43
  negligence and, 46
  pharmacist, 36
  preventive model for, 231, 397
  proneness to, 51
  quality improvement and, 397
  risk of, 231
  slips as, 43
  standards of practice to prevent, 46
  summary overview of, 62
  system contributions to, 51–52
  system failure vs., 49, 62
  types of, 43
  unexpected, 36–37
  violation vs., 45
Evoked set, 165, 407
Expert reviewers, 122
Explicit control, 234–235
Explicit criteria, for prescribing, 161–162, 194, 221
Explicit reviews, 122

F

Face validity, 207
Facilitators, 224, 407
Failures, *see* Latent failure; System failure
Famotidine, 137
FDA, *see* Food and Drug Administration
Feedback, 68, 235, 255
Fee-for-service, 111, 407
Financial access to care, 100–103, 220
FOCUS
  "act" step of, 304–305
  application of, 290–291
  "check" step of, 301–304
  definition of, 290, 407
  description of, 353
  "do" step of, 298–300
  improvement selected for, 296–297
  Ishikawa diagram, 294
  nominal group technique, 294
  pharmacy practice application of, 299–300
  "plan" step of, 297–298
  root causes of variation, 293–294
  team members, 292–293
  validity example, 291–292
Follow-up
  inadequacies in, 33
  need for, 221–222
  pharmaceutical care, 273
Food, Drug, and Cosmetic Act
  adulteration provisions, 133
  drug as defined by, 132
  drug regulations, 133-135
  history of, 131–132
  misbranding provisions, 133
  provisions of, 133
Food and Drug Administration
  adverse drug reactions reported to, 140
  advertising regulated by, 136
  authority of, 145
  clinical trial protocols, 12
  drug approval by, 99–100, 132
  drug research phases, 132
  Food, Drug, and Cosmetic Act, 131–132
  good manufacturing practices, 146
  investigational new drug exemption, 132–133
  nonprescription drugs, 136–137
  regulatory process by, 141–142

safe and effective medications uses system, 146
Formative evaluation, 408
Formulary
closed, 408
definition of, 180, 408
hospital, 182
managed care organizations, 325–327
negative, 408
open, 408
restrictions on, 126, 180–181, 186
terminology, 185
Four bads, 408

G

Gatekeeper, 408
General error model, 44
Generic dispensing, 408
Generic drug name, 408
Good manufacturing practices, 146
Group model health maintenance organization, 312–313, 408–409
Guidelines
clinical practice
definition of, 404
description of, 333–334
health maintenance organization use of, 334–335
definition of, 198
medication use system, 198–199
prescribing, 199
treatment, 199

H

Hansen's disease, 150
Happenstance events, 36–37
Health care
access to, *see* Access to care
accreditation agencies, 400
Employee Retirement Income Security Act effects on, 368
framework for, 8–9
Institute of Medicine findings regarding, 363
managed care influences on, 367, 389
national expenditures for, 103
patient-centered, 117, 362
patient's involvement in, 92, 117, 222, 371–372, 379, 384
performance indicators of, 362
purchasers of, 391–392
purpose of, 390
quality of
assessments, *see* Quality assessments
components, 117–118
definition of, 116
description of, 98–99
domains, 117
improvement in, 120–121
outcomes, 118
process evaluation, 118
standards, 119
structural components, 118
summary of, 127–128
quality problems in, 363
relationships in, 371
team-based approach, 358
trends in, 351
Health Care Financing Administration, 103
Health maintenance organizations
clinical practice guidelines, 334
closed-panel, 312, 404
costs, 316–318
definition of, 409
enrollment in, 315
group model, 312–313, 408–409
IPA model, 314–315, 330
Medicare, 315–316
network, 313, 412
performance measurement in, 318
pharmacy benefit management company interactions with, 325
staff model, 312, 391, 415
Health Plan Employer Data and Information Set, 204, 318, 350, 390, 409
Health-related quality of life
definition of, 80, 90
disease effects, 81–82
domains of, 80–81
drug therapy problems and, 82
factors that influence, 90
illness feelings effect on, 90
measurement of, 81
questionnaires, 81–82
SF-36 evaluations, 81, 95
Heterophilous information source, 171, 409
High adaptive potential, 176
High reliability theory, 60
Hindsight bias, 36, 38
HMOs, *see* Health maintenance organizations
Holism, 409
Homophilous information source, 171
Hospitalizations
events that cause, 40–41

medication use system failure studies, 63–66
preventable drug-related morbidity in
costs of, 22
reduction of, 66
studies of, 15–18, 30–31, 59
HQOL, *see* Health-related quality of life
Human error, *see also* Error
drug-related morbidity caused by, 32, 42–47
studies of, 42–47
system failure vs., 49, 52
tests for, 52

I

Illness
biopsychosocial model of, 242
definition of, 88, 90, 242, 409
subjective nature of, 88
Implicit control, 234
Implicit criteria, for prescribing, 161
Incidence, 1, 13, 410
Incremental cost analysis, 111
Incremental cost-effectiveness ratio, 110, 113
Independent practice association, 410
Indicators
definition of, 200, 410
feasibility of, 208–209
formative use of, 120
medications management system, 227–228
medication use system
applications of, 212–213
content validity of, 211
criteria for, 204–209
definition of, 200
Delphi panel, 209–212, 405
development process for, 209, 399
examples of, 202–204, 210
face validity of, 211
feasibility of, 208–209
Joint Commission on Accreditation of Healthcare Organizations, 204
minimum information need for, 201–202
outcome, 201
process, 201, 390
rate-based, 201
reliability of, 204–206
sensitivity of, 207
sentinel, 201
specificity of, 208
types of, 201, 268
validity of, 204, 206–208, 211
minimum information need for, 201–202
need for, 358
negative, 410
positive, 410
preventable drug-related morbidity
definition of, 56–58
evidence-based, 58
studies of, 20–22
rate-based, 201
rationale for, 202
sensitivity of, 207
sentinel event, 201
specificity of, 208
uses of, 200, 358
Indicator studies, 20–22
Industrialization, 340
Information sharing, 372–373
Initiators, 223–224, 410
Injury
definition of, 410
latent
definition of, 37, 411
drug therapy problem as, 38, 47
example of, 38
Innovation
approaches to, 177–178
diffusion of, 171, 173, 178, 343, 353–354, 369, 405
knowledge of, 173–174
Innovators, 176
Inpatient drug-related morbidity
costs of, 23
examples of, 18–19
studies of, 66–67
Institute of Medicine
attitude changes, 31
Crossing the Quality Chasm, 339, 362, 379, 390, 393
To Err Is Human, 362–363, 379
error defined by, 43
health care statements by, 363
quality as defined by, 118
recommendations of, 7–8
reports by, 339, 362
statistics of, 1, 3
Insulin, 137
Interprofessional cooperation, 222
Investigational new drug, 132–133, 135
IOM, *see* Institute of Medicine
IPA model health maintenance organization, 314–315, 330
Iron triangle metaphor, 98, 361
Ishikawa diagram, 294–296

J

Joint Commission on Accreditation of Healthcare Organizations (JCAHO)
  drug formulary formation, 325
  home care pharmacy standards, 351
  medications use indicators, 204
  membership, 125
  quality standards of, 119

K

Kaizen, 304–305
Kefauver–Harris Amendments, 132–133
Knowledge-based actions, 43–44, 410

L

Labeling
  definition of, 133
  preventable drug-related morbidities described in, 142
Lapses, 43–44, 55, 410
Latent failures
  definition of, 39, 62, 411
  design, 52
  lack of standards of practice to prevent, 46
  operational, 52
  types of, 52
Latent injury
  definition of, 37, 411
  drug therapy problem as, 38, 47
  example of, 38
Length of therapy, 204
Leprosy, 150
Liability, 6
Living with Asthma Questionnaire, 81–82, 96
Low adaptive potential, 176

M

Managed care organizations
  accreditation standards effect on, 392–395
  best practice promotion in, 332–335
  characteristics of, 341–342
  copayments, 328–329
  costs
    containment strategies, 333, 367
    description of, 316–318
  deductibles, 327–328, 405
  definition of, 307, 411
  disease management programs, 333–334
  drug caps in, 329–331, 406
  drug formulary, 325–327
  drug therapy improvements in, 9
  drug use evaluation in, 390
  Employee Retirement Income Security Act effects on, 368–369, 393
  enrollment in, 315
  examples of, 368
  goal of, 375–376
  health care influences by, 366, 389
  health maintenance organizations, *see* Health maintenance organizations
  history of, 307–309, 366
  influences of, 366
  market imperfections, 393
  Medicaid, 316
  medical groups, 316
  Medicare, 315–316
  medication carve-outs, 323–325, 376–377, 384, 387, 404
  medications management system adoption in, 353
  medications use system, 389
  over-the-counter drugs promoted by, 329
  performance measurement in, 318–319
  pharmacists, 389
  pharmacy benefit management company interactions with, 323–325, 354
  physicians
    cooperation among, 376
    drug utilization reviews, 331–332
    prescribing patterns of, 330–331
    utilization controls on, 331–332
  point-of-service plans, 314
  power of, 366
  preferred provider organizations, 310
  prescribing standards in, 348, 389–390
  prescriptions
    information exchange between providers, 330
    limits on, 182, 329–330, 384
    switching to over-the-counter drugs, 329
  preventable drug related morbidities, 345
  problems with, 370
  quality in, 349, 390
  reasons for, 342
  recommendations for, 389–391

reimbursements, 316
scientific basis of, 127
scope of, 307
standards for, 391
strategies for, 324
suboptimization conditions, 113
trends in, 315–318, 367
types of, 309–314
utilization controls in
on patient behavior, 327–331
on physicians, 331–332
Marketing
description of, 132, 139
drug effectiveness evaluations after, 140
drug surveillance after, 145
Medicaid
definition of, 411
managed care organizations, 316
prescription limiting by, 102–103, 329
Medicalization, 90
Medical management system, 286–287
Medical record audit, 195
Medical record review
preventability determined by, 53–54
preventable adverse drug reactions, 13–15
Medicare, 101
definition of, 411
managed care organizations, 315–316
Medication carve-outs, 323–325, 376–377, 384, 387, 404
Medications management system
Acme Zenith Health Plan, 289–290
barriers to improvement, 354–358
current values, norms, beliefs, and procedures compatibility with, 349–351
definition of, 411
description of, 222, 226–227
drug-related morbidities monitored by, 374
functions of, 285–286
goals of, 290
managed care organization adoption of, 353
objectives of, 290
paradigm concepts, 228–229
performance indicators, 227–228
practice level use of, 288
program level use of, 288
psychological barriers to improvement of, 354–358
schematic diagram of, 286
Medications use
accreditation standards for, 350–351, 353
definition of, 159, 411
effectiveness of, 384
environment of, 76, 87
evidence-based, 373
Health Plan Employer Data and Information Set standards, 350–351
objectives of, 76-79
outcomes of, 357
paradigms, 238-241
people involved in, 75–76
pharmaceutical care and, 213–214
pharmacist's role in, 386–387
quality of, 287–288
recommendations for, 384–385, 398–401
safety in, 384–385
simulation model
building of, 246–247
description of, 246
hypothesis development using, 246
logic of, 248
maintenance, 248
output of, 247
preventable drug-related morbidity, 250
results of, 249–253
summary overview of, 253
total cost of care findings, 251–253
state laws, 138
steps involved in, 160
Medications use process
adverse outcomes and, 33–35
definition of, 33, 412
drug-related morbidities in, 36–37
error, *see* Error
improvements in, 33
indicators, 202–204
initiation of, 35–36
preventability and, 58–59
schematic diagram of, 35–36
steps involved in, 229–230
studies of, 63–67
systematic management approach to, 67–69
Medications use system
adoption of, 343–344
advantages of, 345–347, 395
common ground for, 115–116
co-therapists in, 223–224, 231, 263–264, 374, 405
definition of, 218, 412
description of, 34, 197
development of, 378
diffusion of innovation application to, 344
divisibility of, 352
evaluations of, 345–347

facilitators in, 224
incremental approach, 396
indicators
applications of, 212–213
content validity of, 211
criteria for, 204–209
definition of, 200
Delphi panel, 209–212, 405
development process for, 209
examples of, 202–204, 210
face validity of, 211
feasibility of, 208–209
Joint Commission on Accreditation of Healthcare Organizations, 204
minimum information need for, 201–202
outcome, 201
process, 201, 390
rate-based, 201
reliability of, 204–206
sensitivity of, 207
sentinel, 201
specificity of, 208
types of, 201, 268, 289
validity of, 204, 206–208, 211
initiators in, 223–224, 410
managed care organizations, 389
people involved in, 223–224
performance, 198–199
planning of, 375
pre-implementation testing of, 395–396
preventable drug-related morbidity risks in, 347
professional cooperatives in, 348
quality improvement in, 397
relationships in, 223–224
risks for, 347–348
rules for redesigning
anticipating of needs, 375
clinician cooperation, 376
continuous healing relationships as basis for care, 371
customizing of care, 371–372
evidence-based decision making, 373
information sharing, 372–373
overview of, 370–371
patient is source of control, 372
safety, 373–374
sharing of knowledge, 372–373
transparency, 374–375
waste decreases, 375–376
stakeholders in, 342–354
standards, 200
subsystems of, 222
supply side of, 343
testing of, 395–396
trials of, 346
Mercantile system, 341
Mibefradil, 144
Misbranding, 133
Mistakes, 43, 412
Mistimed refills, 203
Mortality, 1

N

National Academy of Sciences/National Research Council, 133
National Committee for Quality Assurance, 127, 204, 318, 350, 353, 390, 412
National Council on Patient Information and Education, 379
National Pharmaceutical Council, 327
NDA, *see* New drug application
Negative indicator, 410
Negligence, 46
Network health maintenance organization, 313, 412
Networks, 171–173
New drug
clinical trials for, 132–133
commercial sponsor of, 133
definition of, 132
Food and Drug Administration approval of, 132
investigational, 132–133
New drug application, 132, 134
Newsletters, 179
90% confidence interval, 303
Noncompensatory decision rules, 167
Noncompliance, 32, 78–79
Nonprescription drugs
drug-related morbidities caused by, 222–223
FDA regulation of, 136–137
side effects of, 137
Normal accident theory, 61
Nutriceuticals, 137–138

O

Objective data, 277
Office visit, 381
Off-label uses, 12, 135, 138–139
Operational failure, 52
Operationalization, 209

Opinion leader, 172–173, 412
Optimal, 411
Orphan Drug Act, 150–151
Outcome(s)
  definition of, 412
  drug therapy, 166, 390
  evaluation of, 124
  indicators, 201, 213
  medications use, 213–214, 357
  studies of, 196, 255–257
Over-the-counter drugs
  advertising of, 136
  contraindications, 382
  facts regarding, 382–383
  Food and Drug Administration regulation of, 136
  interactions among, 382
  managed care organization promotion of, 329
  retail sales of, 137
  side effects of, 382

P

Paternalistic relationship, 83–84, 87
Patient(s), *see also* Consumer(s)
  bill of rights, 369
  definition of, 84
  dissatisfied, 129
  education of, 270, 374, 381, 400
  follow-up with, 221–222
  health care involvement by, 92, 117, 222, 371–372, 379, 384
  history-taking, 266
  influencing of, 59
  information gathering from, 266
  medications use by
    errors in, 58–59
    reasons for, 78–79
    recommendations for, 384–385
    understanding of, 380
  noncompliance of, 32, 78–79
  pharmaceutical care focus on, 9
  responses to signs and symptoms of, 220
  satisfaction of, *see* Satisfaction
  self-monitoring, 221
  well-informed, 385
Patient-professional relationship
  consumer, 84–85, 87
  description of, 83
  example of, 86–88
  levels of, 222
  paternalistic, 83–84, 87
  pharmacists, 218, 382–383
  therapeutic, 85-87
PBMs, *see* Pharmacy benefit management companies
PDRM, *see* Preventable drug-related morbidity
Peer review, 121–122, 208
Penicillin, 137
Performance indicators, *see* Indicators
Persuasion, 174–175
Pharmaceutical care
  definition of, 218, 412–413
  demand for, 343, 353
  documentation of, 277, *see also* Documentation
  follow-up, 273
  market for, 342–343
  medications use management and, 213–214
  microsystems, 9
  outcomes-based focus of, 266
  pharmacist's participation in, 387–389, 401
  physician participation in, 352, 401
  principles of, 219–223, 389
  satisfaction with, 129–131
  systems paradigm of, 242
  total cost of care for, using simulation model, 251–253
Pharmaceutical care system
  consistent process in, 264–273
  co-therapist's role in, 263, 265, 374
  definition of, 219, 225, 413
  flow diagram of, 225–226
  ideal, 246
  medical management and, 286
  monitoring plan, 226
  schematic diagram of, 230
Pharmaceutical industry, 104-105
Pharmacist, *see also* Professional(s)
  characteristics of, 386
  communication with, 4, 382–383
  consistency of care by, 264–265
  cooperation by, 263, 386
  education and training of, 217
  errors made by, 36
  functions of, 388
  in managed care organizations, 389
  medications use recommendations for, 386–387
  patient relationship with, 218, 371, 382–383
  pharmaceutical care participation by, 387–389, 398

- physician interactions with, 387–388, 393–394
- responsibilities of, 270–271, 384
- standards of practice for, 399
- variations among, 384

Pharmacy
- corporate-owned, 381–382
- medicine stocking in, 221
- prescription profiles, 266
- reimbursement basis for, 352
- selection criteria for, 383
- standards of practice for, 399
- variations among, 384

Pharmacy benefit management companies
- definition of, 413
- description of, 323–325, 354, 367, 387
- disease management programs, 334–335
- management of, 392
- performance evaluations of, 392

Pharmacy benefit managers, 349
Physical access to care, 99–100, 103
Physician, *see also* Professional(s)
- autonomy of, 45
- drug therapy objectives, 78
- managed care organization, 330–332
- office visit with, 381
- patient behavior influenced by, 59
- pharmaceutical care participation by, 352, 401
- pharmacist interactions with, 387–388, 393–394
- prescribing by, 163–164
- preventable drug-related morbidity, 7
- standards of practice, 45

Pneumocystis carinii pneumonia, 150
Point-of-service plans, 314, 413
Population, 413
Positive indicator, 410
Positive predictive value, 413
PPOs, *see* Preferred provider organizations
Practice guidelines, 333–334
Preferred provider organizations
- definition of, 413
- description of, 310
- pharmacy benefit management company interactions with, 325

Prescribers
- beliefs of, 166
- inappropriate, 163, 189
- values of, 166

Prescribing
- appropriateness criteria for
  - definition of, 405
  - description of, 158, 220
  - equitability, 160
  - explicit, 161–162, 194, 221
  - implicit, 161
  - proposed types of, 159–162
  - scientific appropriateness, 159
  - specificity, 159
  - studies of, 194–196
  - timeliness, 160
- assessments of, 160–162
- decision rules for, 166–168
- description of, 155–156
- drug choice model, 164–165
- drug use evaluation assessments of, 124
- guidelines for, 199
- improvements in, 177–178
- inadequacies in, 33
- inappropriate, 163, 189
- influences on
  - anomalies in, 184–188
  - description of, 156–157, 178, 364
  - educational, 178–180
  - favored manufacturer's products promoted, 187–188
  - individual education, 179–180
  - mass communications, 178–179
  - prescribing restrictions, *see* Prescribing restrictions
  - small group education, 179–180
- managed care organizations, 348, 389–390
- motivations for, 163–164
- outcomes studies, 196
- philosophical basis for, 158–159
- process evaluation of, 118
- psychological models of, 169–170
- purpose of, 160
- reasons for, 163–164
- restrictions on, *see* Prescribing restrictions
- retrospective review, 157–158
- social psychology of
  - decision making, 163
  - decision rules, 166–168
  - description of, 163
  - problem solving, 163, 165–168
  - reasoned policy and rules, 168
  - unreasoned rules and habit, 168–169
- sociology of
  - adoption, *see* Adoption
  - description of, 170–171
  - diffusion of innovation, 171, 173, 178
  - models, 177–178
  - networks, 171–173
  - relationships, 171–173
- systematic improvement of, 188–189

Prescribing habit, 169
Prescribing newsletters, 179

Prescribing restrictions
burden of proof for, 186
cost shifting to consumers, 188
definition of, 180
drug use evaluation, 183
effectiveness of, 185–186
examples of, 180
formulary, 180–182, 186
literature review, 180–184
objectives of, 186
prescription limits, 182
prior authorization, 183, 185
research regarding, 184–185
Prescription(s)
expenditures for, 104–105
frequency of, 1
limits on, 182, 329–330
managed care organization approach to
information exchange between providers, 330
limits on, 182, 329–330, 384
switching to over-the-counter drugs, 329
management of, 392
Medicaid limiting of, 102–103, 329
patient access to, 220
patient information regarding, 383
Prescription legend, 136
Prevalence
adverse drug reaction, 13
definition of, 413
drug therapy problem, 245
preventable drug-related morbidity, 14–15, 24, 212, 290, 345
Preventability
adverse drug reactions, 59
assumptions and, 58–59
definition of, 54–55, 57–58
description of, 53
medical record reviews for determining, 53–54
medications use process and, 58–59
studies of, 53
system failure and, 55
Preventable drug-related morbidity
attitudes toward, 29–31
attributes of, 54–55
causes of, 34, 219, 352, 364–366
comparisons with medical conditions, 22
costs of, 22–23, 400
definition of, 54–55, 57–58, 209, 414
description of, 1–2, 53
drug abuse vs., 2
drug therapy problems, 219
environmental context of, 362–366
examples of
drug-related deaths, 19–20
emergency department visits, 18
hospitalization, 15–18
indicator studies, 20–22
inpatient studies, 18–19
exclusions, 46
health care policies and programs effect on, 7
health care provision and, 25
hospitalization for, 15–18, 379
indicators
definition of, 56–58
evidence-based, 58
studies of, 20–22
labeling description of, 142
leadership acknowledgment of, 369
length of stay for, 23
in managed care organizations, 345
manifestation of, 357–358, 361
in medications use system, 347
model of, 61–62
motivations for, 53
nonresponse to, 362–366
organizational context of, 362–366
persistence of, 4–7
physician responsibility for, 7
prevalence of, 14–15, 24, 212, 290, 345
preventing of, 3, 400
rate of, 250
significance of, 22
studies of, 14–15, 53
systems approach, 7–8
Primary care, 8
Principle of requisite variety, 235
Prior authorization, 183, 185, 414
Proactive reaction, 356
Problem-oriented medical record, 276
Problem solving
active, 165–168
decision making vs., 163
Process indicators, 201
Process paradigm, 241
Professional(s), *see also* Pharmacist; Physician
cooperation among, 347, 376, 386
culture of, 341
dialog, 278-283
historical development of, 340–341
marketing uses of, 340–342
relationships, 83-88
standards for, 394, 399
Professional covenant, 85
Profiling, 414
Public health education, 365

Q

QI, *see* Quality improvement
Quality
  definition of, 242
  health care
    assessment of, *see* Quality assessments
    chasm in, 364–365
    components, 117–118
    definition of, 116
    description of, 98–99
    domains, 117
    improvement in, 120–121
    outcomes, 118
    patient satisfaction and, 128–129
    problems with, 363
    process evaluation, 118
    standards, 119
    structural components, 118
    summary of, 127–128
  managed care organizations, 349, 390
  rewards for, 363
Quality adjusted life years, 109
Quality assessments
  clinical research validity, 126
  evidence-based approach, 125–126
  explicit reviews, 122
  implicit reviews, 121–122
  market forces effect, 126–127
  methods of, 122–124, 127
  professional consensus approach, 125–126
Quality circle, 292
Quality improvement
  definition of, 414
  description of, 120–121
  error prevention and, 397
  FOCUS
    "act" step of, 304–305
    application of, 290–291
    "check" step of, 301–304
    definition of, 290, 407
    "do" step of, 298–300
    improvement selected for, 296–297
    Ishikawa diagram, 294
    nominal group technique, 294
    pharmacy practice application of, 299–300
    "plan" step of, 297–298
    root causes of variation, 293–294
    team members, 292–293
    validity example, 291–292
  goals of, 287
  tools for, 287–288
  trends in, 351
Quality indicator, 120, 414
Quality of life
  assessment of, 83
  definition of, 80
  description of, 79–80
  health-related
    definition of, 80, 90
    disease effects, 81–82
    domains of, 80–81
    drug therapy problems and, 82, 90
    factors that influence, 90
    illness feelings effect on, 90
    measurement of, 81
    questionnaires, 81–82
    SF-36 evaluations, 81, 95
    therapy objectives, 372
  sexual function, 80

R

Randomized clinical trials, 132, 346
Random variation, 414
Ranitidine, 137
Reasoned rules, 168
Regimens, 158, 268
Relationship
  drug-related, 414
  patient-professional, *see* Patient-professional relationship
Reliability
  coding errors, 301–302
  definition of, 415
  medication use system, 204–206
  professional dialog data, 279
Research
  review of, 253–260
  validity of, 126
Resident pathogen, 47
Retrospective drug use evaluation, 157
Review of systems, 383
Risk
  drug therapy, 12, 380
  error, 231
  financial, 415
  medications use system, 347–348
  pharmaceutical industry, 104
Root cause analysis, 293–295, 391
Rule-based actions, 43–44, 415

S

Safe and effective medications uses system, 146
Safety credibility, 173
Satisfaction
    definition of, 128, 412
    dimensions of, 128
    with drug therapy, 129
    indicators of, 130
    measures of, 129–131
    patient cooperation and, 129
    quality improvement and, 128–129
    reasons for studying, 128–129
Satisficing, 167
Scapegoating, 32, 355
Scientific appropriateness for prescribing, 159
Scientific evidence, 174
Scientific medicine, 91
Senge, Peter, 354
Sensitivity analysis, 113–114, 153–154, 415
Sentinel event
    definition of, 124, 415
    evaluation of, 206
    indicators, 201
Sexual function, 80
SF-12, 95
SF-36, 81, 95
Shewhart cycle, 297–305, 412
Sickle cell anemia, 150
Sickness, 90
Simulation model of medications use
    building of, 246–247
    description of, 246
    hypothesis development using, 246
    logic of, 248
    maintenance, 248
    output of, 247
    preventable drug-related morbidity, 250
    results of, 249–253
    summary overview of, 253
    total cost of care findings, 251–253
Skill-based actions, 43–44, 415
Slips, 43, 55, 415
SOAP notes, 276–277, 281, 415
Social distance, 171
Sociogram, 172
Specialization, 239
Special variation, 415
Specificity of prescription, 159, 415
Specific system, 232
Staff model health maintenance organization, 312, 391, 415
Standards
    accreditation
        definition of, 392, 403
        description of, 350–351, 353
        development of, 399
        managed care organizations effect, 392–395
        professional practice, 394, 399
        providers, 399
    definition of, 200, 415
    medication use system, 200
    practice, 45-46
State laws, 138
Structured implicit criteria, for prescribing, 161
Subjective data, 277
Suboptimization, 113–115
Summative evaluation, 416
Swiss cheese model of error prevention, 231
System
    adaptive nature of, 233
    changes in, 35
    components of, 232-235
    control of, 234–235
    definition of, 34, 49, 416
    elements of, 49
    error proneness and, 51–52
    generic, 232
    ideal, 232
    medications management, *see* Medications management system
    medicine use, 34
    paradigm of, 242, 416
    pharmaceutical care, *see* Pharmaceutical care system
    relationships among, 232
    specific, 232
    teleological, 233
System failure
    causes of, 51
    definition of, 35, 49, 62, 416
    error vs., 49, 62
    example of, 51
    preventability and, 55

T

Teleological system, 233, 416
Terfenadine, 144
Thalidomide, 134–135, 144
Theoretical drug therapy problem, 274–275
Therapeutic drug monitoring, 240

Therapeutic duplication, 203–204
Therapeutic interchange, 416
Therapeutic objectives
  definition of, 277, 416
  description of, 49
  documentation of, 266–267, 276
  monitoring of, 270–271
Therapeutic Outcomes Monitoring model, 265
Therapeutic plan
  definition of, 277, 416
  description of, 266
  evaluation of, 267–269
Therapeutic relationships, 85-86
Timeliness of prescribing, 160
Treatment
  failure of, 416
  guidelines for, 199
  models of, 91–92
Trigger event, 38, 416
Troglitazone, 144
Trust credibility, 405

U

Unapproved uses of drugs, 99–100, 135, 139
Underprescribing, 220
Unreasoned rules, 168–169
Unsafe drugs, 134–135

V

Validity
  content, 207
  criterion, 207
  definition of, 417
  face, 207
  medication use system indicators, 204, 206–208, 211
  professional dialog data, 279
Values, 166
Violation
  definition of, 45, 417
  error vs., 45
  medications use application of, 46

W

Wellness, 88, 90, 130
White-coat hypertension, 74
Withdrawal of drug products, 140–146
World Health Organization
  adverse drug reaction definition of, 13, 39
  health as defined by, 80
Worthless drugs, 133–134